On the Kindness of Strangers

On the Kindness of Strangers
AND OTHER ESSAYS

Musing on
Medicine as a Human Science

Norelle Lickiss

Edited by **Anita Hansen**
Foreword by **Arthur Conigrave**

© Norelle Lickiss 2024

ISBN 978-0-9756406-4-7

Second printing January 2025

All rights reserved.
Without limiting the rights under copyright above, no part of this publication may be reproduced, stored in or introduced into a retrieval system, or transmitted in any form or by any means (electronic, mechanical, photocopying, recording or otherwise), without the prior written permission of the author.

Edited by Anita Hansen

Cover art by Mona Deutscher Lickiss

Design and layout by Kent Whitmore, Forty South Publishing Pty Ltd

Published by Forty South Publishing Pty Ltd, Hobart, Tasmania
fortysouth.com.au

Printed by McPherson's Printing Group, Victoria
mcphersonsprinting.com.au

Dedicated to the memory of
DOCTORS AND NURSES
who have died of COVID-19

and

In memory of
SIR EARDLEY MAX BINGHAM QC
(18 March 1927–30 November 2021)

Foreword

I first became aware of Dr Norelle Lickiss and her work when in the early-mid 1980s I was a junior medical officer and later a registrar in training in the medical discipline of Endocrinology at Royal Prince Alfred Hospital in Sydney. Dr Lickiss was in the process of setting up a palliative care service, primarily for cancer patients. She had already established herself as one of Australia's leading academic physicians at the University of Tasmania, where she had been Foundation Professor of Community Health and Acting Head of Medicine. Soon after I met her in Sydney, I was struck by her decision to treat a patient with advanced cancer, who had developed an associated disorder of calcium metabolism not with agents that correct the abnormal plasma calcium concentration but with agents that suppress the distressing physical responses arising from it. This seemed to go against our medical training (to base management strategies on our understandings of pathological mechanisms), and I will touch on it again below.

In the years that followed, our paths did not cross but I would occasionally hear mention of her work and the power of her presentations from friends and colleagues both at home and abroad. Subsequently in 2017, as Dean of Medicine at the University of Sydney, I had the honour of presenting

Dr Lickiss, freshly graduated Doctor of Medical Science *Honoris Causa*, to the Chancellor of the University, to other colleagues, and to the medical graduates and graduating PhDs of the occasion. She delivered a memorable address that is included in this fine volume, *The Kindness of Strangers*, along with a substantial corpus of other works. I advise the reader of these works to allow the music of the originally spoken words of these essays to seep in, as it did for us that day. These works are best not ploughed through or skimmed over but absorbed. Dr Lickiss is a powerful speaker and advocate: to properly understand this and to benefit requires a little extra time – time of inspiration and great enjoyment!

The following things are abundantly clear from these records: Dr Lickiss cares deeply for the future of humanity; for the role of universities in the development of mind and intellect; for the direction and application of the medical community; for the development of individual doctors and how they practise; and, for those of us engaged in healthcare, for our patients' opportunities to live complete and fulfilled lives, 'to emancipate [the] interior splendour' to quote, after Dr Lickiss, University of Auckland academic, Kingsley Mortimer. It is noteworthy that she richly acknowledges the thinking, both contemporary and historical, that has shaped hers and clearly explains with detailed, frequently powerful and moving, quotations how this came to be.

In the talks, lectures, letters and essays in this volume, which spans 50 years of scholarship and lived experience from the early 1970s to the present time, she draws on her medical practice, her research, her passion for philosophy, and its modern and ancient histories, and on the development of her own thinking. Starting with a uniquely Australian focus, and a concern for the problems that face us across the continent, her discussions encompass global health problems, disease control, and the care and support of all those who need it. The disease ambit considered in these pages is broad, reflecting the roles of the health and medical communities that are called upon to respond. It includes malnutrition and diarrheal diseases, historical curses that continue worldwide even now; disability and the interlinked attitudes of the health profession and our societies to the provision of services for it; the chronic diseases and addictions of the 20th and 21st centuries; cancers; and, yes, the COVID pandemic. In all cases, the emphasis is on quality of care, quality of life, and maximising dignity and opportunity.

If, as a reader of the foregoing, you are curious to understand why Dr Lickiss, the palliative medicine physician, treated the advanced cancer patient with the disturbance of calcium metabolism as she did, you will find the thinking that underpinned decisions of this type, to prioritise the dying patient's lived experience, carefully explained in these essays. You will also encounter a person with an intense dissatisfaction with an overtly unsatisfactory status quo, with a strong commitment to find ways to drive change, and bent upon the consistent application of her own personal energy to the tasks at hand.

Drawing on the philosophical context in which she thought and worked, one is struck by the loyalty and the passion with which she has approached and continues to approach her life's work. The reader shares in her lived experience dealing with Immanuel Kant's three questions beginning with 'What can I know?' and 'What should I do?', on the inner striving of Baruch Spinoza's 'conatus', on the limits that should be applied to liberty with John Stuart Mill, on the primacy of Emmanuel Levinas' answer to the 'call of the other' in directing doctor's responsibilities, on John Henry Newman's understanding of the core role of a university in 'the cultivation of the mind', on Viktor Frankl's insight, from his experience in Auschwitz, to exercise freedom under supreme duress by 'taking an attitude', and much more. In the graduation address I mentioned above, Dr Lickiss drew on the sentiment of another witness to the tragedy of Auschwitz, Oskar Schindler, the German industrialist who is credited with saving the lives of over 1000 people there. When contemplating the people he had *not* saved, Schindler is reported to have expressed this thought, 'I could have done more.' In the mind of Norelle Lickiss at age 90 there is unfinished business, and she hopes that the examples and the ideas expressed in this work might help to inspire the change that is still needed. We can all do more.

—Professor Emeritus Arthur D Conigrave
MD PhD FRACP FRSN

Biology Domain Group Leader, Charles Perkins Centre (D17),
School of Life & Environmental Sciences
The University of Sydney, NSW 2006
Endocrinologist, Royal Prince Alfred Hospital
Camperdown, NSW 2050

Editor's Introduction

This volume sets out to assemble the writings and thoughts (musings if you like) of a very remarkable woman – Emeritus Professor, Dr Norelle Lickiss AO.

A singular woman who has achieved a great deal in her 90 years.

As noted in the Citation for the conferral of Honorary Doctorate of Medical Science, University of Sydney at the end of this book, Norelle Lickiss has, 'undertaken a variety of scholarly activities during her career that span the full spectrum of health care. Her published research has covered such diverse topics as the epidemiologic aspects of myeloproliferative and lymphoproliferative disorders; in vitro drug selection in antineoplastic chemotherapy, and the role of alcohol in the etiology of hypertension.'

But do not imagine this a purely a scholarly tome, Dr Lickiss is – although she would deny it if asked – a deep and contemplative thinker. She quotes from an astonishing range of philosophers and thinkers, from differing backgrounds and eras.

The contents of this volume cover Dr Lickiss's lectures, journal articles, ideas and thoughts from 1973 through to the present. As Dr Lickiss notes in the chapter *Letter to a Young Doctor*, 'These essays are explorations in thought undertaken over several decades'. The articles cover an extraordinarily diverse range of topics; not only health and medicine, but also philosophy, religion, as well as poetry.

In reading the chapters of this book, you can gain an insight to the beliefs and philosophy that informed her practice; the deep respect she has for human dignity – for the individual, the person, who was her patient.

The book is broken into sections, beginning with Dr Lickiss's *Letter to a Young Doctor*, written to a new doctor (or a doctor of any age) from a doctor who has had a lifetime of experience, and now has the luxury of being able to look back and reflect on the position of a medical practitioner and the responsibilities and challenges that come with that role.

The second chapter of the book deals with the oldest of the papers, *Health Problems of Urban Aborigines: with Special Reference to the Aboriginal People of Sydney*, a ground-breaking paper when it was first presented in 1973.

The book then delves into the complex and controversial issues such as; the teaching of deaf children, on individual and patients' rights, the different roles that a doctor has to negotiate.

By section seven Dr Lickiss is exploring 'The Patient as Person' and the human experience of illness.

Dr Lickiss then changes course and discusses her personal reaction to aging. This is a deeply introspective, challenging and personal account of later life.

In the last pieces, Dr Lickiss brings the book up-to-date with her reflections on COVID and how it has changed the world.

Whether your journey as a medical practitioner is just beginning, in the middle, or perhaps nearing the end, or if you are interested in the life of a remarkable doctor, you will find Dr Lickiss's collection of writings and musings thought-provoking, provocative, inspiring, and at times challenging.

I would like to thank – first and foremost Norelle Lickiss, for trusting me with her life's work and her innermost thoughts and ideas, Arthur Conigrave for his help and advice on the medical aspects of this manuscript, and Rosemary Scott for her thorough work in proofreading the text. As they say, all remaining errors are mine.

A Few Notes for Readers

This volume is intended as a 'dip in, dip out' style of reading. It is not intended to be read in one sitting, but rather when you have a few spare moments, or you find a topic that is of special interest. You will therefore occasionally find a topic, or thought, occurs in more than one essay.

It is important to keep in mind when reading this book that the papers span some fifty years or more – medicine, attitudes and language have changed in that time.

Also noteworthy, the majority of the works in this book have previously been published elsewhere, and for that reason I have not changed the text unless an obvious error was detected. I have left the references at the end of each chapter as they appeared when published. I have not replaced American spelling, nor have I updated sexist language (for example, where the patient is always referred to as 'he').

—*Dr Anita Hansen*

Contents

Foreword ix
Editor's Introduction xiii

Prologue 1

1 **Letter to a Young Doctor** *2023* 15
2 **On Our First People** *1973* 24
   Health Problems of Urban Aborigines:
   with Special Reference to the Aboriginal People of Sydney
3 **On Science** *1978* 45
   Science and Community: Educational Considerations
4 **On Limits and Liberty** *1977* 68
   Inaugural Professorial Lecture, University of Tasmania
5 **The Doctor and Education** 118
    i A Consideration of Personal Development
      in Relation to Deaf Children *1971* 118
    ii On Undergraduate Medical Education *1973* 127
    iii The Idea of a University, Now *1978* 138
    iv Address at a Graduation *2017* 150
6 **Medicine and Community** 158
   A The Possibilities and Limitations
     of Medical Practice *1981* 158
     i Doctor as Leader 163
     ii The Doctor as Healer 182
     iii The Doctor as Advocate of the Weak 202

    B   Other Psychological and
　　　　Social Dimensions of Medicine 226
　　　　 i Speech and Comunity *1979* 226
　　　　 ii Psychological Aspects of Cancer *1980* 239
　　　　 iii Care of Aged Persons:
　　　　　　Privilege and Responsibility *1981* 262
　　　　 iv On the Kindness of Strangers:
　　　　　　Notes on the Experience of Care *2006* 278

7 The Patient as Person 303
　　　　i On Human Dignity:
　　　　　　Fragments of an Exploration *2007* 303
　　　　ii Human Experience of Illness *2009* 327
　　　　iii Medical Practice and Spiritual Care *2016* 349
　　　　iv On Facing Human Suffering *2012* 389

8 Palliative Medicine as a Clinical Science 415
　　　　i Symptoms – the Patient as Subject *1986* 415
　　　　ii Palliative Care in a Modern Society:
　　　　　　Giving Structure to Compassion *1993* 429
　　　　iii Palliative Medicine at the Edge?
　　　　　　Questions Worth Asking? *2004–2006* 441

9 Late Musings 473
　　　　i Art, Personal Care
　　　　　　and the Jewish Tradition *2016* 473
　　　　ii Living in the Decade for Dying *2017* 483
　　　　iii After the Decade for Dying (75–85):
　　　　　　What Now? *2018* 498

	iv Spinoza and Medical Practice: Can the Philosophy of Baruch Spinoza Enrich the Thinking of Doctors? *2019*	519
	v The Tasks of Lateness: An Exploration of Living Late *2020*	526
	vi COVID Time *2020*	546
	vii On Poetry *2021*	547
	viii Medicine as Art? Reflections in COVID Time *2021*	554
	ix On Being Bereaved Late *2021*	566
10	**On Hospitality and Medicine: A Note** *2022*	571
11	**On the Occasion of COVID-19 Pandemic:** **Considerations of the Personal** *2022*	579
12	**The View From Here: Late Night Musings** *2022*	601

Epilogue	612
Last Word	615
Dr Norelle Lickiss AO	617
Acknowledgements	620

Prologue

COVID-19 has, since early 2020, applied a blowtorch to humanity everywhere: our ways of being and acting – how we think, work, communicate, endure, suffer and die, and care for each other. Our inequities and injustices are laid bare – and all our social systems.

Particular light has been shone on medical science and practice and the health systems everywhere, as has been the case in previous pandemics. Roy Porter concluded his masterwork on the history of medicine with the words, 'medicine will have to redefine its limits even as it extends its capacities':[1] COVID-19 has surely emphasised both of these tasks, and the media have underlined them both.

But COVID-19 has illuminated more, namely *the ecological frame of medicine.*

Medical historians consistently offer reminders of the profound relationships between disease and society.

Medical science and medical practice are part of the complex human web which includes not only material reality but also the world of thought and symbol. One of the marks of humanness is the creation of symbolic forms: man was styled by Cassirer in the early 20th century as *homo symbolicus.*[2] Medical science and practice relate to the symbolic universe. The 'medicine men' of traditional Aboriginal society, 'men of high degree',[3] were clearly conscious of this, and their practices abundantly demonstrated this dimension. But contemporary Western doctors, in many lands, in the interests usually of 'efficiency', tend to reduce the careful listening to narrative to the noting of check lists, and to replace physical examination of the body with imaging – and wonder at the loss (for patient and physician) of something of the soul of medicine. The failure to recognise the symbolic dimensions of medical practice is a profound deprivation: but the loss is not irretrievable.

Health care – and my focus is on medical practice – is embedded in society. Not only the economy but also prevailing values, political and legal systems and activities all impinge on health care and need to be thought about by doctors. And so do the protests. Angry protests against 'rational' means to control a pandemic are surely the visible face of far deeper societal malaise. What is at stake is not only the flourishing of persons in society but also the capacity of Western medicine, normally supported by adequate societal systems, to facilitate that flourishing. At one level, at least, the pervasive anger may be interpreted as a manifestation of bereavement in the fact of profound loss, not merely economic or consequences of inequity and injustice. A citizen in the midst of an angry protest in Paris (February 2022) mentioned to a reporter the rediscovery of 'fraternity': is this a clue? At the heart of a battle for the soul of democracy?

Bereaved persons and societies are vulnerable to other influences: doctors need to be alert that, as we learned nearly a century ago, dangerous populist leaders may arise in deeply distressed (even bereaved) societies, and widespread moral collapse may follow, even the moral collapse of medical leaders. Moral alertness is essential: history demonstrates that a shift in attitude towards the frail (at any age) or the otherwise marginal may presage serious consequences. Triage type decisions may be essential in desperate situations concerning the allocation of scarce resources, but only on the basis of foreseen benefit, and never made on the basis of the devaluing of the life of one compared with the other.

The time of the COVID-19 pandemic has also illuminated the *primacy of the personal.*

Jacob Needleman, over 70 years ago, pointed out, tellingly, in a communication with the New York Academy of Sciences that 'what medicine lacks is any fundamental notion of the nature of man and any remotely adequate understanding of that to which we refer to as a person.'[4] In COVID time we have seen some aspects of persons and the personal dimensions of existence (and our inadequacies of understanding) demonstrated in high relief. Examples are manifold.

The personal costs of isolation, and the distress wrought by separation from closely bonded others are manifest, as are the effects of loss of place, loss of social roles and dramatic impoverishment: all have high relevance to medical practice.

COVID time has highlighted especially the personal reality of dying: all of us eventually must die, and for some COVID-19 has been the tipping point, but in all circumstances, even when COVID is indeed the 'tipping point', the issue of the *quality of dying* is now writ large. The gross diminishment of quality in dying (and bereavement care) witnessed in COVID time (as in other plagues) is a grievous wound for humanity in our time.

In the face of all of this, and more, doctors may need not new information or facts (we are drowning in information!) but new perspectives, new ways of seeing. We may need to look again at the foundational (and sustaining) pillars of practice.

Now, about these essays!

We humans are lifelong explorers! We are called, above all, to be *thinkers*. John Locke in the 17th century (who trained in medicine) defined a person as 'a thinking intelligent being that has reason and reflection and can consider itself as itself, the same thinking being, in different times and places'.

These essays are explorations in thought undertaken over several decades. There is nothing new, just traces of ways of seeing, prompted often by the challenge of an 'occasion' or a new experience. At a time of bewilderment at an individual and societal level there may be place for reconsideration of old ideas.

Medicine may be perceived generically and formally as not a 'natural science' but 'a human science', a matter considered by philosopher Jean Curthoys as she tried to find rational patterns in some of my circular thinking and writing.[5] Fortunately, some see intrinsic value in a spiral staircase model of thinking (and teaching and writing) going over the same ground at higher and higher (or at least different) levels, and my own thinking – and writing – tends to be 'spiral': a warning for readers.

This collection of writings (*essays* in the primary sense of the word) are relics or traces of mainly unpublished 'occasional' lectures or pieces prepared over several decades, and, especially in later years, of dialogue with oneself, what I have termed elsewhere the 'interior colloquium'. Each bears the marks of the context and time in which it was given. It needs to be stressed that these writings are not academic works but *essays* that attempt to explore matters of concern prompted usually by an occasion, such as a significant meeting, or a requested memorial or keynote lecture. None of these essays are formally philosophical, nor are they concerned with disciplinary boundaries or 'rules': they simply articulate notions emanating during several decades of mainly hospital-based clinical work and teaching, brought to focus by the demands of an occasion or experience.

Ideas are to be grappled with in the raw, so to speak, if worth truly absorbing: some continuity (and repetition) of ideas may be noted, and is hopefully not too tedious; but hopefully also there is evidence of intellectual evolution, as would be expected over several decades. It is obvious that the thoughts of some writers mainly encountered in 1950s, 60s and 70s were absorbed into the mind, and they appear and reappear (I hope not in a boring fashion) in diverse contexts in my own later cogitations: this fact indicates the signal significance of deep intellectual encounters in one's formative years.

I have been privileged to share the human condition with thousands of patients, that is, other persons, often in limit situations, or with young doctors in training for various speciality careers. All these persons – and kind strangers – have been my educators, and have led me to recognise matters needing attention.

It is to be stressed, and it will be obvious, that the writings reflect the temporal and social context which generated them, but no attempt has been made to erase these contextual residues – and it would have been less than honest to do so. Sexist language, now intolerable, is to be found in the early pieces. Several allusions over the decades bear evidence to my continuing concern at the inadequacies of discussions of the responsibilities for care of fellow human beings in all the circumstances of life, however powerless and needy – prior to birth, when frail or disabled, or at the close of life at any age. Care is intrinsically relational, affecting others – and the relational quality of care engenders inevitable tensions concerning possibilities and limits. Recent legislation has clarified (in this society as in many other affluent societies) the legal situation regarding care in many fraught circumstances, notably at the extremes of life: at issue is clarification (in the clinical context) of the circumstances which could justify the deliberate and direct extinguishing of a human life.

Maybe a further comment is needed, in view of serious confusion (not addressed in the essays) concerning the regrettable conflation of 'euthanasia' (in the public mind and also in the mind of some doctors and nurses) with impeccable clinical practice. It is regrettable that bureaucratic procedures have intruded on core elements of sound clinical practice.

The *goal* of medical treatment should be set by the individual patient, guided by his or her habitual ways of coming to decisions (which would ordinarily involve considerations of the well-being if not wishes of involved others); ideally a trusted doctor with responsibilities for care should be partner to the formulation of such goals. If one is guided, as I am, by the perception that it is the role of a doctor 'to affirm life but not to obstruct death', then good clinical practice in all contexts demands attention to the expressed wishes of a person with regard to their life situation. A clearly expressed wish that life not be prolonged mandates identification of clinical processes or procedures which might be obstructing death (now or in the foreseen future), and the development, within trusted clinical relationships, of strategies to minimise their effect, with attention to the overall quality of life, and of course, the precise management of troublesome symptoms (with specialist help if needed) and unfailing care. Such clinical activity calls for a high level of clinical competence as well as adequate resources. (Decisions to avoid 'obstructing death' whilst affirming life are far removed from 'euthanasia' or 'physician assisted suicide'– terms which should be restricted to the administration of a lethal substance with the specific intention of causing death: such clarification gives precise focus to careful discussion concerning the issue at stake.) A clinical landscape embracing careful decision-making as outlined above, should be the norm wherever relevant patients are to be found – in emergency departments, hospital wards, in specialist institutions, and in the community: a massive administrative and educational challenge.

But it is essential to distinguish legality from morality. Whilst necessarily accepting what Alastair MacIntyre called 'the varieties of moral possibility',[6] there is need to recognise that the complexity of the manifold moral issues remain. Indeed, far richer discussion is needed regarding what we owe to one another in all circumstances, not as an issue of rights but as an exercise of responsibility. At a time when previously trusted institutions are failing to model moral rectitude, the integrity of doctors has never been more desperately needed. I remarked many years ago that a doctor whose morality is defined by the law is a danger to society: I think it is still true.

These essays range widely, reflecting the multitude of matters which come to mind in the course of clinical practice and educational activities of many forms and in many contexts. As the years rolled on I have been more and more concerned with generic issues in medicine, notably with the notion of 'person' at the core of the human science which medicine is, and with the task of medicine in the human community, as well as the experience of care. Maybe a word here or there may interest persons contemplating the same ground.

2023 Comments

Each of the older essays could merit a 2023 commentary (if not revision) – but such an exercise would be too tedious. However some comment may be in order concerning three essays, notably *On Limits and Liberty* (1977), *Psychosocial Aspects of Cancer* (1979), and *On the Occasion of COVID-19 pandemic: Perspectives on the Personal* (2022).

The inaugural professorial lecture, *On Limits and Liberty*, was a rather naive and limited expedition of a clinician outside her turf. Little did I dream in the mid 70s that medical expertise and wisdom (and civic injunctions which accepted it) would be the object of widespread angry protests 50 years later in the most affluent democracies. Freedom is the catchcry of the current protests focussed on medically relevant matters.

Isaiah Berlin in his landmark essays on liberty[7] (which at that time I had not read) offers thoughts (to non-philosophers) which resonate with our clinical experience. He undertook, he said:

> [T]o examine some of the fallacies resting on misunderstanding of certain central human needs and purposes – central, that is, to our normal notion of what it is to be a human being; a being endowed with a nucleus of needs and goals, a nucleus common to all men, which may have a shifting pattern, but one whose limits are determined by the basic need to communicate with other similar beings.

Berlin's legacy has been examined closely by scholars, with some serious criticisms of his positions[8] but his relevance and accessibility to thoughtful doctors is noteworthy.

Berlin is noted for his insistence on ethical pluralism, and the concept that not all apparent 'truths' are reconcilable.

Kelly in her appraisal noted that, 'Berlin held that there is a minimum of civilized values on which compromise is not possible. But on others collisions can be softened, claims balanced, compromises reached.'[9] He was committed to a radical humanism – with commitment to the human source of values. Kelly noted that this was a view which mirrored that of a 19th century Russian thinker, Alexander Hertzen. Berlin wrote of Hertzen that, 'he believed that values were not found in an impersonal, objective realm, but were created by human beings, changed with the generations of men, but were nonetheless binding on those who lived in their light'.

In the third essay, *Two Concepts of Liberty*, Berlin famously distinguished two notions of freedom: negative freedom – the area within which one may act unobstructed by others, and positive freedom – derived from the wish on the part of the individual to be self-determined. He wrote (carefully) concerning freedom:

> The fundamental sense of freedom is freedom from chains. From imprisonment, to struggle for personal freedom is to seek to curb interference, exploitation, enslavement by men whose ends are theirs, not one's own … Nevertheless freedom is not the only value than can and should determine behaviour.

In Berlin's fourth essay (*John Stuart Mill and the Ends of Life*) he specifically considered civil liberty in the light of Mill's ideas. It is noteworthy that Mill's ideas (reinforced by Immanuel Kant) have left a lasting legacy and, often poorly grasped, are central to the two most controversial medical issues of the present – the pressure for physician assisted suicide/voluntary euthanasia and matters concerning vaccination against COVID-19. Discussions on these matters often embody seriously inadequate notions of liberty and autonomy: at the heart of the errors are not merely the failure to recognise such limitations, but also failures to have an adequate understanding of person as intrinsically and essentially relational and embedded thus in community – a central notion in these essays.

It is relevant to observe that Bernard Williams, in his deliberation on some of the ideas of Berlin, noted that values with a long history defy easy definition: he gave as examples, liberty, equality and justice.[10] The same could particularly be noted concerning autonomy (at the core of 'positive' liberty) and the value of choice almost as an end, not means; bywords in popular argumentation.

It could be useful to point out that some of the ideas of Baruch Spinoza, a 17th century philosopher who is regarded by many as a forerunner of the European Enlightenment, may subtly enhance the sense of freedom of mind and heart, even of hard pressed 20th century doctors. Spinoza is mentioned here and there in these essays.

There is much to ponder.

A remark is also in order concerning including the 1979 essay: *Psychosocial Aspects of Cancer*. It reflects the thinking of the time. This piece is the edited response to a request made to me by the Australian Cancer Society to probe this area in the face of considerable community conjecture in the 70s concerning the relationship between 'Mind and Cancer' regarding causality, implying possibly a direct influence. Since the 70s the immunological effects of experiences such as bereavement have been much clarified. Access to information has been revolutionised by the digital revolution, and bodies such as the Cochrane Collaboration undertake extensive reviews of any conjecture. Furthermore, there may be now more appreciation of the complexity of causality of biological phenomena: Oxford cardiac physiologist and evolutionary biologist, Denis Noble, has eloquently explored such matters.[11] Is there still a place for a solitary curious clinician to explore conjectures, even now, with a vast repository of information at the fingertips?

A comment may be in order regarding the essay, *On the Occasion of COVID-19 Pandemic: Perspectives on the Personal,* ponderous indeed, but I hope not totally opaque or useless.

Thomas Fuchs, Professor of Psychiatry and Philosophy at Heidelberg, has recently published a weighty exposition of much relevance to ideas in the 'intellectual infrastructure' of the essays in this collection. He begins his discussion of the section on psychiatry and society with the following lines:

> The British psychiatrist Sir Martin Roth once described psychiatry as 'the most humane of the sciences and the most scientific of the humanities' ... This aphorism expresses the hybrid character of psychiatry, but also its unique bridging position. Located between the natural sciences and the humanities, being theoretical and applied science in equal measure, focussing on human beings in their physical, psychological, and social disciplines.[12]

It is my contention that medicine *as a whole* is a human science (or at the very least a bridge between 'natural sciences' and 'humanities'), and therefore that an adequate concept of the personal should be embedded in *all* aspects of medical practice: diagnosis, therapy, prognosis, care: *all* clinical decision-making needs to be rooted in a profound awareness and adequate understanding of the personal in all its dimensions. A clear view of the human good must be embedded in the mind of every clinician, lest judgement stray and (laudable) curiosity or addiction to more and more precise information (of no personal value to the patient) takes the place of care: 'flat-of-the-curve' medicine, indeed. How wise is it to define precisely the probability of the presence of a morbid degenerative condition for which there is no well placed hope of remedy? What is the value of truth as such in the face of possible personal deconstruction? The personal centre may not hold. Yet medical science is advanced by the wondering mind and the taking of risks by both patients (phase 1 trials) and doctors (think Jenner). Who can exercise the wisdom (as of Solomon) in such circumstances? Who can bear this burden? How? At the very least there needs to be in all clinicians (junior and senior) *awareness* of the calculus of harm and good and attentiveness to the need to strive for good, to have a professional *bias* towards the personal, adequately understood. A balancing act which is not beyond the wit of those privileged to belong to a tradition founded on both care and curiosity. It is a hard task – to embed this conviction, this bias, in the depths of the mind and heart of every medical scientist, every medical student and every clinician (especially doctors, nurses, paramedics). As Thomas Fuchs notes, what is involved in such a vision of clinical practice is a 'burden and a task'. But it is the core of what medicine can be, and what authentic clinicians may become: guardians and restorers of human dignity and the possibility of authentic human flourishing. And our leaders (even our politicians) and our diverse cultures, globally, nationally, and locally need such support – and even leadership – desperately.

 My perspective is particular and privileged. I have known, not the direct effects of war or famine or pestilence, but enriching encounters throughout my professional life, notably with the indigenous people of Sydney in the 60s, and since then with thousands of patients, and hundreds of students and trainee doctors, mainly but not only in Australian metropolitan public teaching hospitals. But also I have had enriching encounters with experienced doctors and their nurse colleagues (mainly cancer specialists, clinical academics and administrators) in other places in non-Western contexts, notably in Indonesia, Japan, China and Iran, and in professional relationships with colleagues near and far, some enduring many decades.

These essays express 'the view from here' – in this locus of being and doing: it is the only view possible to me. One of the advantages of ageing is the opportunity to see further, backwards at least, and the view from here is fulsome.

So my particular perspective has obvious limitations. However, it is my hope that the exposition of some of these old (but maybe not outdated) ideas may stimulate the new thinking which needs to occur as the humanity emerges from the present hard times.

Finally, Samuel Johnson (as noted by Roy Porter) described medicine as the 'greatest benefit to mankind'. In a world so distressed, is it possible that doctors (young and old), embedded as we are in the depths of society, sharing in human fragility – and knowing it so well, may find again the capacity, everywhere, to be unalloyed benefit, even a blessing, to mankind? It would be my hope that a glance now and then at some paragraphs in some of these old essays might stimulate new thinking, facilitating the reaching out towards such an ideal.

References

1. Porter R., *The Greatest Benefit to Mankind: A Medical History of Humanity from Antiquity to the Present*, Harper Collins, London, 1997.
2. Cassirer E., *An Essay on Man*, Yale University Press, New Haven, 1944.
3. Elkin AP., *Aboriginal Men of High Degree: Initiation and Sorcery in the World's Oldest Tradition* (1977), Inner Traditions, Rochester, Vermont, 1994.
4. Needleman J., 1969, 'The Perception of Mortality', *Annals New York Academy of Sciences*, 164:733–738.
5. Lickiss N., *Medicine as a Human Science*, Jean Curthoys (ed), Ginninderra Press, Port Adelaide, South Australia, 2022.
6. MacIntyre A., quoted in Owen Flanagan, *The Geography of Morals: Varieties of Moral Responsibility*, Oxford University Press, New York, 2017, p5.
7. Berlin I., *Four Essays on Liberty*, Oxford University Press, Oxford, 1969.
8. Dworkin R., Lilla M., Silvers RB. (eds). *The Legacy of Isaiah Berlin*, New York Review of Books, New York, 2001.
9. Kelly A., 'A Revolutionary Without Fanaticism', in Dworkin R., Lilla M., Silvers RB. (eds). *The Legacy of Isaiah Berlin*, New York Review of Books, New York, 2001, pp 3–30.
10. Williams B., 'Liberalism and Loss', in Dworkin R., Lilla M., Silvers RB. (eds), *The Legacy of Isaiah Berlin*, New York Review of Books, New York, 2001, pp 89–103.
11. Noble D., *Dance to the Tune of Life: Biological Relativity*, Cambridge University Press, Cambridge, 2017.
12. Fuchs T., *In Defense of the Human Being: Foundational Questions of an Embodied Anthropology*, Oxford University Press, Oxford, 2021, p181.

1

Letter to a Young Doctor
2023

Congratulations, doctor, after such a journey on such a road! And now you are at the end of the beginning, and beginning again! When you are not working maybe at least for a while, you would rather just sleep, perchance to dream. And you have no time to read, except clinical stuff, in summary if possible, or a note of what you have to do, or menus when you have time to think of really eating 'out', or messages from your long suffering family or friends. But maybe there will be time one day to dip into pools of ideas, about this and that, of some relevance to what you have to do and what you have become. And maybe you will find this little book, and dip into it!

    Let me make a confession: in trying (in my old age) to get these thoughts together I have not done a literature review on any of it! So if you are looking for assertions based in, say, level one or two evidence, forget it! I have two reasons (excuses). First, I have not the time! If I sought to review publications available on even one of the issues we reflect on, it could take all my remaining life! But there is a more cogent reason which bears careful cogitation: not everything that is known about critical aspects of medical practice has been written down, and not all that is written down is written in Western European languages, and not all of these writings are accessible now for examination by me (or the Cockrane collaboration, for that matter). Can you see that there is serious reductionism going on, with continuing neglect of valuable resources? What has been discarded as not fitting guidelines or seeming irrelevant or of no value might be useful after all! Be innovative! Mine literature of the past again (like a gold miner hearing about an abandoned mine) – you may find gold!

You are young, and in a new place, on a new path, facing a new threshold, with potentiality to be changed into actuality – like Michelangelo's sculptured 'prisoners' emerging from the rock: gaze at them in the Academia if you go to Florence. But who is the sculptor who will shape your becoming? You! As you respond to life, to all that happens, every day. Do not be afraid!

You are a doctor! But 'doctor' is a relational term (like 'parent' or 'child'). You, now, have a new and particular relationship, defined by law, with your fellow humans: the relationship of radical availability to anyone in your vicinity needing your skills. It is not for you to turn your back, or call any person 'enemy': every man or woman is neighbour to you! It is for philosophers to articulate the nature of human flourishing and the right paths for attaining it. It is for doctors to assist other humans whose flourishing is threatened or damaged by matters amenable to good medical practice. We as doctors belong to the world of the particular.

You are called to beneficence, never to harm. And called you are, with a particular responsiveness! And it is a vocation, a calling. Desmond Manderson, in a memorable address at a symposium of the Sydney Institute of Palliative Medicine in the 90s, gave us a rare insight into the philosophical basis of medical practice related to the thought of the philosopher Emmanuel Levinas. This basis is not adequately understood as law, or social contract, but as a response to the call of the other in need. Any decent and brave man or woman will go to the aid of another in need – say drowning in a river – but a doctor has such a response as a core requirement of life. You may be conscious of this already, through the long days and nights you already experience in your first years after medical school: as the years and decades roll on, you will be more and more conscious of this. Another way of looking at it is that a patient places an obligation on you to care, not out of a concept of 'human rights' but because of your radical love for mankind (cf. Henri Bergson – for whom the main purpose of human rights is to initiate all human beings into love.) Yes, there are limits to availability and to appropriateness on each occasion (and you must observe them), but the fundamental orientation of your being now needs to bear the mark of radical availability. Think about this.

The path is new, to you, but though the soil on it, even the stones, may be new, the path is old, and many generations have trod this way before you, maybe speaking different words, carrying many different tools, but responding with the same urgency to help another in need – and humankind has not changed much. So tread lightly, be aware, listen carefully with respect, and you will know that you are not alone, not ever; the past generations of doctors will be present to you, even in you, urging you on, especially when the going gets tough. Think of them. And be present where you are.

You are entering a new world, with structures, language, culture, customs, demands, currents, stresses, wild places, sanctuaries – all of which you thought, as a student, you not only knew but understood. But you did not! And now you must, as a novice, learn. You may be swamped by an ocean of information – evidence, guidelines, protocols, other clinical resources – much of it on-line, at your fingertips. But how to manage it, sift it, prioritise it, interpret it, use it! And not turn into an obedient machine. You have not been educated to become a monkey pressing buttons on cue, or a slave to 'guidelines' or 'protocols' (however useful as tools in your hands), but a wise person capable of interpreting facts, and (with due regard to fundamental values) making wise decisions with respect to this (unique) person in this place at this time.

You have limited time for reading, and when tired, may well prefer totally non medical stuff. This little book is organised into chunks mostly digestible in one bite, although you may want to go back over some paragraphs at a second sitting: it is certainly not designed to be read through. For this reason some central ideas are repeated – you will find out which ones. I may dare to say that when you notice this, you can surmise that I think (rightly or wrongly) that the idea may be a significant one, of lasting value, but of course that is just my opinion. And you will be the judge. Much will be so simple that you find it obvious ... OK! Maybe it simply took me a long time to learn what is obvious now to you!

You will also notice that there is nothing new here, nothing at all. Maybe old ideas are expressed in new ways, or perspectives which have not already occurred to you may pop up. Maybe talk to colleagues about these.

Or some ideas may simply want you to rebel and recast your own ideas even more vehemently; that would be very good! As Karl Popper asserted, progress in knowledge is not made by assertions/hypotheses being confirmed (or praised) but by being shown to be incorrect, that is, through constructive criticism. Ideas are like ships, and as Thomas Aquinas wrote: 'Ships are safe in harbour but that is not what ships are built for'. Ideas need to be tested, not just looked at. You will build better ideas in the future and incorporate them into better clinical practice: you must.

On a sombre note, be aware of the moral failings of medical practitioners in the twentieth century, by immoral research projects (USA Downs syndrome children and prisoners re hepatitis). And, never forget that in one of the most medically advanced nations on earth, from the mid-1930s until mid-1945, the doctors failed the people. Leo Alexander, medical observer at the 1948 trial of Nazi doctors at Nuremberg, after a careful analysis published shortly afterwards (*New England Journal of Medicine* 1949), wrote:

> Whatever proportions these crimes finally assumed, it became evident to all who investigated them that they had started from small beginnings. The beginnings at first were merely a subtle shift in emphasis in the basic attitude of the physicians. It started with the acceptance of the attitude, basic in the euthanasia movement, that there is such a thing as life not worthy to be lived. This attitude in the early stages concerned itself merely with the severely and chronically sick. Gradually the sphere of those to be included in this category was enlarged to encompass the socially unproductive, the ideologically unwanted, the racially unwanted and finally all non-Germans. But it is important to realise that the infinitely small wedged-in lever from which this entire trend of mind received its impetus was the attitude toward the non-rehabilitatable sick.

It is, therefore, this subtle shift in emphasis of the physicians' attitude that one must thoroughly investigate. Maybe you can see already that your own attitude to the most frail patient you encounter – in the wards, clinics or ER – even the dying one, the one you cannot cure, but only care for with profound respect, skill and kindness, as best you can – this attitude will define your quality as a doctor as well as a human being: it is no slight matter. Be sensitive to any slight shift from profound respect, in yourself, your colleagues, your students – do not be a bystander: we have seen enough of that. 'A man is a man is a man' – let the famous words of Gertrude Stein (who would not have meant her words to be sexist!) ring in your ears! In ER especially on a bad night! It might be worth mentioning Tennessee Williams play, *A Streetcar Named Desire* (which your grandparents may have thought avant garde!): a young woman of the streets at one point becomes desperately in need, mentally ill – and becomes dependent on 'the kindness of strangers': maybe just like you!

Some of this is poignantly relevant, for all is not well with medical practice in our time. There are gross global inequities yet every person is of equal value, and we try to respect them as such when in clinical encounter, anywhere. And even within an affluent country there is disquiet, with runaway costs making the present system unsustainable, and no clear solutions. New ideas are breaking the surface and some of these ideas will survive. It is my hope that reflection on some of the ideas raised in these pages will help shape your thoughts as your generation succeeds where mine has failed – to ensure a sustainable system for applying the stores of medical knowledge and resources to human flourishing, with no neglect of the most marginal and weak, at a local, national and global level.

In sum, you are in a new place, not just because of what you know or can do, but because of the person you have become. As you will see, 'person' is a relational concept: you have a new relationship with us fellow humans, and with your own self. You are not your own anymore, yet you have become richer in yourself, and each day, as you open to the persons and experiences which are along your path, and if you reflect on them so that you live and act from your 'centre' and your 'whole', you will continue on the way to becoming what you can be in your place and time. You will 'personalise' where you are, not by art on the walls, or cartoons on your car, but by expressing personhood, in fitting relationship not only to objects in your vicinity but by dialogue, even just with your eyes, with everyone you encounter, especially your patients. I suggest you read Martin Buber's *I and Thou* and *Between Man and Man*, or *The Knowledge of Man* written long before you were dreamed of. They are not easy bedside reading, but are books which could change your life.

'No man is an island, sufficient to himself' ... We are all together as humans, sharing various corridors together as we live, grow and eventually, at whatever age, approach the end of our lives. We are, each of us, obligated to attend to each other, to help each other, with varying degrees of obligation, often related to proximity. But you, you are obligated to any person, as a human person, not merely as family, friend, or assigned charge. You, as doctor, are called to respond differently to any person in need in front of you – friend or foe, if you are the competent one on the spot, and always respecting the dignity of that person in all times and places.

Medicine is a human science. You may think that this is a non-issue! But in recent centuries, as knowledge increased, divisions were made between the 'Natural Sciences' – like biology, botany, geology, and the 'Human Sciences' such as literature, music, philosophy and so on. The first group were characterised by observation, experimentation, and the latter by thought, argument, and so on. The German philosopher, Willhelm Dilthey, gave much attention to the criteria by which an area of knowledge could be classed as a human science.

This old debate is relevant because if medicine is thought about as primarily biology or a 'natural science', then the core element is lost. Medicine is not adequately understood as simply applied (brilliant) biological science, however essential this may be to the edifice of thought which is medical science. Medicine is about humanity – individual men and women, and human communities, whose flourishing is either threatened, limited or thwarted by illness. Philosophy, as part of the wondering which is its initiating spark, is about the understanding of human flourishing and its impediments. Medicine is about the understanding of the impediments to and consequences for human flourishing derived from sub optimal or malfunctioning of the human body (including the brain), and the correction (where possible) of these impediments and consequences. It is truly a human science, and if the humanness at its core is lost, the biological science may be seriously misdirected. The critical links with other human sciences such as philosophy are surely clear; philosophy should assist us not only in conceptualising human possibility (and limits), but also in delineating the features of right action.

There are matters which call for your examination and reflection. Henry Sigerist, the medical historian of the early twentieth century, stressed the interplay between medical practice and the age in which it occurs. We are living in a time of continuing depersonalisation of human services – in the interests of efficiency – but be aware, very aware (even afraid, very afraid) of the cost, and the danger of efficiency becoming an end, not a means, for health care. The fundamental pillars of medical practice, and most of its problems, have to do, not with fashion, but with abiding issues, even though the prevailing thought currents do shape the context of medical practice and the priorities and poignancy of the anxieties and even fears which arise. The context of medical practice now differs from medical practice 60 years ago when I was in your situation, but the fundamentals have not changed. Some of these will be briefly examined or at least mentioned so that you may think about them and build up your own conceptual frame for your practice.

Late at night when you are weary after a difficult day and wonder whether what you are doing has any significance at all, so immense is the tide of human distress, especially if one dares to think of the images of famine or war, you may want to recall as I have done many times, sometimes wistfully, the words of Kingsley Mortimer, a former Professor of Anatomy at the University of Auckland: 'The task of medicine is to emancipate man's interior splendour'. The particular is the place of our endeavours, even in the midst of a multitude. Just be what you can be, and do whatever you are able, faithfully – and be at peace.

2

ON OUR FIRST PEOPLE
1973

HEALTH PROBLEMS OF URBAN ABORIGINES: WITH SPECIAL REFERENCE TO THE ABORIGINAL PEOPLE OF SYDNEY

Edited version of a paper presented to the Royal Australian College of Physicians, Adelaide, May 1973.
Soc. Sci. & Med., Vol. 9. pp. 313 to 318. 1975.

Abstract

Australian people of Aboriginal descent are becoming increasingly urbanized: probably one fifth of the total of 120000–140000 live in the capital cities, including at least 12000 in Sydney. Patterns of ill health are becoming more defined despite difficulties in data collection: at least in the more readily identifiable Aboriginal households, there are trends towards high childhood morbidity (mainly due to infections and trauma), growth retardation and childhood delinquency, together with parental alcohol-related problems.

Such patterns are common in situations of stress and social disintegration and an attempt is made to try to discern the major stresses contributing to the Sydney situation. Urbanization involves, for the immigrant from country towns or settlements, a transition into a more impersonal situation where relationships may be fragmented, transactions more complex and the range of everyday options widened to a confusing degree. Culture contact carries its own stress, although colour-based discrimination may be less marked in the city environment than in country towns. Stress associated with residential mobility from country to city and within the city a notable feature may be somewhat buffered by the kinship network existing in the city and the relative paucity of neighbourhood bonds. Value dissonance may contribute to stress: there is apparent dissonance between value systems of past and present Aboriginal society as well as between contemporary urban Aboriginal subcultures and the metropolitan non-Aboriginal subcultures. Such conjectures point to the need for interdisciplinary research.

It is clear that alleviation of the most obvious manifestations of ill health by clinical expertise (available in a culturally accessible situation) should be accompanied by culturally appropriate radical therapy in the form of efforts at community development in order to reverse the underlying cultural disintegration.

Australian people of Aboriginal descent, *in toto* in the vicinity of 120000–140000, are becoming increasingly urbanized.[1] According to Census data, which tend to underestimate numbers of part-Aboriginal people, there has been an increase in the percentage of urbanized Aborigines from 23 in 1966 to 43·5 in 1971 whilst the percentage of all Australians rose from 82 in

1966 to 85·6 in 1971. Difficulties of definition of Aboriginal in terms of the Census and an increasing tendency to identify as Aboriginal may contribute to the rise in enumerated urbanized Aborigines, but the trend is clear. Probably one fifth of Australians of any degree of Aboriginal descent currently live in the capital cities and currently probably at least 12000 live in Sydney; the figure could be much higher.[2] There is increasing awareness of metropolitan Aboriginal people.[3]

Demographic data on the Aboriginal people of the Sydney region has always been sparse. The numbers of the Aborigines in the Sydney area at the time of the founding of the Colony proved difficult to ascertain. [Governor Arthur] Phillip, in a letter to Lord Sydney, 15 May 1788, wrote that: 'it is not possible to determine with any accuracy the number of natives, but I think that in Botany Bay, Port Jackson, Broken Bay and the intermediate coast they cannot be less than 1500'.[4] Sadly, disease rapidly took its toll and a letter of 1790 from Phillip to Lord Sydney carried the estimate that half of the native population of the Sydney area had died from smallpox.[5] Further decline in numbers occurred. The Honourable Richard Hill, M.L.C., in 1892 wrote a pamphlet concerning the Aborigines of New South Wales, describing therein the Sydney he knew as a 'young fellow' 60 years previously.[6] In his young days hundreds of Aborigines were living in the Sydney district and he lamented that in 1892 nearly all were dead and, he wrote, 'drink has been the principal cause'. Other sources indicated that during the 19th century immigrating Aborigines were not entirely welcome in the Sydney area. JH Bell[7] indicated that from 1878 onwards South Coast Aborigines began wandering to Sydney and set up camp near Circular Quay in the heart of the city; after the appointment of the Protector of Aborigines in 1880 an attempt was made to remove the Aborigines from Sydney but 26

South Coast Aborigines were permitted to remain at
La Perouse, some 10 miles beyond the central urban area.
This policy at least made the presence of Aborigines not
obvious to the casual observer. In 1824 C Hedley noted that 'an
Australian Aboriginal is almost as much of a curiosity in the
streets of Sydney as he might be in London'.[8] Contemporary
well-informed Aborigines,[9] estimate that at the time Hedley
wrote there were about 1000 persons of Aboriginal ancestry
resident in the Sydney region. It is clear from informants that
a considerable movement of Aboriginal people from country
areas to Sydney took place during the economic depression of
the 1930s. The war of 1939–1945 contributed to the growth of
the Aboriginal population of Sydney as Aborigines involved
in the services became aware of the attraction of city life and
subsequently brought their families to Sydney. Over the last
two decades the urban drift has rapidly accelerated under
the influence of economic pressures (there are more work
opportunities in the city) and social pressures (colour-based
discrimination is less in the city, housing is of better standard
and urban kinship groups offer support).

This paper attempts to offer first a perspective of the major
health problems followed by an approach to the understanding
and alleviation of these problems chiefly by means of an
analysis of the stresses or health educators.

I

Health problems of Sydney Aboriginal people have been
serious, certainly ever since the foundation of the colony, and
contemporary problems cannot be dissociated from those of the
past.

Investigation in Sydney in 1968–1970 reported elsewhere[10]
indicated trends which are clear, even accepting the possibility

of slight bias towards more readily identifiable Aboriginal households. Five major health problems emerged:

1
High childhood morbidity

With very frequent hospitalization in early childhood, mainly for infection (respiratory or gastrointestinal) or for trauma.

2
Depressed growth indices

With a tendency for the growth-retarded children to live in a household where alcohol abuse was a feature, where marital disruption had occurred and/or where residential mobility was marked. Factors such as income per capita in the household, legality of marriage of biological parents, eosinophilia or hypergammaglobulinaemia were not correlated with poor childhood growth indices.

Some aspects of the observed life style of the children may be relevant to these first two problem areas.

  i Despite the observation of Captain Watkin Tench in 1793[11] that the 'natives around Port Jackson are in person rather more diminutive and slightly made ... than the European' it is almost certain that nutritional, not genetic factors, are paramount in the growth retardation of these children. The evidence for this surmise is circumstantial but weighty; questioning of the mothers re the children's eating patterns was supplemented by direct observation of many meals and it was clear that meal times, at least in the inner city households, tended to be haphazard; low amounts of first class protein were eaten and a high carbohydrate intake was the rule.

  ii Morbidity from infections may be related to overcrowding; 26 per cent of the 120 children studied lived in situations where there were three or more persons per room available to the household – a figure indicating accommodation pressure well above the Australian average. High fertility contributes to the situation.

iii Trauma is made more likely by frequently observed hazardous leisure activities, such as climbing round old cars and buildings or playing in the street, as well as by poor lighting and storage arrangements in dwellings, making scalding and poisoning more likely.

iv Observed high residential mobility may be of considerable influence, e.g. 39 per cent of 120 children had three or more places of residence in the previous 3 years and during the first 9 months of observation 15 per cent moved at least once. The Sydney Aboriginal people, or at least the more easily identifiable Aborigines, are frequently urban nomads with shallow neighbourhood roots and lack of continuity of contact with helping agencies; such factors make health care more difficult unless the life style is understood and appropriate measures taken.

v Similarly, complex household structure with diffusion of child care responsibilities and with ultimate authority vested frequently in the grandmother, if accessible, even if not in the same dwelling, is an important cultural fact of relevance to health care planners and health educators.

3
Childhood delinquency

'Health' describes 'not a state but a potentiality ... the ability of an individual or a social group to modify himself or itself continually, not only to function better in the present but also to prepare for the future'.[12]

Aboriginal people share this broad concept of health and consider childhood delinquency one of their gravest urban problems. Discussion of this problem has been pursued elsewhere at length.[13] Let it suffice here to note that it became

clear that delinquency is an iceberg phenomenon, with overt
delinquency the visible tip of a mass of illegal acts which
are important constituents of the recreation pattern of poor
Aboriginal children, just as lorry skipping was the delight
of British dockside children in Liverpool.[14] It was also clear
that more serious illegal acts can be precipitated by personal
stress (for example, aggressive behaviour can be precipitated
by emotionally traumatic domestic upheavals) or can manifest
the search for something which will 'hold' as [Donald Woods]
Winnicott[15] described, or can be an attempt at role-playing in
a desperate search for identity. There were notable problems in
father-son relationships with, presumably, problems in finding
suitable models during the adolescent years. It was noted also
that delinquency has its own mortality – one lad died during a
prank with a car, another died tragically during involvement in
a legal process.

4
Alcohol related problems
Captain Tench in 1789 wrote of the Aborigines of the Colony
that 'spirits they could never be brought to taste a second
time'.[16] It seems, however, that very soon the taste of alcoholic
beverages became much sought after, and within a generation
excessive drinking became a serious social problem among the
Aboriginal people in contact with Europeans. Even Governor
Phillip's protege, Bennelong, became a problem drinker and
died in 1813 in a brawl.[17] By 1819 the drunkenness of the
Aboriginal people was a byword, according to some French
visitors.[18] One Daniel Wheeler, a Quaker, made a 'religious visit
to New South Wales and the South Seas' in the 1830s and wrote
in 1839 an account of the 'effects of the introduction of ardent
spirits' among the native peoples. He noted, when visiting
Aborigines in Sydney in 1834, that 'their debased condition

is greater than can well be conceived, and such as to render every attempt to assist them fruitless: if money is handed to them it is immediately exchanged for rum, or if clothes, they are forthwith sold or exchanged for whatever will procure strong drink, such is the curse entailed upon them since their acquaintance with the British'.[19]

Even the Aboriginal aristocracy was not immune from the problem: King Boongarre was wont to visit Europeans, often by boat, to solicit 'the loan of a dump, on pretence of treating his sick gin to a cup of tea, but in reality with a view of treating himself to a porringer of 'Cooper's best', to which His Majesty is most royally devoted'.[20]

In the early years of the colony, Aborigines withdrew from European contact by voluntary segregation. However, as the settlement expanded, Government policy[21] enforced segregation by limiting contact of Aborigines with whites and by forbidding the sale of liquor to Aborigines from 1810. The laws were not consistently administered: even Macquarie 'continued to give the native liquor until the very last day he spent in the colony. Yet his actions were in direct contravention of his own laws'.[22] Moreover, the closest associations of the Aborigines tended to be with those segments of the European society most given to heavy drinking, for example the itinerant white bushmen, such as drovers and shearers, who 'were mostly unmarried, rarely owned more than a horse and swag, and at the end of a period of work, spent their earnings in the nearest bar in a spent of revelry and mateship. Aborigines found this mode of living more congenial than the middle class values of thrift, diligence, cleanliness, sobriety and settled domesticity pressed upon them in later years'.[23] The prohibition of the supply of liquor to Aborigines was official Government policy in New South Wales until 1963 when the Aborigines' Protection Act was amended (with abolition of Section Nine).

During this period some Aborigines were able to obtain exemption certificates giving full citizenship rights if they were of good behaviour, had no recorded convictions, were in constant employment and had satisfactory living standards and domestic relationships. The matter of exemption was a bone of contention in the Aboriginal community and liquor was obtained surreptitiously during the period of prohibition: the present decade, witnessing the passing of such social systems, is in some ways a period of reaction.

It is hazardous to attempt to give current rates of problem drinking among Aboriginal people; data are not available. It is relevant that probably 10 per cent of white Australian males aged 21–64 have a drinking problem.[24] A high proportion of Sydney Aboriginals appeared to be young adult males; [Fay] Gale in Adelaide demonstrated this trend on the basis of detailed demographic data.[25] Young urban Aboriginal males often have difficulties in finding a marriage partner (Aboriginal women do not experience such difficulties) and are readily involved in a subculture where heavy drinking is the norm. Despite the absence of reliable figures for the frequency of drinking problems among Aboriginal men it is obvious to any in contact with Aboriginal people and to the Aboriginal people themselves that alcohol-related problems loom large.

Any approach to alleviation of the situation, by for example provision of functional equivalents of drinking[26] demands understanding of the role of alcohol within the life style of the urban Aboriginal people. It became clear during the Sydney household study during which many relevant discussions and observations took place, that Aboriginal men drink for recreation, for company, as a relief from stress (work, marital or racial), in some cases 'to feel a man' and for the pleasure of intoxication in a secure environment.

Many of these reasons are in no way specific to the Aboriginal subculture.[27] Some of the discernible roles of the public drinking place are, however, important and more specific. A considerable amount has been written about the social role of the public house elsewhere. [Ernest] Moore wrote nearly 80 years ago of the American scene that the saloon:

> ... supplies legitimate needs and is alone in supplying them. It transforms the individual into a socius, where there is no other transforming power. It unites the many ones into a common whole which we call society and it stands for this union amid conditions which would otherwise render it impossible, and intemperance is but its accident.[28]

It appeared that in Sydney the public house was a social centre of great importance for Aboriginal men (and to a lesser extent for Aboriginal women) in the absence of viable alternatives. It was a place of communication in a subculture where telephones were largely unused and where places of residence or work were transient and far less reliable places for finding a man than was the public house which he frequented. Further there appeared no other social situation in which integration of Aboriginal and non-Aboriginal Australians could take place with such ease. The needs for recreation, communication and racial integration are deep social needs and failure to fulfil them will prove costly. Alternatives to the public house are urgently needed but difficult to establish in the face of such a strong tradition. Alternatively, earlier diagnosis of problematic drinking is essential – also a difficult goal requiring intensive community education as well as culturally appropriate personal counselling services available at times of high life stress such as during secondary schooling, early years at work or early years of marriage as well as at diagnosis of a problematic drinking pattern.

5
Psychopathology – a note

Bostock in 1924 wrote that 'the Aboriginal has not reached an evolutionary stage in which the neuroses and certain of the psychoneuroses, hysteria and the phobias can exist'.[29] There is evidence that such an extraordinary view has been disproved. Psychiatric admissions do occur but, as may be expected, the proportion of disturbed persons reaching psychiatric facilities appears to be very low. Several instances of obvious psychopathology were noted during contact with the Sydney Aboriginal households:

i Depression in young mothers with heavy childcare burdens, expressed in feeling of inadequacy, often associated with anxiety concerning child control in the city, sometimes expressed desire to die and occasionally associated with alcoholism.

ii Anxiety often expressed in psychosomatic symptoms in teenaged girls beginning secondary school, often with a vast cultural gulf between home and school.

iii Behaviour disturbances in toddlers, e.g. in one child who had had marked discontinuity of mothering observed during a period of readjustment to another mother figure and subsequent gross anxiety observed in an infant present during serious domestic violence.

It is obvious that formal psychiatric studies are urgently needed in order to facilitate appreciation of the level of psychopathology in urban Aboriginal people and of the interplay of etiological factors, in order to devise possible fruitful programmes for prevention and optimum management of psychopathology. It is essential to appreciate the value systems within which the urban Aboriginal lives – the superficial observer will certainly underestimate the influence of Aboriginal tradition on the so-called detribalized contemporary urban Aboriginal people.

II

Such appear to be the major health problems in the urban Aboriginal scene as seen in Sydney at least. Health impairment is highly significant at a time when valid social progress is a critical need, for as Herophilus wrote in 300 BC:

> When health is absent, wisdom cannot reveal itself, art cannot become manifest, strength cannot fight, wealth becomes useless, and intelligence cannot be applied.

What should be the approach to these problems?

A National Seminar on Aboriginal Health Services held at Monash University, Melbourne in 1972 may prove a turning point. It was clear that a conceptual advance was needed and such an advance with grave implications was articulated in an editorial prompted by the Seminar:[30]

> It is only now that the question is being raised: is not the conduct of the Aboriginal people basically common to all human groups under stress? It would appear that the ill health and other problems of the Aboriginal people are symptoms of an underlying state of social and spiritual disintegration. Improvement in health can come only from an approach based on this underlying cause and not simply from the provision of better health services.

In the spirit of this far reaching statement, it may be fruitful to try to analyse the stresses to which urban Aboriginal people, as seen in Sydney, are exposed and then to look more closely at the concepts of social and spiritual disintegration in order to understand a little more of the aetiology of the observed health problems.

a)
STRESSES OF METROPOLITAN ABORIGINAL PEOPLE
1
The stress of low-socio-economic status,
commonly the experience of urban Aborigines

There is a freedom in being poor but severe poverty presses. Between the poor and the higher socio-economic groups there is a cultural gap, with the poor being conscious in some respects of a restricted range of options with often frustrations attendant on non achievement or non-possession of what is seen as desirable.

The financial situation of Aboriginal households was seen to be the resultant of several factors – income, output or spending pattern and reserve mechanisms embodied in kinship networks. The resultant was a stable equilibrium in some cases; in others there was a clear upward or downward trend during the period of contact. Lack of kinship contacts (with deprivation of economic reserves) was seen to be associated with economic instability – an isolated urban family had great difficulty in surviving as an economic unit.

An adaptation to poverty stress may be the observed lack of future orientation expressed in many ways: absence of the concept of insurance provision, poor appreciation of training programmes involving years of low wages prior to increased earning capacity, need for instant gratification and failure to store desirable and necessary goods. This failure of future orientation has many obvious health care implications.

2
The stress of urbanism

The city life has always attracted many men and its advantages are many. However, for the immigrant from a village type of society – and Aborigines in settlements and in small towns live in a cohesive network of relationships somewhat reminiscent of a village – the city offers also much stress.

　i　There is fragmentation of interpersonal contacts – business or social relationships are segmented, involving not a person's whole self but a part of their expertise, time, etc. and may appear impersonal in comparison with village-type contacts.

　ii　Confusion is caused by a wide range of options requiring complex choices, for example the supermarket scene. The public transport systems are seen by some Aborigines as too complex to use – and one observed them spend large sums in taking taxis long distances across the city.

　iii　Services may be relatively inaccessible because of cultural barriers; for example it was noted that Aboriginal women often fail to use well-baby clinics or some other health services and the reasons are largely cultural, not lack of awareness of need. Culturally appropriate services probably with Aboriginal staff are necessary for recent immigrants to the cities: the recently established Aboriginal Medical Service in Sydney is meeting some of these needs.

　iv　The city offers susceptible youths ready models of social deviance and facilitates their involvement with a marginal subculture, with psychosocial and legal consequences which are far reaching.

3
Migration stress

Rural-urban movement together with high intra-city mobility may be expected to lead to stress. In fact any such stress appeared to be buffered in the Aboriginal people by the presence of kinship groups in the city with the preservation of kinship visiting patterns irrespective of place of residence and by the shallowness of neighbourhood roots-moving was in this sense not the uprooting it might be for a middle class child closely integrated into a neighbourhood community.

On this point, [Erik] Erikson wrote relevantly: 'It is in disrupted developmental time that man loses his best roots, not in abandoned localities'.[31] So, whilst the urban Aborigine at least in the early years of urban living tends to be decidedly nomadic, the network of significant relationships has a permanence independent of residential location – and this may make the Aboriginal child less subject to migration stress than a middle class child without a firm kinship network and relying instead on neighbourhood roots.

4
Culture – contact stress

JH Bell (1964) wrote of the part-Aborigines of Sydney, 'today these part-Aborigines ... are assimilated ... no vestiges of traditional Aboriginal life remain and there is no idealization of traditional ways ... The part-Aborigines have no sense of separate identity'.[32] Ten years later certainly large numbers of the Aboriginal people of Sydney are conscious of being different and vestiges of traditional Aboriginal life certainly do remain.[33] It is also clear that race-based discrimination does occur in the city. It was of interest to note that appreciation of discrimination was inversely related to darkness of skin in a group of delinquent boys (most of whom had lived at some time in the city). The lighter the skin colour, the more the awareness of discrimination. If this was not a chance finding, it may suggest that the nearer to white in colour the more aggravating the gulf in achievement of readily perceived goals, just out of grasp; maybe with darker skin colour passivity was more likely, possibly made even more likely by the circumstances in which darker lads were reared, e.g. settlements or reserves. Militancy may be more likely on the edge of achievements, not in a situation where even the shaping of goals is folly.

5
The stress of value dissonance
RG Hausfeld[34] has recently highlighted the role of value dissonance in the genesis of morbidity as assessed by the Cornell Medical Index. His concepts may be open to further development as follows.

It could be claimed there are two aspects of value dissonance in the lives of urban Aborigines:

i dissonance between present Aboriginal value systems and past Aboriginal value systems and

ii dissonance between present Aboriginal value systems and those of the dominant culture.

The first source of dissonance may be the root of the sadness so noticeable in the contemporary Aboriginal people of Sydney. The second gulf may be the root of misunderstanding and aggression (active and passive). The urban Aborigine in general lacks the work ethic, the achievement ethic, the individualist ethic, the materialist ethic and the future orientation of the WASP society and is therefore considerably alienated. If value dissonance – in its two faces – is a potent cause of sadness as well as misunderstanding and aggression, what can be done? Can the Sydney Aborigine of today return to his canoes? No – but a more detailed understanding of Aboriginal history may integrate

past and present more satisfactorily so that nostalgia is replaced by salutary pride and appreciation of the relevance of traditional Aboriginal talents for solving the problems of the present.
And the achievement gap? This situation calls for a rethinking of educational goals and programmes within the context of community development.

b)
FURTHER CONSIDERATION OF SOCIAL DISINTEGRATION

The editorial already quoted noted an underlying state of social and spiritual disintegration.

In the urban situation the historical and sociological data together with available medical data are consistent with the following simple schema with its implications not merely of correlation but causality.

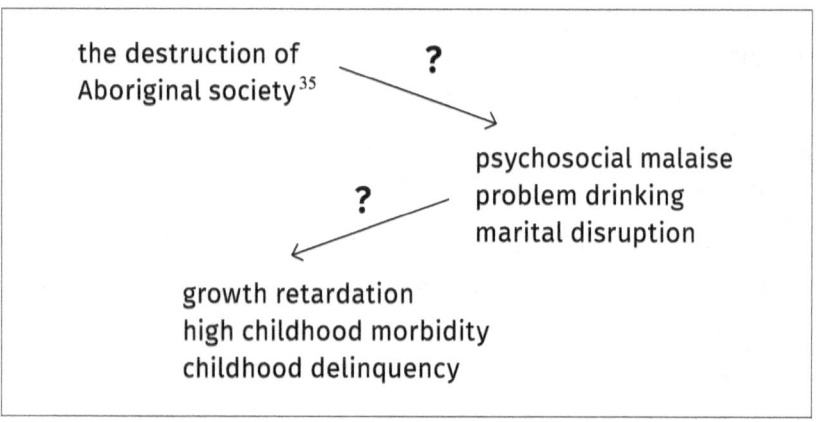

If such an aetiological hypothesis can be sustained the implications are wide.

i Therapy of the current situation must be interdisciplinary and multilevel: traditional medical measures alone are inadequate to solve what is a pattern of disturbed ecology.

ii Radical therapy implies the reintegration of Aboriginal society by all the means known to the development sciences.

iii Symptomatic therapy has an essential place – at the individual level and at the group level.

The individual should have adequate clinical expertise available when preventive measures have failed – the family may require a broad range of therapeutic measures: in the present justifiable clamour for more adequate preventive medicine the role of the clinician must not be decried.

c)
SPIRITUAL DISINTEGRATION?

The editorial previously mentioned claimed that the health problems are symptoms not only of social but also 'spiritual disintegration'. What does this mean? How can one prove or measure the spiritual disintegration of any man, especially of a man existing across an ethnic frontier? Assessment is difficult and maybe data derived from instruments such as questionnaires is questionable indeed. Nevertheless the notion reflected in the editorial may have a point.

Hausfeld has made observations concerning loss of value and belief systems. Maybe it is the world view or 'construction of reality' which is at stake. Some degree of spiritual disintegration may be necessary for spiritual growth and changing constructions of reality may be basic in profound social change. The forging of a new synthesis involves the freeing of the building materials from former contexts if not the introduction of entirely new building materials.

We cannot measure the spiritual disintegration of the Aboriginal people any more than it is possible to measure the spiritual disintegration of non-Aboriginal Australians. What one man might call disintegration, another might call freedom of the tyranny of false belief. Certainly there is no indication that the spiritual disintegration or lostness of the urban Aborigine is more intense than that of the urban white except that the Aborigine is perhaps more conscious of his lostness: even this is debatable.

III

In times past it was possible for physicians to remain apart from social problems. Those competent in curative medicine are essential links in a health programme in which many disciplines are involved; adequate understanding of the whole is essential if the physician is to contribute optimally in the task of alleviation of Aboriginal health problems and the promotion of the health of Aboriginal people.

The Aborigine of Sydney at the time of the founding of the colony, knew who he was and whither he was walking, understood his social role and appreciated his significance and dignity. In him past and present were integrated as his feet trod the land which had belonged to his people for thousands of years. It is different now. The urban Aborigine of today (like other urbanites) is involved in a search for self, seeking for the vision of the self he truly can be and the means to make himself according to that likeness. The road is hard and there is no other way.

REFERENCES

1 Broom L. and Lancaster Jones F. *A Blanket a Year* pp. 48–51. Australian National University Press, Canberra, 1973.
2 Stevens F. Aborigines. In *Australian Society: A Sociological Introduction*, (edited by Davies A. F. and Encel S.) 2nd Ed. Cheshire, Melbourne, 1970.
3 Rowley C. D. *Outcasts in White Australia*. Australian National University Press, Canberra, 1970.
4 Phillip A. Letter to Lord Sydney (1788). *Historical Records of Australia* **I**, I, 29, 1790.
5 Phillip A. Letter to Lord Sydney (1790). *Historical Records of Australia* **I**, 2, 299, 1790.
6 Hill R. 1892, Notes on the Aborigines of New South Wales, (pamphlet). In: *New South Wales Commission, World's Columbian Exposition, Pamphlets* Vol. 2. Government Printer, Sydney, 1893.
7 Bell J. H. *The La Perouse Aborigines: a study of their group life and assimilation into modern Australian society*. Ph.D. thesis (Anthropology), University of Sydney.
8 Hedley C. The Aboriginal people of Sydney *Mid-Pacific Ma*g. **28**, 55, 1924.
9 Groves, Personal communication, 1970.
10 Lickiss J. N. The Aboriginal people of Sydney with special reference to the health of their children: a study in human ecology. M.D. thesis, University of Sydney, 1971; and Health problems of Sydney Aboriginal children. *Med. J. Aust.* **2**, 995, 1970.
11 Tench W. *A Complete Account of the Settlement at Port Jackson*, (1793) reprinted with *A Narrative of the Expedition to Botany Bay*, (1789) as *Sydney's First Four Years* (edited by Fitzhardinge L. F.) pp. 274–275. Angus & Robertson, Sydney, 1961.
12 Dubos R. Human ecology *W.H.O. Chron.* **23**, 499, 1969.
13 Lickiss J. N. Social deviance in Aboriginal boys *Med. J. Aust.* **2**, 460, 1971.
14 Mays J. B. *Growing up in the City: A Study of Juvenile Delinquency in an Urban Neighbourhood*. Liverpool University Press, Liverpool, 1954.
15 Winnicott D. W. The antisocial tendency. In *Collected Papers: Through Paediatrics to Psychoanalysis*. Tavistock, London, 1958.
16 Tench W. *A Narrative of the Expedition to Botany Bay* (1789). In *Sydney's First Four Years (op. cit.)*.
17 Bridges B. Aboriginal and white relations, 1788–1855, M.A. Thesis (History) p. 101. University of Sydney, 1966.
18 Arago J. (1819) *A Frenchman sees Sydney in 1819*. Translated from the Letters of Jacques Arago (edited by Ward and Harvard) p. 286.
19 Wheeler D. *Effects of the Introduction of Ardent Spirits and Implements of War amongst the Natives of the South Sea Islands and New South Wales*. Harvey & Darton, London, 1839.

20 Cunningham P. (1828) *Two Years in New South Wales*, Vol. I, 3rd edition. Quoted in *The Sydney Scene*, (Birch A. and Macmillan D. S.) p. 49. Melbourne University Press, Melbourne, 1962.
21 Bell J. H. The La Perouse Aborigines ..., *op. cit.* 1959; and Bell J. H. Official policies towards the Aborigines of New South Wales. *Mankind* **5**, 345, 1959.
22 Bridges B. *op. cit.* p. 285.
23 Hiatt L. R. Aborigines in the Australian Community. In *Australian Society: A Sociological Introduction* (edited by Davies A. F. and Encel S.) p. 274. Cheshire, Sydney, 1965; Saint, E. G. Bacchus transported. Purporting to be an historical impression of alcoholism in *Australia Med. J.* Aust. **2**, 548, 1970.
24 Rankin J. G. The size and nature of the use and misuse of alcohol and drugs in Australia, Abstracts, 29th International Congress on Alcoholism and Drug Dependence, Sydney, 1970.
25 Gale F. *Urban Aborigines*. Australian National University Press, Canberra, 1972.
26 Lemert E. M. Alcohol values and social control. In *Society, Culture and Drinking Patterns* (edited by Pittman D. J. and Snyder C. R.) Wiley, New York, 1962.
27 Sterne M. W. Drinking patterns and alcoholism among American Negroes. In *Alcoholism* (edited by Pittman D. J.) p. 66. Harper & Row, New York, 1967.
28 Moore E. C. The social value of the saloon. *Am. J. Social.* **3**, I, 1897.
29 Bostock J. Insanity in the Australian Aboriginal and its bearing on the evolution of mental disease *Med. J. Aust.* (Suppl., July) **5**, 459, 1924.
30 Editorial. Health for Aborigines; a new approach? *Med. J. Aust.* **2**, 693, 1972.
31 Erikson E. H. Identity and Uprootedness in our Time. In *Uprooting and Resettlement*, p. 44. World Federation for Mental Health, London, 1960.
32 Bell J. H. The Part-Aborigines of New South Wales. Three Contemporary Social Situations. In *Aboriginal Man in Australia* (edited by Berndt R. M. and Berndt C. H.) p. 396. Ure Smith, Sydney, 1964.
33 Lickiss J. N. Aboriginal Children in Sydney. The Socio-Economic environment. *Oceania* **41**, 201, 1971.
34 Hausfeld R. G. Value Orientations, Change and Stress. Ph.D. thesis (Anthropology), University of Sydney, 1972.
35 Rowley C. D. *The Destruction of Aboriginal Society*. Australian National University Press, 1970.

3

On Science
1978

Science and Community: Educational Considerations

Stanhope Oration.
Annual Conference of Australian Science Teachers' Association, Hobart August 1978.

The New Biology: What Price Relieving Man's Estate? This is the title of an article published in *Science* in 1971 by Leon Kass. In his introduction Kass writes:

> A full understanding of the new technology of man requires an exploration of ends, values, standards. What ends will or should the new techniques serve? What values should guide society's adjustments? By which standards should the assessment agencies assess? Behind these questions lie others: what is a good man, what is a good life for man, what is a good community?[1]

Kass discusses the biomedical technologies in three groups:
1. control of death and life (by technologies of medicine),
2. control of human potentialities (by the technology of genetic engineering),
3. control of human achievement (by neurological and psychological manipulation).

After a lengthy exposition of the situation, warnings that 'questions of use of science and technology are always moral and political ...' and that power is in the hands of a few, and pointers towards what needs to be done (recovery of humility, regulation, caution), Kass concludes in a fashion which may serve as a point of departure for this oration:

> But caution is not enough. Nor are clever institutional arrangements. Institutions can do little better than the people who make them work. However worthy our intentions, we are deficient in understanding. In the *long* run, our hope can only lie in education: in a public educated about the meanings and limits of science and enlightened in its use of technology; in scientists better educated to understand the relationships between science and technology on the one hand, and ethics and politics on the other; in human beings who are as wise in the latter as they are clever in the former ...

'In the long run, our hope can only lie in education ...' So the gauntlet is thrown down and the educator is challenged and the prospect is more than fearsome. Why?

To one involved in one form of scientific education there appear to be major problems and these may benefit by some delineation in order that we may undertake some exploration towards solutions. While these may be more palpable to one involved in medical science, some elements may be found in the situation of those immersed in other scientific streams. The problems appear to me to be: fear, guilt, powerlessness, futility, confusion. Let me enlarge.

Fear

[Edmund] Leach in the Reith lectures 1967 said 'Men have become like gods. Isn't it about time that we understood our divinity? Science offers us total mastery over our environment and over our destiny, yet instead of rejoicing we feel deeply afraid.'[2]

It is as if our generation has not yet recovered from two major shocks of the mid 40s: the realization at the sight of the gas chambers and so on, of Auschwitz, of the potential for evil in human behaviour, and the appreciation after Hiroshima and Nagasaki of the destructive possibilities of technology. Even the memory of these events, secondhand for most of us, revives a sense of horror, awe and, I believe, fear. On the one hand our trust in the basic goodness of mankind seems to have been shaken: on the other was shaken our trust in the benevolence of the scientific revolution.

Guilt

The reports to the Club of Rome:* *The Limits to Growth*,[3] *Mankind at the Turning Point*,[4] *The Goals of Mankind*,[5] and *Reshaping the International Order*,[6] and the writings of responsible economists, biologists, ecologists, and humanitarians, and the mass media, constantly bear witness to the gross maldistribution of the benefits of modern scientific technology as well as the simple fruits of the earth.

We know there are 100 million seriously malnourished children on the earth while over-indulgence in the foods of

---

* The Club of Rome is a non-profit, informal organization of intellectuals and business leaders whose goal is a critical discussion of pressing global issues.

affluence is a significant health problem in Western society. We know that affluent Western nations allot something over $100 per capita annually in health care whilst poor countries cannot spend as many cents. In order to live with such harsh inequality and ignore the warnings of the Club of Rome we must be exercising communal repression. The phenomenon is so serious (and so extraordinarily irrational) that one of the latest projects of the Club of Rome is the investigation of the mechanisms of these psychological blocks.[7]

Powerlessness

There is a sense in which the community appears powerless in the face of the advance of technology – there are confrontations, strikes, aggression (and all have been seen recently in Australia) rather than a sense of sharing in the decision-making to permit technology to be developed. What can be done tends to be done, and just for that reason, on the assumption that every technological advance is in the long term for the good of man – and so it may be. However, the elementary principles of social psychology, if not justice, dictate that wherever possible the public (the masses as Mao [Tsetung] called them not disparagingly) share decisions of community significance. Although the matter is in a real sense political, all involved in science are potentially involved in controversy concerning technological advance in relation to the good of man.

Futility

The powerlessness has another dimension – that of futility – for the validity of medical science as an unlimited boon to the community is proving questionable.

In an Australian Medical Association prize essay published August 1978,[8] a fifth-year medical student of the University of

Sydney, Peter Root, castigates current medical practice in terms of what he calls 'the three social pathologies of modern medical practice'. He attacks first the economics of medical care – the market structure and the lack of evaluation of expensive efforts – 'In other words, much of today's high technology medicine is built on shoddy and statistically dubious empirical foundations'; second, he deplores the fact that the current medical system is oriented toward health-crisis intervention, not crisis prevention, and third, deplores, in the tradition of Ivan Illich (Austrian philosopher), the expropriation of health and social control – 'we need a shift in emphasis from a sickness-care model to one of health support, an appreciation of the need to control disease processes rather than just react to them'. Thus, an articulate student (and one of many) rejects, albeit with overstatement, the conventional body of wisdom which medical science has become and points to the need for a new paradigm. Other more sophisticated and experienced writers are supporting this approach, referring particularly to the 'flat of the curve' medicine currently practiced in the West, where vast rises in expenditures are producing insignificant or even no improvement in the life expectancy of our people.[9,10] The myth of the miracles of modern medical science is buried beneath the mass of the diseases of affluence. Our increasing technology has not been matched by an improvement in lifestyle – rather the reverse is the case. We have learned to transplant hearts, but we have not learned how to apply even what is known about the prevention of heart disease. We are seeking more and more radical treatments for cancer and seeking 'breakthroughs' every day, but we have failed to remove from our environment a potent proven carcinogen known to cause 90 per cent of our lung cancer and to contribute much to cancer of bladder, larynx and some other organs. We are learning to support a man's failing liver in all sorts of ways, even by using animal livers, but we seem to be powerless to prevent the alcohol abuse responsible for most of the liver disease in our men in their prime. The doctor in an intensive care ward can usually prevent a young woman dying of drug overdose but walks away with no sense of triumph when it is for the tenth time and it is rather the same with motor accidents except that even ephemeral success is less likely. Medical science in its brilliance is powerless in the face of social disaster and the shine of the latest instrument is not causing the glimmer of enthusiasm which it did in my time as a student.

There is another aspect of futility which has roots which are far more deep, for there is a more profound ethical dimension to the social failure in this case. The problem may be illustrated by the sadness of Ian Donald, Emeritus Professor of Midwifery, University of Glasgow. His name was a byword for generations of students of obstetrics and yet the last section of his little book *(Life, Death, and Modern Medicine)* is entitled 'Was my life worthwhile?'[11] In his booklet he talks of what he calls 'God-baiting research' and refers to work he saw going on in Sweden:

> The procedure is to put live babies aborted by abdominal hysterotomy late in the middle trimester into tanks of artificial liquor and then maintain them alive on cardiopulmonary bypass. These babies could be seen making crying grimaces and gestures as the effect of various drugs was noted in their circulation.

Finally, as he questions the possible misuse of his own research into early intra-uterine life, he ends with the sad words of the poet [GK Chesterton]:

> I tell you naught for your comfort
> Yea, naught for your desire
> Save that the sky grows darker yet
> And the sea rises higher.

Such sadness in an eminent medical scientist must be a warning that all is not well. The elimination of the unwanted for the sake of the good of the rest was the justification of Auschwitz and the shadow of this argument lies over us still. The shadow is there when technology is applied to make intra-uterine diagnosis of a possibly deformed foetus, or when abortion is rightly or wrongly considered as the wisest solution to an unwanted pregnancy: the dilemma is highlighted in a prominent teaching hospital in Australia where in the same building foetuses – even mid trimester (three to six months gestation) are deliberately destroyed and in another unit, high technology and devotion seeks to save tiny premature foetuses who are *wanted*.

In the face of such problems outlined above – and there are many more – information saturation, lack of direction, value confusion, polarization of sciences and humanities, apart from the sheer stresses of being an educator, there appears to be the likelihood of settling down with resignation to the fact that the adolescent dream of the joy of scientific discovery and sheer delight in the wonder of things has proved a mirage, and the harmony we hoped for is lost in contradictions and tensions on all sides. However, the present crisis may be in fact a growth phase, and as a pointer to the way through the morass, we may note the words of Chairman Mao Tsetung:

> The world consists of contradictions. Without contradictions the world would cease to exist. Our task is to handle these contradictions correctly. As to whether or not they can be resolved entirely to our satisfaction in practice, we must be prepared for either possibility; furthermore, in the course of resolving these contradictions we are bound to come up against new ones, new problems. But as we have often said, while the road ahead is tortuous, the future is bright.[12]

As part of seeking the way through contradictions, I wish to explore in three directions, seeking as it were for light: science and creativity, the interrelationship of the sciences and the humanities, and the question of goals.

Science and creativity

In considering what is essential to man, thinkers throughout the ages have reached varying conclusions. Plato and Aristotle stressed the fundamental need for intellectual understanding. In more modern times the voluntarists tended to treat freedom and autonomy as ends rather than as means, seeing autonomy as the final realization of man's nature. Determinist views of man reject the concept of freedom and choice entirely, and interpret all thinking, acting, and making to the interplay between basic drives and environmental influences. Freud saw man as 'driven', whilst modern behaviourists such as Skinner see man as wholly malleable. Marx conceived of man as primarily a productive animal: 'We can distinguish men from animals as soon as they begin to *produce* the means of life.'[13]

More recently man is being more clearly seen as inventor, and some writers see this concept as a unifying focus for consideration of man in the face of many other models reflecting particular perspectives or capacities. [Philip H] Rhinelander of Stanford University wrote:

> It is my belief that a unifying focus may be found if we stress man's capacity for inventiveness, recognizing that such inventiveness is displayed not merely in man's arts and crafts, but in his ability to establish complex symbol systems, to make and modify social systems and to build elaborate normative systems to guide his own behaviour. The root of man's inventiveness seems to lie in his capacity – evidently correlated with his highly developed

brain – to envisage *possibilities* beyond the actualities of immediate experience.[14]

Man's capacity for symbol-making finds one of its highest expressions in language, one of the most important and remarkable of human inventions. If we consider the model of man as inventive symbol-maker as probably the richest model we have and accept that language is the most remarkable symbol-system invented by man, it is clear that language (written or spoken) is close to the core of what is human.

Language is crucial in the development of science considered as that body of laws, concepts and ordered observations which man has created. The view is taken here, after [Karl] Popper, that the world of ideas is man's creation. It may be wise to quote Popper at some length in order to reveal the richness of his position on this point. In his recent paper 'How I see Philosophy' Popper wrote:

> I follow common sense in holding that there exists both matter ('World 1') and mind ('World 2'); and I suggest that there exist also other things, especially the products of the human mind, which include our scientific conjectures, theories and problems ('World 3').[15]

In his autobiography first published in 1974, he wrote:

> It would be easy ... to regard the whole of World 3 as timeless, as Plato suggested of his world of Forms or Ideas. We only need to assume that we never invent a theory but always discover it ... I propose a different view – one which, I have found, is – surprisingly fruitful. [*I regard World 3 as being essentially the product of the human mind* ...] More precisely, I regard the World 3 problems, theories and critical arguments as one of the results of the evolution of human language, and as acting back on this evolution.[16]

Near the end of his autobiography, he reiterates the autonomy of World 3 in a telling fashion:

> As with our children, so with our theories, and ultimately with all the work we do: our products become largely independent of their makers. We may gain more knowledge from our children or from our theories than we ever imparted to them ...[17]

Connected with this insight of the world of ideas and concepts as a *human creation* are several other concepts which offer food for thought. Popper sees World 3 having a history:

> It is the history of our ideas: not only a history of how we invented them, how we made them, and how they reacted upon us, and how we reacted to these products of our own making.

Further he notes:

> This way of looking at World 3 allows us also to bring it within the scope of an evolutionary theory which views man as an animal. There are animal products (such as nests) which we may regard as forerunners of the human World 3.[18]

Finally, as a close to his autobiography, Popper notes:

> If I am right that we grow, and become ourselves, only in interaction with World 3, then the fact that we can all contribute to this world, if only a little, can give comfort to everyone.[17]

I believe Popper gives us a key to the rediscovery of a truly human joy – that of inventiveness. The well-springs of human creativity are expressed not only in the arts, but also in the invention of symbol systems and in the making of theories and finding solutions to problems, at all levels from the carpenter's solution to the problems of joining wood to the theorist's conceptualisation of the movements of the stars. His theories concerning the advancement of science stress the key role of criticism in facilitating invention.[19]

Human work and life, even leisure, is so often concerned with the formulation of theories or solution to problems. If we can only recover the sense that such things, and the necessary criticism entailed, far from being obstacles to getting on with living, are in fact the exercise of human inventiveness, life might even be fun again.

The expansiveness of Popper's views prepares well for the consideration which follows of the interrelationships of the humanities and sciences.

The interrelationship between the sciences the sciences and the humanities

The sciences and the humanities may each find their focus in man – in man understood as far as possible in his totality. In seeking to elucidate the interrelationships it is useful to look first at an ecological model of man.

Ernst Haeckel in 1870 coined the word 'oecology' to describe the study of some aspects of the relationship of an organism with the outer world.[20] The application of this concept to the study of man has become widespread over the last few decades in connection with several disciplines, notably medicine, geography, sociology and anthropology, each discipline giving to the term 'human ecology' a particular nuance.

A child has been described by a contemporary paediatrician as a unique ecological experiment.[21] He envisaged the child at the centre of an environmental continuum which included the family primarily and other aspects such as race, geography, culture, nutrition and poverty. It may be that [John] Apley's useful model of child ecology could be adapted and enriched to take into account the dimensions of history and inheritance, biological and cultural.[22]

The environmental continuum can be seen to include persons, physico-chemical elements (including nutrients, toxins, heat, light, buildings, soil and so, on).

Behind or beneath, so to speak, each person lies a unique history with all its aspects: genetic endowment, cultural inheritance, intrauterine and extra-uterine nutrition, and total life experience. The pattern of the past influences and is embodied in the shape of the present. The person then is seen in time and space as in a dialectical relationship with the environmental continuum, with the past continually influencing the present, and the present contributing to the shape of the future.

In the perspective of this model of man (and it is only one of many models), several of the sciences and humanities may be seen to be interrelated: genetics, anthropology, biology, earth sciences, natural sciences, archaeology, history, linguistics, psychology, geography, sociology and so on. It appears clear in this view that an understanding of one of these intellectual disciplines is inadequate without some perception of all of the other disciplines. A balanced understanding of man as situated in community, and in time and space, is crucial if authentic scientific progress is to be made.

Biological/cultural

This appeal for a holistic view of the humanities and sciences has been made by many persons in many places. A report in 1971 of an *ad hoc* group of OECD on new concepts of science policy[23] recommended as follows:

> New social concerns raise issues with different linkages to science, and also different linkages within science. For example, science has received social support over the last 15 years primarily because of its role as a source of technology, but in the future it will be equally important

in providing a wider intellectual base for the control and orientation of technology – a more subtle and more complicated role. Similarly, the new problems call for much stronger linkages between the natural and social sciences or behavioural sciences. For example, in the field of health, the focus of attention is shifting from the biology of individual diseases to socio-medical pathologies such as drug addiction, alcoholism, and environmentally induced diseases. In education, the development of new techniques of learning may call for closer linkages between engineering and the behavioural sciences.[23]

The need for scientists to be grounded in the humanities is matched by the need for experts in humanities to understand the concerns of science. [Jacob] Bronowski in his wisdom warned: 'The world today is made; it is powered by science; and for any man to abdicate an interest in science is to walk with open eyes towards slavery.'[24]

There is, then, no more time or place for the two cultures in polarization: the humanities and the sciences must be interlocked because of their rootedness in the human reality.

The implications for education are considerable. The scientist of the future (including the medical scientist) must have, not as a luxury but as sheer necessity, an equally adequate understanding of the social sciences, politics, ethics – and the concept that these are mere soft options in which a poor standard is adequate is a dangerous myth. A scientist of the future who does not have a clear understanding of human behaviour (including his own), of social organization, of social forces, of the processes of social change (including disintegration and recovery) will be sheer danger to the human community. Even the concept of scientific (or medical) teams does not allow for one of the members to be socially and sociologically ignorant, for the team function may be impaired by such inadequacy. The discernment and introduction of beneficial technology demands human wholeness, first in the educators if such wholeness is to be imparted with the transmission of knowledge.

The question of goals

Francis Bacon (1561–1626) in the *Novum Organon* wrote:

> There is another powerful and great cause of the little advancement of the sciences, which is this: it is impossible to advance properly in the course when the goal is not properly fixed. But the real and legitimate goal of the sciences, is the endowment of human life with new inventions and riches.[25]

Medical science has become accustomed to pleas for a sense of direction:

> The momentum of modern medicine has provoked a philosophical dialogue forcing all the parties to it to consider certain questions that not too long ago seemed more clear and settled; those questions concerning the value of human life, the basis of human dignity, the goal of human existence, and the corollary duties of medicine to be governed by these assumptions.[26]

René Dubos went so far as to say that: 'The fundamental difficulty in formulating a program for the genetic improvement of man is that we do not know what we want to become or where we want to go'.[27] Is it true that we do not know what we want to become or where we want to go? We do have a clear idea of the main lineaments of the portrait, or we think we have, at least abolition of crass inequality. The late Paul VI, in the encyclical *Progressio Populorum* (on the Development of Peoples, 1967) articulated the aspirations of many:

> Freedom from misery, the greater assurance of finding subsistence, health and fixed employment; an increased share of responsibility without oppression of any kind and in security from situations that do violence to their dignity as men; better education in brief, to seek to do more, know more and have more in order to be more ...[28]

Such human aspirations can be facilitated by true advancement of science, but the wholehearted adoption of such goals on a world scale would change the face of Western science. Contemporary Western science is built on the principle of inequality – inequality in the availability of the earth's resources – and a wholesale restructuring of global scientific policy (largely as urged by the Club of Rome) would be mandatory.

At another level, the goals of human effort are not so clear. What is human effort for? What is my effort for? For me as an individual? That is one possibility open to me – to direct all my effort towards my own gain. There are others: effort may be directed not for the sake of the self, but for the family, for the nation, for the species, or towards what? Maybe my goal is to contribute to World 3 ideas, theories, concepts ... or is it to grow towards the absolute?

If I declare that my life is ultimately at the service of the nation I am seeing myself as a means, not an end, and am in danger of doing likewise to others, going against the principle of Immanuel Kant that man must never be seen as means but as end only. Or is Kant outmoded on this point? Are we in need of a new concept wherein the individual man can be seen as part of the whole while never as a means to what is less than man? This concept becomes crucial in the consideration of the adaptability of man. Science in the broadest sense is called often to assist in adapting man to conditions within the environment, or indeed within the self, normally considered inimitable to human survival. The condition is the *given* and the presumption is that man must adapt. It is considered that much of the ill health of today is wrought by maladaptation to twentieth century lifestyle and we may have it all wrong. In all this we may need to remain questioners of whether man's adaptability is being used to perpetuate that which is not for his benefit. Dubos warned us that:

> Man is so adaptable that he could survive and multiply in underground shelters even though his regimented subterranean existence left him unaware of the robin's song in the spring, the whirl of dead leaves in the fall, and the moods of the wind – even though indeed all his ethical and aesthetic values should wither …[29,30]

Each man, then, each one of us who is a teacher must clarify the goals of his or her life, and the hierarchy of values which motivate us, and be prepared to be part of what Schumacher called 'metaphysical reconstruction'. Science as the body of ideas, concepts and ordered observations forming part of World 3 may be initially given direction by those who create them but, as Popper insists, World 3 has its own autonomy and ultimately is directionless (and a potential monster) unless given direction deliberately by man.

There is much talk of values,[31] their nature, their origin, their shape, their influence, and much of the talk is confused (and some say mere 'hot air'). But however great the confusion in concept, the debate about values is crucial and the interrelationship with ethical issues has become clear.

The Club of Rome is well aware of the situation. A report of a technical symposium of the Club of Rome held in Tokyo in 1973 is explicit:

> There is an obvious need for an overarching, globally integrated vision of a desirable, and at the same time feasible future. A vision that is also a *moral* vision ... A new balance between individual rights and collective obligations, between freedom and social discipline, between economic efficiency and justice, has to be found ... Real concern for man's present predicament and for his options for a civilized future in a crowded and limited world inevitably forces man to confront himself and the ultimate questions of life and death, the meaning he chooses to give his own life and that of the human race.[32]

It may be relevant here to look briefly at the analysis made by Lawrence Kohlberg of the stages of human moral development: I am indebted to [Ronald] Duska and [Mariellen] Whelan[33] for a guide to his thought.

Kohlberg, currently professor of education and social psychology at Harvard, followed a group of fifty American males (aged ten to twenty-eight) for eighteen years, using as a basis of his research the response of the subject to certain moral dilemmas. Initially, he identified six generally distinguishable orientations or perspectives which became the bases of his six stages of moral development. Over the eighteen years Kohlberg found that each subject went through the same sequence of stages and subsequent work has shown that the sequence is found in several diverse cultures. In brief, the stages of moral judgement are:

Stage 1   The punishment and obedience orientation – the physical consequences of an action determine its goodness.

Stage 2   The instrumental relativist orientation – right action consists in that which instrumentally satisfies one's needs and occasionally the needs of others.

Stage 3   The interpersonal concordance of good boy/nice girl orientation – good behaviour is that which pleases or helps others and is approved by them.

Stage 4   The law and order orientation – right behaviour consists of doing one's duty, showing respect for authority and maintaining the given social order for its own sake.

Stages 1 and 2 are termed 'pre-conventional' and stages 3 and 4 'conventional'. The following two stages are termed 'post-conventional' and are marked by a clear effort to define moral values and principles which have validity apart from the authority of those holding those principles.

Stage 5   The social contract legalistic orientation – right action is defined in terms of general individual rights and in terms of standards which have been critically examined and agreed upon by the whole society.

Stage 6   The universal ethical principle orientation – right is defined by the decision of conscience in accord with selfchosen ethical principles appealing to logical comprehensiveness, universality and consistency. These principles are abstract and ethical, not concrete moral rules like the ten commandments. At heart these are universal principles of justice, of the reciprocity and equality of the human rights, and of respect for the dignity of human beings as individual persons.

The Swedish State Commission on Sex Education 1974 issued proposed guidelines for sex education in the Swedish school system, introducing the concept of fundamental values, reminiscent of Kohlberg's sixth stage. A guideline is offered in *Instruction on Values* as follows:

> By the terms of the curriculum for the basic and the comprehensive school, instruction shall be given both on the fundamental values and on values which are in dispute, which are termed controversial values. In handling the fundamental values teaching should not be objective but should take sides and aim to promote certain ideas. Examples of such values are the 'inherent value of man, the inviolability of human life and thus the right to personal integrity'. Examples of controversial values are the various fundamental political philosophies, and different attitudes to certain questions of sexual morality. In the case of controversial values teaching should be objective.[34]

The idea implicit in the Swedish Commission's noble attempt is that men agree on what values are fundamental, or are subsumed under agreed fundamental values: however, the classification of the inviolability of human life as a fundamental value could lead to the right of the foetus to life to be recognized as fundamental and not controversial, a conclusion probably unintended by the Commission.

The discussions of Kohlberg and the Swedish Commission raise unavoidably the origin of values and the matter of absolutes. For Bronowski 'The values by which we are to survive are not rules for just and unjust conduct, but are those deeper illuminations in whose light justice and injustice, good and evil, means and ends are seen in fearful sharpness of outline'.[35]

It is said that to every man is given illumination from within. From a god within? From without? From interaction with World 3? It has been said, too, that the question is not 'do you believe in God?' but 'in what god do you believe?' It can be argued that every man has an absolute before which or before whom he is prepared to bow. The shape or name of that absolute in the case of the scientist may be the fear or the hope of the community. It must be the concern of every true scientist that in the end the goal towards which scientific effort is directed will be such that there may be an end to the fear, guilt, powerlessness and futility, which overshadow us.

The scientific progress of the last three centuries has given shape to a garment which having served its time may be now outmoded. There are abundant signs that in the terms of Thomas Kuhn [36] a new paradigm is needed – we need a scientific revolution. It may be that the unilateral development of science; impelled from within by the inventiveness of man, needs to be moulded by extrinsic influences. Kuhn, however, might suggest that in his terms 'the resolution of revolutions' ('selection by conflict within the scientific community of the fittest way to practice future science') may still prove in the ultimate the way through the present crisis, rather than to offer goals from without to science. If such a model is to prove satisfactory, then the conflict within the scientific community must be vital, with none of us failing to throw what light we can on the values debate – even if that light at times generates heat.

Whatever be the means a new concept of science (if not of the scientist) must be born. To patch the old is not good enough, but it is of the very nature of man the inventor to bring forth something new, and now is the time, for the sake of us all.

References

1 Kass, LR. 'The New Biology: what price relieving man's estate?' Science 174 (1971) 779–88. Kass was writing as executive secretary, Committee on the Life Sciences and Social Policy, National Research Council, National Academy of Sciences, Washington DC.
2 Leach, E. *A Runaway World?* Reith Lectures. BBC London 1967, 1.
3 Meadows, D.H., Meadows, D.L., Randers, J. and Behrens, W.W. *The Limits to Growth.* First Report to the Club of Rome, Earth Island Limited, London 1972.
4 Mesarovic, M. and Pestel, E. *Mankind at the Turning Point.* The Second Report to the Club of Rome, Hutchinson, London 1975.
5 Laszlo, E. *The Goals for Mankind.* Report to the Club of Rome on the New Horizons of Global Community, Dutton, New York 1977.
6 Tinbergen, J., Dolman, A.J. and von Ettinger, J. *Reshaping the International Order.* A Report to the Club of Rome, Hutchinson, London 1977, 19–20.

'We have today about two-thirds of mankind living – if it can be called living – on less than 30 cents a day. We have today a situation where there are about one billion illiterate people around the world, although the world has both the means and technology to spread education. We have nearly 70 per cent of the children in the Third World suffering from malnutrition, although the world has the resources to feed them.

'We have maldistribution of the world's resources on a scale where the industrialized countries are consuming about twenty times more of the resources per capita than the poor countries. We have a situation where, in the Third World, millions of people toil under a broiling sun from morning till dusk for miserable rewards and premature death without ever discovering the reasons why'.

7 Boniecki, G.J. 'Is Man interested in his Future? The psychological question of our times.' *International Journal of Psychology* 12 (1977) 59–64.
8 Root, P. 'Medicine in the Year 2000.' *A.M.A. Gazette* 17 Aug. 1978, 14–18.
9 Enthoven, A.C. 'Shuttuck Lecture – Cutting Cost without Cutting the Quality of Care' *New England Journal of Medicine* 298 (1978) 1229–38.
10 Maxwell, R., *Health Care: The Growing Dilemma*, 2nd edition. McKinsey, New York 1976. See also Hetzel, B. *Health and Australian Society*, 2nd edition, Penguin, Ringwood 1976.
11 Donald, I. *Life, Death and Modern Medicine.* Social Responsibility Series, Order of Christian Unity, London 1974.

12 Mao Tsetung. *Selected Works*, vol. V, Foreign Languages Press, Peking 1969, 306.
13 Marx, K. *Capital and other Writings*, ed. Eastman, Modern Library 1 (quoted in Rhinelander, *vide infra*, p.71) 1932.
14 Rhinelander, P.H. *Is Man Comprehensible to Man?* Freeman, San Francisco 1974, 97.
15 Popper, K. 'How I see Philosophy.' in *Philosophers on Their Own Work*, vol.3 (ed. A. Mercier and M. Svilar) Peter Lane, Berne, Frankfurt am Main, Las Vegas, 1977, 147.
16 Popper, K. *Unended Quest: An Intellectual Autobiography*. Fontana, Collins, Glasgow 1976, 186.
17 *Ibid*, 196.
18 *Ibid*, 187.
19 There are quite specific points in which, according to Popper's theory of the advancement of science, the community of scholars plays an essential role. Popper points out, notably in his book, *Objective Knowledge*, (Oxford 1972) that in logic a scientific law is conclusively falsifiable although it is not conclusively verifiable. Popper urges, therefore, that we do not systematically evade refutation, but we formulate our theories as unambiguously as possible so that they may be exposed to refutation. Where an observation is made which refutes the theory by methodology which is truly rigorous, then we must search for a new hypothesis which may then be tested by devising confrontations between its consequences and new observable experience. Criticism, then, is to be prized and the competent criticism of the scientific community is part of the process of growth of science.
20 Haeckel, E. 'Ueber Entwickelungsgang und Aufgabe der Zoologie', *Jenaische Zeitschrift für Medicine und Naturwissenschaft* 5 (1870) 353, cited by Bates in *Anthropology Today: Selections*, ed. by Tax, Chicago 1962, 222.
21 Apley, J. 'An Ecology of Childhood.' *The Lancet* 2 (1964) 1.
22 Lickiss, J.N. 'The Aboriginal People of Sydney with Special Reference to the Health of their Children: A study in human ecology.' M.D. thesis, University of Sydney 1971, 6.
23 The Secretary-General's *Ad Hoc* group on New Concepts of Science Policy, Science, Growth and Society: *A New Perspective*, Organization for Economic Co-operation and Development, Paris 1971.
24 Bronowski, J. *Science and Human Values*, revised edition, Harper and Row, New York 1965, 6.
25 Bacon, Francis. *Novum Organon*, I: 80, quoted in *Great Treasury of Western Thought* (ed. M.J. Adler and C. Van Doren) Bowker Company, New York 1977, 1110.

26 Stumpf, S.E. 'Some Moral Dimensions of Medicine.' *Annals Internal Medicine* 64 (1966) 460.
27 Dubos, R. *Man Adapting.* Yale University Press, New Haven 1965, 278.
28 Paul VI. *On the Development of Peoples.* Vatican Translation St. Paul Publications, Homebush, Sydney 1967, 7.
29 Dubos, *op. cit.* 434.
30 Schumacher, E. 'The Greatest Resource – Education' in *The Small is Beautiful.* Blond and Briggs, London 1973, 92.
31 Laszl, E. and Wilbur, J.B., *Human Values and Natural Science.* Proceedings of the Third Conference on Value Inquiry (held at State University of New York 1969) Gordon and Breach, New York 1970.
32 Siebker, M. and Yoichi Kaya, *Report from Tokyo.* The Technical Symposium of the Club of Rome. Tokyo 1973, typescript January 1974.
33 Duska, R. and Whelan, M. 'Kohlberg's Theory of Moral Development' in *Moral Development. A guide to Piaget and Kohlberg*, Paulist Press 1975, 42–79.
34 Swedish State Commission on Sex Education 1974, *Proposed guidelines for Sex Education in the Swedish School System*, quoted in Royal Commission on Human Relationships Final Report, vol. 2, Australian Government Publishing Service, Canberra 1977, 81.
35 Bronowski, *op. cit.* 73.
36 Kuhn T.S. *The Structure of Scientific Revolutions.* 2nd Edition. International Encyclopedia of Unified Science, University of Chicago Press, Chicago, 1970.

4

ON LIMITS AND LIBERTY

1977

INAUGURAL PROFESSORIAL LECTURE,
UNIVERSITY OF TASMANIA

Edited version of Inaugural Professorial Lecture, Hobart, Launceston and Burnie, Tasmania. 1977.
Occasional Paper, University of Tasmania.

A man who follows an intellectual profession must pause time after time in the midst of his activity as he becomes aware of the paradox he is pursuing. Each of these professions stands, indeed, on paradoxical ground. When he pauses, something important has already happened. But this happening only becomes significant if he does not content himself with taking such fleeting upheavals of a well-ordered world into the register of the memory. Again and again, not too long after the completion of the thus interrupted activity, he must occupy himself, in strenuous yet dispassionate reflection, with the actual problematic to which he has been referred. With the involvement of his living and suffering person, he must push forward to greater and still greater clarity of that paradox.

—*Martin Buber*[1]

In 1859 John Stuart Mill commenced his essay entitled *On Liberty* with the following words:

> The object of this Essay is to assert one very simple principle, as entitled to govern absolutely the dealings of society with the individual in the way of compulsion and control, whether the means used be physical force in the form of legal penalties, or the moral coercion of public opinion. That principle is, that the sole end for which mankind are warranted, individually or collectively, in interfering with the liberty of action of any of their number is self-protection. That the only purpose for which power can be rightfully exercised over any member of a civilised community, against his will, is to prevent harm to others. His own good, either physical or moral is not a sufficient warrant.

Some paragraphs later Mill further notes:

> Each is the proper guardian of his own health, whether bodily, or mental and spiritual. Mankind are greater gainers by suffering each other to live as seems good to themselves, than by compelling each to live as seems good to the rest.[2]

Contemporary medical practice is in a sense at an impasse, confronted on every side by problems of choice, involved, albeit unwillingly, in the decisions being made by the human community today concerning the very shape of the future. Such decisions presume but also appear to threaten liberty – and this in an age where freedom is so treasured that limitation of freedom implies for many some limitation of humanness. It appears, however, that a tension between liberty and its limits is perceptible in several current health issues. Mill has, as it were, in his own exaltation of liberty, thrown down the gauntlet and serves admirably as a point of departure in an exploration of one of these issues, namely, the evolution of disease patterns in Australia in the last one hundred years, medical care problems and certain global health issues.

Mortality and Morbidity Trends in Australia

Information concerning mortality and morbidity patterns in the Australian colonies tends to be fragmentary in the early part of the nineteenth century. Registration of deaths became compulsory in Van Diemen's Land in 1839, in Western Australia in 1841, in South Australia in 1842, in Victoria in 1853, and in New South Wales (then including Queensland) in 1856. Information concerning disease patterns and survival trends has been recently usefully summarized by [CM] Young.[3] Life expectancy at birth a century ago was approximately forty-six years for males and fifty years for females; at that time nearly twenty percent of deaths of males and eighteen percent of deaths of females occurred below the age of five years.

Young has also demonstrated that reliable data regarding births, deaths and migration coupled with national census data enable age-specific mortality rates to be traced for each year since 1921. Recent less formal studies of the Australian mortality experience are also now readily available.[4,5]

Morbidity (or illness) patterns as distinct from mortality patterns are rather more difficult to establish and the design of the study (e.g. population based on health care services/doctor-based) influences the pattern remarkably. The Royal Australian College of General Practitioners has recently published an Australia-wide doctor-based morbidity survey.[6]

Significant contributions to the documentation of the Tasmanian health scene have been made in recent years not only by historians such as [Michael] Roe[7] but also by senior medical students of the University of Tasmania.[8] From these data several general trends emerge:

1. There was in Australia a steady and impressive decline in infectious diseases, notably tuberculosis, during the last decades of the nineteenth century and the first four decades of the twentieth century as a result undoubtedly of improved social conditions (including nutrition); medical measures, including case finding, antibiotics and immunization, had most influence since that time and accelerated the improvement.

2. Maternal and infant mortality fell steadily since the turn of the twentieth century, exhibiting the influence of both social and specific medical factors.

3. The last three decades have seen the emergence of ischaemic heart disease, lung cancer, and motor vehicle accidents as causes of mortality in almost epidemic proportions; there are, however, recent signs suggesting a levelling off of the situation with respect to ischaemic heart disease as has already been noted in ischaemic heart disease elsewhere.

4. Life expectancy in Australia has, under the influence of all these trends, improved overall in the last century, especially at birth and early childhood, but improvement has been considerably less for the middle-aged, especially men, because of the emergence notably of ischaemic heart disease. [Keith] Windschuttle[9] demonstrated a rising mortality rate for 15–24 year old males 1960–1975, mainly due to accidents, and to a lesser extent suicide.

5   On a world scale Australia ranks tenth when mortality rates are compared, including prenatal, infant, maternal, men 35–44, 45–54, and women 35–44, 45–54, according to methods used by [Robert] Maxwell.[10,11] Countries with more favourable mortality situations are (in order) Sweden, Norway, Netherlands, Switzerland, Denmark, England and Wales, Finland, Belgium and Spain.

These trends are disturbing and are reasonably attributable at least in part to life-style factors, notably cigarette smoking and alcohol abuse, rather than to deficient health care, but both areas require careful consideration. Rabbi Heschel noted of U.S.A. 'according to my own medical theory, more people die of success than of cancer'.[12] It may also be true in Australia.

'Epidemiological evidence from many countries implicates tobacco smoking as an important causative factor in lung cancer, chronic bronchitis and emphysema, ischaemic heart disease, and obstructive peripheral vascular disease. It also shows that smoking plays a part in the causation of cancer of the tongue, larynx, oesophagus, pancreas and bladder; abortion, still-birth, and neonatal death; and gastroduodenal ulcer.' So commences a recent World Health Organization report on smoking and its Effects on Health (1975): and Expert Committee reviewed in considerable detail the evidence relating smoking and disease and recommended national and international action.[13] [Richard] Doll's classic study of many thousands of British doctors over twenty years confirms these observations.[14]

Attention is being paid to the economic losses engendered by smoking. James Hedrick in 1972[15] drew the attention of U.S.A. to a Canadian study undertaken in 1967. The Canadian costs were classified on a fourfold basis; costs of providing medical care; income lost because of illness; future income forgone because of death, and value of property lost in fires caused by smoking (excluding forest fires). Total costs were estimated by an accepted method and 'attributability' percentages were developed to represent the proportion of total costs of the diseases considered attributable to smoking. The Canadian estimate of annual costs calculated on this basis was $387.5 million.

The Canadian study omitted the costs of paramedical and ambulance services, and of drugs and laboratory services not provided as part of hospital services. The study also omitted consideration of diseases other than lung cancer, coronary heart disease and chronic bronchitis and emphysema, whereas it can be shown, as Hedrick points out, that they account for only two-thirds of the total excess mortality associated with cigarette smoking and Hedrick suggested extrapolation of mortality costs accordingly, raising the total annual cost to $526.5 million. Despite limitations, the Canadian approach has merit and indicates that present Australian economic losses (with approximately half the population of Canada) attributable to smoking must be several hundred million dollars per annum, if cigarette smoking rates in the countries are comparable.

Alcohol abuse is recognized as now a major Australian health and social problem. It is well established that despite local variations and some inaccuracies of data, alcohol abuse is, as Everingham, then Minister of Health, stated in 1974 at the opening of the significant Alcoholism in Industry Conference:

> [A] direct cause of the following: occupancy of one in five hospital beds, one in five battered children, one in five drownings and submersion cases, two in five divorces and judicial separations, almost half of the serious crimes of the whole community, half the deaths from road crashes ... loss of more years of life that from heart disease, or cancer or mental illness, the only three categories of illness which cause more premature deaths

than alcohol abuse does. The so-called alcoholics make up one in twenty men, one in one hundred women and this has been estimated overall to include one in twenty-five of Australia's work force.

[Basil] Hetzel and other commentators on the Australian health scene have expounded on the situation.[4,5,16] Detailed clinical and pathological studies have given abundant evidence of the damaging effect of alcohol used in excess on gastrointestinal tract, brain and heart. Recent estimates suggest that alcohol abuse costs the Australian community at least $1000 million annually, and the social costs are almost incalculable.[17]

[Eric] Saint, in a paper entitled suitably enough 'Bacchus Transported',[18] outlined the history of alcohol abuse in Australia, commenting on the cultural situation (including serious shortage of female companionship) which led to emergence of an ethic of mateship or masculinity etched in heavy drinking patterns. Several Tasmanian medical students[19] documented the early Tasmanian experience, indicating that Bacchus was alive and well early in the history of Hobart Town. Brewing commenced in Van Diemen's Land soon after 1820 and proved very profitable. Early Hobart had 150 taverns and beer shops and alcohol-related problems were rife.[20] Against this background temperance movements emerged strongly: witness the Tree of Dissipation published in the Tasmanian Colonist.[21]

Records indicate that the health and social problems in Tasmania were obvious and grave. The roots of alcohol abuse in Australia are very deep and the ways in which it is manifest are in continuity with the past. Transmission of patterns of alcohol abuse occurred not only between coexistent communities (the effects of alcohol were devastating among the aborigines early in the nineteenth century[22]) but also successive generations of Australians have, as it were, inherited the patterns of the past. The phenomenon of cultural inheritance or social heredity with reference to alcohol abuse is very clear in Tasmania.[23]

However, despite these observations it cannot be held that the alcohol abuse of today in Australia is merely a relic of the past – a relic noted more because of increased contemporary sensitivities. It is clear that far from decreasing, the problem is increasing. The total number of persons in difficulty with alcohol is related to the average level of alcohol consumption of the community;[24] sales of alcoholic beverages in Australia show unrelenting growth and widespread reports indicate that alcoholism is being confidently diagnosed at younger and younger ages, well recognized now in late teens.

Despite the epidemiological evidence concerning the prevalence of alcohol abuse in the Australian community, the recent national morbidity study[6] showed a very low rate of mention of alcoholism, indicating either that the diagnosis is very difficult, a general practitioner is loath to make the diagnosis, or affected persons are not in contact with general practitioners.

Diagnostic criteria have been clarified since the publication of the findings of the U.S. Criteria Committee, National Council on Alcoholism.[25] Since there is evidence that alcohol abuse can be controlled or cured if diagnosed prior to gross physical or social damage (the analogy of the curability of tuberculosis when diagnosed prior to gross manifestations is significant), the more precise understanding of the early signs of the disorder becomes critical. Not only is it necessary for the community to become convinced of the value of early diagnosis, but also other community-wide conceptual changes may be essential. The social isolation of the person experiencing difficulties with alcohol is aggravated if the community stigmatizes alcoholics: it may be necessary to stress that such a person is not intrinsically 'different' but is near one end of a normal distribution curve of drinking habits: 'Heavy users belong to same population as the moderate users – they are not a distinct group as has been maintained. There is, in other words, no such person as a born alcoholic, biochemically different in some way so that he has an insatiable urge to drink'.[26]

Society stigmatizes those affected by that which it fears: leprosy, mental illness, cancer – all these have in their time carried this burden and, whilst the 'life of the party' (who may be a broken person inside) is welcomed, the situation tends to be changed once an alcohol problem is diagnosed. It may also be true and needs to be realized by our community that problematic drinking may be self-limiting, and that the realization that a drinking problem has developed should not engender fear and compound anxiety or depression in the sufferer, with inevitable further delay in diagnosis and progress in the disorder. It is said that the medical profession is ambivalent towards alcohol abuse. Certainly alcoholism is well-known amongst doctors, and medical students may be at special risk. The results of a recent study of thirty-six male and five female doctors in treatment in U.K. indicate that the recovery rates may be considerably better than expected: at a mean follow-up period of sixty-three months, five had died (of cirrhosis or suicide) but seven were fully recovered and ten nearly so; nine persisted in almost continuous dependent drinking.[27] The ambivalence of doctors may merely reflect in general the ambivalence of society, but it is noteworthy that there may be historical roots even within academia, for Arnaldus de Villanova, a professor of medicine at the University of Montpellier in the late 13th century, contributed to the lore regarding the preparation of spirits and wrote the following:

> Limpid and well-flavored red or white wine is to be digested twenty days in a closed vessel, by heat, and then to be distilled in a sand bath with a very gentle fire. The true water of life will come over in precious drops, which being rectified by three or four successive distillations, will afford the wonderful quintessence of wine. We call it aqua vitae, and this name is remarkably suitable, since it is really a water of immortality. It prolongs life, clears away ill-humours, revives the heart, and maintains youth.[28]

Morbidity and mortality due to abuse of substances other than alcohol and cigarette smoking are even more complex: ranging from self-administered drug overdose, chronic problems engendered by abuse of analgesics, and the wide range of drug-induced disorders resulting from medically prescribed drugs. There is a large literature on all these subjects and all are highly socially significant, both because of consequences to the individual and the immediate family (or other close associates) and the serious economic consequences for the health care system. There are several hundred admissions to Tasmanian public hospitals each year for drug overdose (total population 400,000). Most Australian series indicate that drug overdose is disproportionately common in women under thirty years: a reflection on the serious degree of distress in young Australian women, the causes of which demand attention, and need prevention. Any measures taken must be effective long before adulthood for habitual taking of drugs such as analgesics is well established in childhood.[29]

Other life-style factors justifying consideration are exercise (or lack of it) and diet: evidence is pressing that both are highly relevant to health, but have been discussed, together with other less tangible factors such as 'stress', by many authors.[30]

Even though cursory, this glance at Australian mortality and morbidity patterns with clear evidence of life-style induced diseases of immense economic and social significance raises problems with respect to individual liberty in the terms supported by Mill: the social damage done to others directly or indirectly (by means of costs borne by the whole community) raises ethical issues. Is there a limit to an individual's right to choose a life-style which will seriously increase the costs borne on his behalf by the community and reduce his own contribution to the creating and sustaining of that community? Is it ethically justified for a person to embark on a smoking career (or persist in it) without contributing to the public purse in proportion to the costs his smoking can be foreseen to engender? Is the community free to continue advertising of alcohol and tobacco use? What of the morality of the huge national revenue from excise? And so on. The ethical debate has hardly begun with respect to these issues. The individualist ethic expounded by Mill must, I believe, give way to a communitarian ethic in which the adoption of a life-style which is not only self-destructive but also costly to one's fellows requires acceptance of [some] responsibility for the consequences.

The question of how freely an individual man or woman chooses knowingly a self-destructive life-style raises further issues. Do these life-style-induced disorders testify to the concept that our society is indeed a bound society, not a community of free men? If so, why? And how can liberty be reborn among us? If the cause of this 'unfreedom' is communal, then in a sense the argument has run a full circle and it is fitting that society bear the costs of the failure of its members to live freely in self-possession, as celebrants of life. It appears that we have ourselves, collectively, by the decisions made in the past, the routes chosen and the situations tolerated, created limits for our own liberty.

Medical Care Problems

George Bernard Shaw in his preface to *The Doctor's Dilemma* – the play was first produced in London in 1906 – wrote: 'It is not the fault of our doctors that the medical service of the community, as at present provided for, is a murderous absurdity ...'[31] On that note (ignoring Shaw's expansion of his theme) we may dare to look at some aspects of the medical care situation.

Medical care once was simple with very few effective remedies and plenty of room for tender, loving care. Hippocrates excelled in clinical description and prognosis but we have little evidence of his therapeutic effectiveness in situations where self-healing is not common. But some early sources do mention remedies which could hardly have endured if there had been no evidence at all of hope of effectiveness, for example, in an Egyptian papyrus there is a remedy that 'to make the hair of a bald-headed person grow: fat of lion, fat of hippopotamus, fat of crocodile, fat of serpent, fat of ibex, are mixed together and the head of a bald person is anointed therewith.'[32]

The therapeutic revolution of the last few decades, especially of the last ten years, has altered expectations of doctors and patients alike with respect to the approach of illness. The burgeoning of hospitals, the increasing concentration of staff within them, the continually increasing demands for training and equipment to realize the potential of each new medical advance, has brought about an economic situation our forefathers did not imagine.

Health costs in Australia are rising exponentially with the total over $4000 million annually. The problem is similar in other western countries, although each country has its own particular problems of distribution of health care and methods of meeting costs. [Robert] Maxwell undertook a health survey of U.S.A. and European countries in the face of growing awareness of the limits being approached in health care costs.[33]

Maxwell, by way of preamble, outlined the paradox of health needs:

> The fundamental paradox of health care is that medical advances so often breed further needs and increase future requirements for care ... In short, every inch of ground gained is won with greater difficulty and at higher cost than the last. It is the familiar phenomenon of diminishing returns, with one vital difference: no new gain, however costly, can ever be dismissed as marginal if it promises some real reduction of human suffering. There is, in the nature of things, no possibility of saturating 'demand' for the reduction of mortality and the relief of pain. In every nation the demand for health care is growing and the balance of needs is changing towards less tractable problems associated with handicap, affluence and age.

In every country studied health expenditure has been rising faster than the Gross National Product, no matter how fast the latter has risen. The proportion of the GNP spent varied from four and a half percent in U.K. to about six and a half percent in Sweden and U.S.A. It is clear that a limit situation is approaching and the trend to increase health spending in response to demand cannot go on indefinitely. At the time of the Maxwell study Sweden had decided to halt the rise in health spending by budget cutting – a measure Maxwell notes to be an inadequate answer to the problem. Effort is required to concentrate on how to increase the cost effectiveness of health care delivery systems, especially with regard to hospitals, since it was noted that hospitals, with associated physicians' fees, generally consume half the total health care expenditure. It was also noted that 'countries with the strongest continuing tradition of general practice seem to manage with fewer doctors while maintaining, comparatively speaking, good standards of health care'. One point of interest also was that doctors sharply increase their productivity when they delegate to highly trained health professionals other than doctors, e.g. in private medical practice in Germany it was shown that the doctor was able to delegate in such a way that he and a team of five less highly trained auxiliaries could handle the same patient load as six physicians working on their own.

The Maxwell enquiry considered many other facets of the health care delivery system: patterns of supply of health professionals, their geographical distribution, patterns of use of hospitals and the cost effectiveness of the systems prevailing in the various countries. It was clear that 'each country requires a means of confronting and resolving the question of priorities'.

In every health care system there are organizational problems which the Maxwell enquiry lists as: (1) barriers to patient access (simple non-availability, financial problems, the complexity of the system); (2) inflexibility of resource use (e.g. by boundaries between hospital services and services outside hospital, professional demarcation; (3) ill-defined responsibilities with inadequate planning; (4) excessive complexity and cost.

The Maxwell enquiry concludes that 'four kinds of shifts in strategy will be widely called for', and details these as:

1. Greater attention to, and expenditure on, prevention and health education.
2. Building and maintaining stronger systems of primary care.

    Specialization has been the foundation stone for skilled care of specific, acute illnesses. But such conditions,

though intensely important, represent only a small fraction of the total incidence of disease. Something like nine out of ten cases can be dealt with quite satisfactorily by a well-trained general practitioner or specialist in primary care.
In the absence of such a practitioner, what happens to these nine cases? The patient has to decide to which specialist to turn, many cases are seen by specialists that do not require their skill and are outside their main field of competence, and there is little continuity in the doctor/patient relationship. In consequence, the quality of care suffers, and resources are wasted. The greater the proliferation of medical specialties, the more doctors will be needed to deal with a fluctuating caseload. Only when the specialized skills are really required is this an acceptable price to pay for higher quality care.

3   Upgrading the treatment of long-term illness and handicap.
4   Streamlining the acute hospitals as an integral part of the total pattern of provision.

The first step, which depends on strengthening the primary and long-term care services, is to relieve the pressure of inappropriate admissions and to allow earlier discharge of patients who no longer require acute medical care. The right use of a major acute hospital's skills is possible only when the acute hospital no longer has to make good the deficiencies of other parts of the health system.

The Maxwell report has been discussed at length, not because the points it makes are new or unexpected but because it represents, from an international perspective, a sound recent synthesis of the health care dilemma and contains within the questions it asks and the conclusions it reaches the shape of a very vital problem indeed, namely, how can the contemporary doctor retain professional freedom in the face of forceful recommendations which, if adopted, would inevitably impinge on his liberty to practise medicine where and how he prefers in accord with his professional competence and within the very special relationship relating doctor and patient? In short, there appear to be limits to the liberty of a medical practitioner today, differing from those limits which may have prevailed and been accepted a century ago. If so, how can a doctor today rediscover professional freedom?

The rediscovery of true professional freedom, a crucial point, relevant to the malaise and indeed conflict sometimes encountered among doctors in our society, may be facilitated, I believe, by having a sense of history, by perceiving the breadth of the medical task and by grasping Popper's principles of how knowledge grows and progress is achieved. These will be considered in turn.

A Sense of History

'Let the past serve the present' said Chairman Mao (a comment given prominence at the Chinese Exhibition recently seen in Australia [1970s]). The physician of today needs to understand the evolution of his art and its practice in order to grasp the full significance of his social position today and so more freely exercise his task.

Henry Sigerist in his historical writings has demonstrated that 'the present-day physician is only the latest in a long series of different types of physician, and that current modes of practice are relatively new and hardly immutable'.[34]

In primitive society the medicine man was sorcerer, priest and physician in one and this still prevails in some areas, with wide variations with respect to the time devoted to medical practice and the manner in which the community remunerated him.

In ancient Greece, the physician was a craftsman and primarily itinerant. Sigerist[35] noted: 'The Hippocratic physician was paid for his services, and since society despised people who worked for money his social position was not very high. Yet among all the craftsmen he was held in the highest esteem because health was considered one of the greatest goods'.

Physicians in early Rome were slaves usually and, those who new how to treat disease brought a good price on the market, as much as a eunuch. The situation changed in imperial Rome and doctors were frequently salaried (e.g. in the army) or in private practice where competition was fierce and unscrupulous.

In the Middle Ages physicians were clerics at first but later laymen and sought salaried positions as body-physician to a nobleman or as a municipal doctor with rigid codes of ethics governing private practice. The prevailing ethos was profoundly influenced by mediaeval ideals of service.

With the evolution of the new economic order in the sixteenth century, physicians for a long time sought to resist its consequences:

> [A]s heretofore they sought salaried positions as body-physicians or in government services, in order to be independent and free to serve the poor or to devote part of their activities to research or similar occupations ...
>
> The physicians' attempt to preserve mediaeval ideals of service in a world ruled by iron economic necessities was heroic but was doomed to failure. The situation became still more complicated during the nineteenth and twentieth centuries when, as a result of industrialization, the needy population increased tremendously and at the same time the cost of medical care was rising, largely because of the progress of medical science. Against his

will and in spite of desperate resistance the physician
found himself in a harshly competitive business. When
this was generally recognized, although it was not openly
admitted, medical societies were organized, and codes
of ethics and etiquette were promulgated to safeguard
the profession against some of the worst features of
competition ... Physicians still looked back to mediaeval
ideals, still were willing to attend indigent patients
free of charge, but an untenable situation arose. Unless
special adjustments were made, either large sections of
the population would remain unattended or the medical
profession must be ruined.[36]

It appears that understanding of the evolution of the role of doctors (apart from surgeons who evolved in a different manner) does give the doctor of today a sense of freedom, whilst recognizing not only the realities of economic pressures but also the instinct within him that there is a pressing obligation to serve the people irrespective of their economic circumstances. The conviction that every human person (especially the poor and powerless) is worthy of compassion and of the application of skill, I believe, lies deep, maybe in the subconscious, of every doctor, sometimes to his discomfort (where there may be otherwise inexplicable guilt feeling, depression or anxiety where this obligation is not expressed in the totality of his life).

We are shaped by our history and our cultural inheritance as surely as by our genetic inheritance, and the grasp of our rich cultural heritage as doctors can be a source not of bondage but of freedom.

The Nature of the Medical Task
A sense of the breadth of the medical task can enlarge our sense of freedom by the added perspectives it brings to doctors as individuals and as members of a fraternity at the service

of the people. Once again it is the historian Sigerist who has articulated the contemporary medical practice. He noted that:

> For thousands of years the treatment of the sick was considered the primary task of medicine while today its scope is infinitely broader. Society has given the physician four major tasks, which although they can hardly be separated since there are no sharp borderlines, yet may be discussed separately for simplicity's sake.[37]

Sigerist discerned these tasks as: the promotion of health, the prevention of illness, the restoration of the sick, and rehabilitation. His view of each of these tasks was broad, deep and sensitive. 'Sigerist made us aware of the fact that medicine is the study and application of biology in a matrix that is at once historical, social, political, economic, and cultural. The practice of medicine is a part of sociology, and a product of sociological factors'.[38]

It is possible (and one suggests this tentatively) that the unifying theme running through Sigerist's schema of the fourfold tasks of medicine and subsequent variations of it, whatever the terminology or variation of emphasis, is that of human liberation. The doctor is involved in freeing other human beings from the threat of infirmity, from the effects of illness limiting function, and from the consequence of such illness. Finally, in the face of incurable illness, the doctor has as his task the freeing of a human person to express his humanness within the limitations imposed by his situation, being with him in his dying as a free human being transcending, as it were, his limits of time and space, all the while knowing that he himself is mortal.

Another perspective in which the medical task may be viewed is that of human ecology. The term ecology was coined in 1870 by Ernst Haeckel (or possibly by earlier writers)[39] to describe the interaction of an organism with its environment. A human being can be considered as an individual with a multitude of organic functions, and indeed internal medicine as a discipline is specified by its focussing on these functions and so there may be (and need to be) specialists in cardiology, neurology, rheumatology, gastro-enterology, respiratory medicine, etc., charged with the task of enlarging our knowledge of disorders of certain body systems. These special branches of medicine must be closely integrated with that type of medical practice which focuses specifically on the person as a whole, interacting with the persons who make up his personal field, and understood only in his total social context and with awareness of his personal history: the community then is seen as made up of unique individuals with interlocking life cycles. Such perspectives of man, in sickness and in health, can be called ecological and may assist the medical student (and fully-fledged doctor) to a more profound grasp of his professional task amidst the family of man.

Karl Popper and the Liberty of Doctors
If a sign of significance of a philosopher is the seminal nature of his ideas, in that his concepts stimulate progress in thought in a broad range of other disciplines, then Karl Popper, currently in retirement in England and with, according to Magee,[40] some of his finest work still to be published, is a highly significant philosopher in our times. His thought is rich and out of this richness may be distilled many lines of enquiry of relevance to medical practice. The remarks here made must be regarded as comments of one who has recently discovered Popper and there is no doubt that if one were spared the years to ponder on his thought, new perspectives would emerge making the present remarks exceedingly naive but I hope not erroneous or valueless.

Popper's theory concerning the growth of knowledge [41] is refreshing indeed and seems to weave the history of human thought into an exhilarating pattern. He rejects the traditional or orthodox view of scientific method first described by [Francis] Bacon in the seventeenth century. That approach on which we are nurtured at school, involves multiple observations which once systematized are the bases on which scientists generate hypotheses; the individual scientist then seeks by evidence to confirm his hypothesis and, if successful, he contributes another scientific law ... and investigation begins at a new frontier between knowledge and ignorance.

Popper pointed out that in logic a scientific law is conclusively falsifiable although it is not conclusively verifiable. Popper therefore urges that we do not systematically evade refutation but we formulate our theories as unambiguously as possible so that they may be exposed to refutation. Where an observation is made which refutes the theory by methodology which is truly rigorous then we must search for a new hypothesis which may then be tested by devising confrontations between its consequences and new observable experience. It is a liberating thing to turn the mind not to defending (even irrationally) what one holds to be correct but to devising means whereby it could be shown to be false or inadequate. 'The man who welcomes and acts on criticism will prize it almost above friendship: the man who fights it out of concern to maintain his position is clinging to non-growth.'[40] Popper insists further that the wrong view of science betrays itself in craving to be right.

Popper's concepts here can readily be applied to medical investigation at the laboratory bench as was done by scientists such as [Peter] Medawar and [John] Eccles. What is less obvious is that these concepts are applicable also to clinical medicine: in a sense every clinical diagnosis is an hypothesis raised in the face of the data available. Clinical problem-solving frequently proceeds by means of investigations (often costly in personal and financial terms) to confirm the diagnosis (hypothesis). Clinical medicine becomes an even more challenging scientific task if one deliberately seeks for evidence which would refute the diagnosis (hypothesis) rather than sustain it. Such a procedure may be a more direct route and as such may be more rapid and less stressful for the patient whose problem has to be solved. In many instances these concepts are obviously quite irrelevant, but in some of the diagnostic problems of modern clinical practice their application can be most relevant and fruitful. On the broader front of medical care organization a proposed medical care system is (if planned at all) basically a hypothesis generated in the face of data concerning needs, resources and foreseeable trends. It could be fruitful to seek deliberately for additional data which would demonstrate that the proposed plan (hypothesis) is inadequate, incorrect, 'false' rather than approaching the 'truth' in relation to the context within which it has been generated. A policy, then, according to Popper, is a hypothesis which has to be tested against reality and corrected in the light of experience. Once again, the search for multiple pieces of evidence which would confirm the policy may be far less valuable (even though emotionally more comfortable) than the search for one soundly-produced piece of evidence which would refute it.

Popper's concepts demand that we objectify our theories, our ideas, so that they can be adequately criticized. Any criticism, proposed change or a solution to a problem has to be formulated in language before it can be tested or even discussed. It is then an objective proposal and can be 'argued about, attacked, defended, used, without reference to the man who put it forward'. In the present turmoil of medical practice where conceptual growth is desperately necessary rather than sterile controversy, Popper's concepts may prove the wanted key.

There is a further area of Popper's thought put forward in *The Open Society and its Enemies*[42] as the general guiding principle for public policy: 'Minimize avoidable suffering'. Popper bases this on his observation of, as it were, a logical asymmetry: we do not know how to make people happy (as the policy 'maximize happiness' demands) but we do know ways of lessening their unhappiness (minimize unhappiness'). 'Instead of the greatest happiness for the greatest number, one should demand, more modestly, the least amount of avoidable suffering for all; and further, that unavoidable suffering, such as hunger in times of unavoidable shortage of food, should be distributed as equally as possible.' The relevance of this concept to health planning at the national, regional or local level is singularly obvious, and liberating indeed, capable of giving impetus to the creative spirit of the doctor.

> Scientific creation is not free in the same sense as artistic creation for it has to survive a detailed confrontation with experience; nevertheless the attempt to understand the world is an open task and, as creative geniuses, Galileo, Newton and Einstein are on a par with Michelangelo, Shakespeare and Beethoven.[40]

A sense of history, an appreciation of the breadth of the medical task and a capacity to welcome sound criticism: these things may lead to a rediscovery of the true freedom of the professional man. Much more could be said – the interaction of clinicians with countless human beings in their birth, living, suffering, ageing and especially in their dying, should add a personal dimension to the freedom of the doctor as a human being – for [Albert] Camus (who styled himself in his acceptance speech for the Nobel Prize as 'rich only in his doubts') wrote in his notebooks: 'There is only one liberty, to come to terms with death. After which, everything is possible'.[43]

Global Health Problems

We do live today in a global village and it is imperative that we look beyond the health scene of the well-developed nations (as Maxwell did not) towards the health situation of less industrialized developing nations. We are *not* free to look only at the local scene, for the community of man is one and to be a man is to be part of the whole, and a conscious part of that. The sheer human reality demands this quite apart from ethical considerations or higher moral (or religious) aspirations associated either with the concepts of the roots of the solidarity of the human race or the nature of inter-human obligations. The situation has been well documented by the World Health Organization, but the message is clear that the health problems are part of a total problem set. Alexander King, Director-General of Scientific Affairs, O.E.C.D., Paris, and Founder Member of the Club of Rome outlined the problems thus:

> The problems themselves in their wide spectrum which ranges through disparities between developed and underdeveloped countries, inflation, unemployment and monetary problems, islands of poverty in seas of prosperity, race, environmental deterioration, individual alienation, crime and violence, have a number of features in common. They seem to appear in all countries at a certain level of development irrespective of the political system. They are extremely multi-variant in their elements and they all seem to interact in ways that are only dimly understood. There is a tendency to refer to this cluster of problems as 'the problematique', a series of difficulties so intimately interrelated that it is increasingly difficult to identify discrete problems and apply discrete solutions. To tackle elements of the problematique appears increasingly to be an attempt to remove symptoms of a disease which has not been fully

diagnosed with the consequences that interactions within the system may add to further difficulties in other parts which are not obviously recognized as being due to the initial remedial action.[44]

Against this background (with the cautions implied) should be noted the disturbing health data.

Disorders of communicable disease still ravage the developing world. The Fifth Report on the World Health Situation (1975) covering the period 1969–72[45] records once more the serious impact of communicable diseases (notably tuberculosis where the annual rate of risk of TB infection was still often more than 0.5 percent – up to 2 percent in some countries). Cholera remains a problem, but smallpox since 1975 may have been eradicated. Sexually-transmitted communicable diseases are high in the developed world (but reaching epidemic proportions in parts of the West). Malnutrition remains a serious cause of death both directly and indirectly. It is known that tens of millions of children under five years in developing countries are suffering from moderate to severe protein-calorie malnutrition,[46] a condition that may lead either to death or at least deprive the children of their full physical and mental potentialities. Eye damage induced by vitamin A deficiency and nutritional anaemia are widespread to a degree hard to imagine by a Westerner: both seriously limit human freedom to realize potential.

Health expenditure is trivial per capita by Western standards but patterns of expenditure can be disastrous if Western models are followed (e.g., by placing much of the resources in hospitals using doctors as points of primary contact, failing to give priority to preventive and curative activity at the grass roots of the system). It is of interest to see that in the limit situation in which Western style medical care organization finds itself, the models of health care appropriate to the developing world have some features worth close consideration, particularly the notion of using health professionals such as nurses, health visitors and others at the highest level of their potential and training. Such a policy ensures that the doctors (who inevitably are far more expensive) can exercise to the full their capacity to solve difficult administrative and clinical problems, their ability to help plan the deployment of health services and devise the most fruitful programmes, their minds and hearts being continually stimulated by the patients referred to them for problems not solvable by their colleagues.

The Club of Rome* has made available two major reports prepared for it on the total global situation, the first *The Limits to Growth* under the leadership of Professor Dennis Meadows.[47] The computerized model projected into the future current trends in a limited number of quantifiable elements of the 'problematique' – population growth with the consequent demands for food and agriculture, capital and industrial growth, raw material depletion and pollution, taking account of their gross impacts, and predicted virtual collapse of world population and society within the next one hundred years. It was asserted that dramatic changes in such variables as population growth and resource usages are essential *now* to alter these disastrous trends. It is widely accepted that despite criticisms of methodology and estimates the *Limits to Growth* portrait must be taken seriously. The second Report to the Club of Rome, entitled *Mankind at the Turning Point* (and dedicated 'to future generations') was prepared under the direction of M Mesarovic and E Pester.[48] This study set out to look at

---

* The Club of Rome is a nonprofit, informal organization of intellectuals and business leaders whose goal is a critical discussion of pressing global issues.

five major regions of the world and the interactions between them and significantly includes a telling chapter on 'Limits to Independence'; after analysing by computer scenarios created by conflict and another scenario of cooperation with much better conditions than those in a state of conflict for all concerned, the report goes on:

> No computer can predict whether men will be rational enough to follow this path; however, the computer does give rational men all the evidence they need to convince other men that the emergence of a new world system is a matter of necessity, not preference, and that that system must be built on cooperation. Cooperation is no longer a schoolroom word suggesting an ethical but elusive mode of behaviour: cooperation is a scientifically supportable, politically viable, and absolutely essential mode of behavior for the organic growth of the world system.

The chapter concludes that we must acknowledge 'the dawn of an era of limits to independence even for the strongest and biggest nations of the world'. In the epilogue the Report notes:

> If the human species is to survive, man must develop a sense of identification with future generations and be ready to trade benefits to the next generations for the benefits to himself. If each generation aims at maximum good for itself, *Homo Sapiens* is as good as doomed.

There are many other areas which could have been explored (and have been explored by others) where the basic problem appears to involve a definition of a limit to human freedom: the transplant area, the limitation of family size, the rights of the battered child or wife to protection, the limits to sexual freedom, decisions re application of costly technology and .the priorities involved in the face of finite resources and, finally, the right to be born once conceived and the right to die in dignity. It may be profitable, however, to shift the focus away from health-related situations on to the notion of liberty itself, which like a will-o'-the-wisp intrudes into the scene, disturbs it, sometimes finds itself overcome or retreats leaving behind in the scene it has left a certain nostalgia or frustration.

Intrinsic Limits to Human Liberty

I must warn the physiologists, pathologists, biochemists, anatomists, high technologists of all types, philosophers, sociologists, psychologists, and all empiricists, that as Dag Hammarskjöld wrote in quite another context: 'Here ends the known. But from a source beyond it, something fills my being with its possibilities'.[49] The exploration out beyond the empirical will inevitably reflect the shape of a life and will bear the imprint of ideas experienced from within and without during the adventure of being (or growing) human.

The liberty of man, its definitions, its origins, its expressions, its value, its limitations, its burdensomeness, its glories ... have been considered through the ages by philosophers, poets, theologians, psychologists, politicians in a way which almost bespeaks fascination, almost like that of a jeweller gazing on the beauty of an opal in the sunlight ... In our time man has even been described as 'incarnate liberty'.[50]

Freedom is not merely the absence of restraints but the capacity to respond to life, to create, to go even beyond the apparent limits of possibility. We may consider the individual as involved in a life cycle, or better, as the sociologists might put it, a trajectory, constantly in process. For convenience in our exploration of limits to human freedom we might focus in turn on different phases in that ongoing process (though not in quite the detail nor from the same perspectives as in Shakespeare's seven ages).

Birth, Childhood and the Growth towards Maturity

Is man born free? The answer must be that in most senses he is not. A person is a 'situated' being, born into a predetermined context; we cannot choose whether to be born or not, nor can we choose the temporal or social milieu in which we come to be.

Further, human beings are physically and metaphysically incomplete and sociality is intrinsic to man. The human baby, quite apart from obvious physical needs such as warmth, food and shelter, needs human beings in order to emerge as a self. The self may be regarded as a social structure arising in social experience but sociality is not merely a product of external forces or so-called interaction; rather, interaction and the emergence of complex social structures are, at least to some, derived typifications of the essential sociality of men.[51] The emerging self is limited but also fulfilled by its social roles and social expectations.

As [Ralf] Dahrendorf noted, there is a dialectical paradox of freedom and necessity. 'It is an entirely speculative question whether anyone would be capable of shaping his entire behaviour on his own, without the assistance of society. Since complete freedom has its drawbacks ... it is at least conceivable that a human being stripped of all roles would find it very difficult indeed to make his behaviour meaningful.'[52] Others would stress, however, that this derived world of social expectations is not the whole world of Self, not the world of the Thou.

Sociologists recognize that being confined to the social self as the object of their study they are in danger of overstressing the constraints human interaction places on man and minimizing his real freedom. 'Is man a social being whose behavior, being predetermined, is calculable and controllable?

Or is he an autonomous individual with some considerable measure of freedom to act as he chooses?'[53]

Dahrendorf asked 'Is there a necessary contradiction between the moral image of man as an integral, unique, and free creature and his scientific image as a differentiated, exemplary aggregate of predetermined roles?' Dahrendorf went on to discuss the problems raised by Kant and recognized that by transforming man into what he called *homo sociologicus* sociology could be a supporter of unfreedom. He concludes his serious re-examination of the nature of sociology as follows:

> Only if the sociologist selects his research projects with an eye to what may help liberate the individual from the vexations of society, if he formulates his hypothesis with a view to extending men's range of free choice, if he does not shy away from supporting political changes designed to increase individual freedom, and if he never forgets the superior rights of Herr Schmidt the person over his role playing shadow – only then can he hope to use the insights of sociology to protect man the inhabitant of the earth from the boundless demands of man the inhabitant of a country. Only then can the sociologist cease being a brake and becomes motor of a society of free men ...[54]

Another slant on the complex issue of individual freedom in relation to societal reality was offered by John MacMurray in the Gifford lectures delivered in the University of Glasgow in 1954 and published in 1961. In an analysis of community which he considered as a unity of persons as persons (as distinct from society which is an organization of functions with each member a function of the group), MacMurray noted: 'The self-realization of any individual person is only fully achieved if he is positively motivated towards every other person with whom he is in relation'.⁵⁵ Later, he brought out the same point worth quoting at length:

> We need one another to be ourselves. This complete and unlimited dependence of each of us upon the others is the central and crucial fact of personal existence. Individual independence is an illusion; and the independent individual, the isolated self, is a nonentity ... It is only in relation to others we exist as persons; we are invested with significance by others who have need of us; and borrow our reality from those who care for us. We live and move and have our being not in ourselves but in one another; and what rights or powers or freedom we possess are ours by the grace and favour of our fellows
> ... This mutuality provides the primary condition of our freedom ...⁵⁶

I feel MacMurray goes too far, but in association with the comments of Dahrendorf and others against the background of Kant we must recognize, I think, that man as man is not born free nor does he grow in absolute autonomy, but by being incorporated into the community of men and the fulfilling of social roles he emerges as a total self endowed with liberty though subject to constraint.

It hardly needs stating that the health, physical and mental or social, of the emerging self will be determined not only by biological (genetic) and cultural inheritance, but also by the physical and, above all, psychosocial health of the persons with whom he has significant interactions. It is to be expected and not to be wondered at that the psychosocial problems of one generation are manifested in the next generation.

So man is not born free, nor is his development free from the constraints of his context, but it is essential to recognize that whilst a man's social circumstances may influence his development and even the shape of the emerging self, and profoundly limit his range of options with all sorts of consequences, these things do not destroy freedom, for freedom is intrinsic to man. Wise men of our own day have emphasized that bondage, even unjustifiable evil bondage, does not destroy freedom. Victor Frankl in his writing on the experience in concentration camps wrote that 'everything can be taken from a man but one thing: the last of human freedoms – to choose one's attitude in any given set of circumstances, to choose one's own way'.[57] [Kahlil] Gibran made a similar point rather more obliquely, as a poet may:

> You shall be free indeed when your days
> are not without a care, nor
> your nights without a want and a grief,
> But rather when these things girdle your life
> and yet you rise above
> them naked and unbound.[58]

These sentiments though framed in language referring mainly to maturity of life are relevant also to the young, especially in the light of the current very legitimate stress on the influence of environment on personal growth.

Maturity

Once the self has emerged into what society terms maturity, what of freedom then? How is it expressed and what are its limits? Formal statements of the basic expressions of human freedom are embodied in various formulations of human rights. Some of these may be worthy of comment.

The human being has a right to express the impulse to love, in freedom. No one can be constrained to love, and 'any limitation on the human impulse to love ultimately destroys the life, of the human person'.[59] Simone de Beauvoir, in her (to me) sensitive analysis of womanhood notes that her situation in our society is such that love is in a sense dangerous for women but noted: 'On the day when it will be possible for woman to love not in her weakness but in her strength, not to escape herself but to find herself, not to abase herself but to assert herself – on that day love will become for her, as for man, a source of life and not of mortal danger'.[60] D.H. Lawrence expressed the situation of both men and women most poignantly: 'If only our civilization had taught us ... how to keep the fire of sex clear and alive, flickering or glowing or blazing in all its varying degrees of strength and communication, we might all of us have lived our lives in love, which means that we should be kindled and full of zest 'in all kinds of ways and for all kinds of things'.[61] There appears to be in our times need for rediscovery of truly free sexual love, not sexuality in bondage expressing blind undirected instinct but sexuality as free discovery of the wonder of humanness in the other and the rebirth of real love of the self. Doctors have repeatedly expressed deficiency in education in human sexuality and recognize the special training of other professionals; but because of the trust placed in many doctors, knowledge and skills are obviously needed and our medical students are seeking to acquire them.

The mature human being has the freedom to procreate in addition to love. Under what circumstances is the liberty to bear children to be limited? And is this always to be voluntary limitation or under what circumstances should procreation be prevented involuntarily? These questions are critical on the global scale, as we have noted and in the smaller scale even locally, when family limitation may be essential in the interests of parents, children or society. There is no doubt in my mind that limits are clearly justified: even the case for prohibition of any procreation could be argued in the case of grave genetically determined disease transmitted in a Mendelian dominant pattern of inheritance. Whether however, coercion, compulsion or, for example, involuntary sterilization would ever be ethically justified is at present problematic.

What of the right of a man to work and to possess? These human freedoms are basic though less immediate than those previously discussed, and one recognizes easily that social circumstance (as in economic recession) may limit or even abolish the exercise of these rights. Right and freedom are not synonymous but the possession of right (implying obligation of another to respect it) is in fact closely allied to an expression of human liberty to act or not to act in a given manner. These questions will not be further discussed here.

Freedom of action implies exercise of power. If there are limits to power, what are these? Popper quotes 'the famous story of the hooligan who protested that, being a free citizen, he could move his fist in any direction he liked; whereupon the judge wisely replied: "The freedom of the movement of your fists is limited by the position of your neighbour's nose."'[62]

One obvious limitation to our liberty with respect to power is then the possession of complementary rights and powers by our fellow human beings, but I would like to take this discussion rather further. In his prologue to the great collection or code of ancient Babylonian law, the king Hammurabi (c.1728–1686 BC) states that it is his purpose 'to make justice appear in the land, to destroy the evil and the wicked, in order that the strong might not oppress the weak'.[63] In the long history of mankind it has become ever more clear that humanity finds its richest expression in the defence of the weak and this characteristic has been most explicit in those involved with the sick, the doctors by whatever name they have been called down through the ages. Doctors have power but it is never fitting for it to be used at the expense but rather for the defence of those without power.

It may be worth recalling the narrative of the problems once encountered by a very gifted young man, obviously of attractive personality, high intelligence and gifts of healing shown later in his life, for the sick thought it worth coming to him day and night. In the story with mythical overtones this young man went out into the desert and was tempted first to turn stones into loaves, to throw himself down from the Temple and remain unhurt (because of the protection of angels, as if an insurance policy were held), and finally to bow down before Satan in order to gain the kingdoms of the world: all three temptations are in fact related to the use or gaining of power. In fact, Jesus of Nazareth chose not to use his power for himself (turn stones into bread) nor to demonstrate his power by public display, nor to seek material power at the price of denial of his true self, but instead adopted the role of the servant, fulfilling in fact the strange but poignant Hebrew prophecies of the suffering servant. The point is that we who are doctors may be in danger of abusing our very real power and forgetting that above all we are servants of the people. It is this that sets doctors apart from tradesmen or even other professionals: that a doctor is one who responds to human distress and serves the weak and powerless, whether this state is temporary (a broken leg or appendicitis can make one powerless) or chronic. It is fitting that doctors should be seen to be on the side of those oppressed by any form of tyranny, or violence and I believe that this commitment of the doctor to the powerless should lead to the defence of the unborn: maybe the ground swell of concern even among those who have conscientiously supported the recent liberalizing of abortion is related to this deep medical instinct. [Bernard] Nathanson, one of those instrumental in establishing the abortion service in New York State and author of a study of 25,000 abortions, wrote in a telling article in a prominent American medical journal in 1974:

> In pursuing a course of unlimited and uncontrolled abortion over future years, we must not permit ourselves to sink to a debased level of utilitarian semiconsciousness. I plead for an honest, clear-eyed consideration of the abortion dilemma – an end to blind polarity ... The issue is human life, and it deserves the reverent stillness and ineffably grave thought appropriate to it. We must work together to create a moral climate rich enough to provide for abortion, but sensitive enough to life to accommodate a profound sense of loss.[64]

Before leaving consideration of the limits to power it may be worth reiterating Kant's principle that man must act 'as to treat humanity, whether in your own person, or in that of another, in every case as an end, never as a means only',[65] a principle which should, with the principle that the powerless are to be defended, assist in the clarification of several ethical issues arising in contemporary medicine.

There are limits then to man's power. There are limits also to his knowledge. Popper warned us that our 'concern in the pursuit of knowledge is to get closer and closer to the truth, and then we may even know that we have made an advance, but we can never know if we have reached our goal'.

Bronowski has reminded us in *The Ascent of Man*[66] that we must live without absolute certainties: there is a limit to knowledge, all knowledge, and this principle of uncertainty was translated by Bronowski into the principle of tolerance. Above all we are limited in our knowledge of the future. The future is *open,* as Popper has stressed, not predetermined in such a manner that we either have certain knowledge of it, or that human activity is a mockery or sheer absurdity.

There are limits also to human integrity. Knowledge however profound, and emotional balance however fine do not ensure that we will act with integrity. We are at the heart of a mystery here. 'The basic lines of the phenomenon are drawn in the creation narrative', wrote Claus Westermann in the course of a fine analysis, 'man is such that under certain circumstances he can be seduced ... Both man's ability to defect and the intention of the one who causes him to defect points to man's limitation. That is what he is, and no ethic, no religion, no political power can alter the situation in any way ... The narrator also wants to say that it is not possible to come to terms with the origin of evil. There is no etiology of the origin of evil'.[67]

Bronowski recognized that in true human progress integrity is crucial. 'The Ascent of Man is not made by lovable people. It is made by people who have two qualities: an immense integrity and at least a little genius'.[68] Lack of integrity is, in a sense, bondage.

It is obvious that other aspects of the human condition limit the capacity of man to exercise his freedom. By ill-health options may be reduced, dreams shattered and the future seem closed. Mental illness, especially despair (possibly articulated in recent times most poignantly by [Gabriel] Marcel), profoundly binds the sufferer such that there seems 'no exit'.

In the face of limitation of human freedom by illness the doctor may, if therapy is available, have the privilege of being in a small way a liberator, one who frees a human being to get on with the task of exercising social roles, building the earth, giving life meaning. Such therapy may well be through a wide range of means: the provision of a simple aid to enable an arthritic person recover mobility and go out again, or the prescription of the correct drug in the face of a precise indication for it, a surgical procedure, simple counselling or supportive psychotherapy.

We know the range of human morbidity in our culture today; the conditions for which doctors are consulted and the therapies offered also range widely. However, it would not be inappropriate to mention a form of therapy which appears to be directly related to the release of human potential in the face of the commonly seen stress or life style induced disorders: anxiety states, intractable cigarette smoking, alcoholism and so on. The approach also has value in assisting those with incurable incapacity or near to death and needing, to live in liberty, the maximum of their resources. [Herbert] Benson, Associate Professor of Medicine at Harvard, and his associates, on the basis of careful physiological studies, devised a simple meditative technique which appears to release persons from the physiological effects of stress and impressively increases well-being.[69] [R] Beattie[70] has made available for scrutiny a number of Hobart case records and the results are so impressive that it is obvious that there is appearing a new adjunct to conventional medical therapy of potential value to the community. 'The longest journey is the journey inwards'[71] but the human liberations achieved thereby may give our culture the new beginning it seems to long for, and may already be witnessing.

> There is a revolution coming. It will not be like the revolutions of the past. It will originate with the individual and with culture, and it will change the political structure only as its final act. It promises a higher reason, a more human community and a new and liberated individual. Its ultimate creation will be a new and enduring wholeness and beauty – renewed relationship of man to himself, to other men, to society, to nature and to the land. Today we are witnesses to a great moment in history – a turn from the pessimism that has closed in on modern industrial society; the rebirth of

a future; the rebirth of a people in a sterile land. If that process had to be summed up in a single word, that word would be freedom.[72]

Ageing

Finally, as maturity blossoms into late middle age and old age, what of liberty then? To the Platonist who would regard the body as a prison for the real self, there would be assertion of increasing liberty by the very fact that strength is slipping away. Being more earth-bound, most doctors will insist that ageing does bring restriction of liberty in many ways – and there is consequent need to safeguard the health of the elderly in such a way that freedom of choice is maximised, restraint minimized and opportunity given for them to respond to life in all its fulness, to persons, to places, to beauty. 'It is the function of medicine to emancipate man's interior splendour'[73] and this may be nowhere more true than in the elderly and the dying, in the last phase of human growth, needing to express somehow what they have become.

It is relevant to recall that as life passes, what one becomes is increasingly what one has given. 'Only that can be really yours which is another's, for only what you have given, be it only in the gratitude of acceptance, is salvaged from the nothing which some day will have been your life.'[74] All health professionals (and the community at large) appear to have the obligation to safeguard and indeed to create opportunities whereby the ageing (or ailing person of any age) can give himself or herself to other persons in some way by loving and expressing love, of serving others, helping others in distress, of giving the self in the countless ways learned in the course of a lifetime, and in the new ways learned in the course of incapacity. The liberty of the ailing and of the aged to give themselves, to grow, to seek, to find new dimensions of the human mystery is, as it were, intrinsic but the opportunities for exercise of that liberty can be given by others, including the doctors. The idea that all that the elderly need is a means to 'pass the time' is a tragic misconception of the purpose and value of time (a personal view of course).

Acceptance of the fact and even the proximity of mortality may bring with it profound freedom. However, in accepting death [Maurice] Merleau-Ponty (in discussing Hegel) urges that this acceptance 'cannot be separated from the decision to live and to get a new grip on our fortuitous existence'[75] and the poet [Rainer Maria] Rilke, who said it was the poet's mission to bind life and death together, wrote 'Whoever rightly understands and celebrates death, at the same time magnifies life'. In Freudian terms [Norman] Brown held that the acceptance of death, its reunification in consciousness with life, cannot be accomplished by the discipline of philosophy or the seduction of art but only by the abolition of repression: 'Man who is born of woman and destined to die is a body, with bodily instincts. Only if Eros – the life instinct – can affirm the life of the body can the death instinct affirm death, and in affirming death magnify life'.[76] These concepts are surely in accord with [Erik] Erikson's description of integrity by which he means a sense of wholeness of life and acceptance of one's place in space and time (in contradistinction to despair) which is the task of the last phase of life.[77]

Death then is indeed a limit, but a limit in which:

> ... the inner light becomes wholly extensive, not a glow cast upon the field as in sociology, but a ray beamed out of the dome. In other words: if in view of death, against the above death, the inner man comes wholly into the open – if the hostile prick of death, the blow of doom, involves the most central application and rebirth of inwardness – death serves as the master-test of our journeyman years.

> It tests the height we have reached, the value of our inner metapsychics; it examines its strength, its utility, durability, and suitability in mobilization and in the most terrible reality: it introduces a factor alien to the subject and thus summons us directly from the subjectively ideal sphere, from the freely suspended realm of ideal self-definitions, to the 'cosmic' realm of danger and diffusion, and of the gathering from the bustle of this world of death in which the self finally proves itself, after all.[78]

The human person, then, in his birth, growth and dying is not wholly free. He is situated instead in the world, bound in a sense by time, place and social context and yet somehow human persons are conscious of a core of freedom, of responsibility, of accountability, of indeterminism, of a self thrusting towards life or death. The basic mode of human freedom has been called by [Max] Muller transcendental freedom[79] and his analysis gives depth to the foregoing: man has the faculty of distancing all things from himself and the possibility of absolute reflection, and of this transcendental freedom man can never be deprived (witness its expression in [Viktor] Frankl). The human person cannot remain thus distanced but rather has the task of giving himself out of this distance, his own concrete form. Man becomes truly a person by going freely out of himself into the work to be done. Muller argues 'Hence the first step in the realization of freedom must be alienation. But since self-possession is the essence of human freedom, the "objectivation" of freedom in work must be followed by a further movement: the return which is the fetching in of the work in the act …' Such concepts and their implications give a philosophical basis for the perceived enriching effects of simple meditative techniques, of the need for quiet and gentleness if human freedom is to blossom into the fruitfulness of lasting works. 'The task and potential greatness of mortals lie in their ability to produce things – works and deeds and words – which would deserve to be and so that through them mortals could find their place in a cosmos where everything is immortal except themselves.[80] If it be true that it is the task of medicine to reveal man's interior splendour then it is a privilege indeed.

Limits of Human Possibility

Attention has been paid to some concerns of human health and the tension between liberty and limit which frequently lies at the root of a difficulty in solving major health problems. Some exploration has been made of the limits imposed on human liberty and the role of medicine in recognizing and alleviating some of these limits. It remains to look again at the limits in another light: to examine the limits of human possibility. 'In our time, what is at issue is the very nature of man, the image we have of his limits and possibilities as man'.[81]

Some years ago [82] I expanded on this theme or rather area of exploration and I still know now no richer portrayal than that I dwelt on then, namely, the early chapters of Genesis. The portrait of man in these chapters is a diptych, first, a glimpse of the ideal human existence in Semitic terms, followed by a glimpse of the actual state of man, in alienation from the earth, self, woman and so on. It is distinctly probable that in the writer's mind the second is the portrait of existence as known and the first an instinctive, intuitive grasp of human possibility, springing no doubt from the consciousness of the richly sensitive human group within which these traditions arose. The story is then a presentation of the tension between human actuality and human possibility. Prescinding here from formal theological considerations, we may discern the following major tensions:

1 Man in actuality is a toiler on the earth, subject to joyless labour, subdued by the harsh earth, yet he has the potential

to be master of the earth, called even to name the animals – a Semitic way of expressing power over them and the capacity to be giver of meaning. Man at odds with the earth, shut out from the garden, shares common origin with the things of earth (Genesis speaks of mud and so on; the biologist speaks of evolution from primordial forms), and so is radically made to be at peace, in harmony with the earth.

2 Man's interpersonal relationships are in actuality not all harmonious, and his sexual relationships, in particular, are marked frequently by interpersonal tension, and yet there is in him the desire, and the primordial vocation, to be at peace with men and to enjoy sexual harmony.

3 Man, real man, is afraid of complete openness to the ultimate dimensions of reality, shut in on self, in a hell of pseudo-autonomy, yet he has the possibility of radical openness to all that is, in communion not only with nature, his fellows, but also with the ground of all being.

Genesis portrays the seeking to be God in a way unfitting for man as the reason for the discrepancy between the actuality and possibilities of man and this is an interesting point, but for the moment this discussion concentrates on the possibilities of humanness. The creation myths expressed the consciousness not only of the Semitic but also of the non-Semitic world[83] and may represent the earliest quintessence of human reflection on humanness and its ambiguities and possibilities.

It is not reasonable, in considering the human condition, to ignore the fact of Jesus of Nazareth, a man who the Marxist [Ernst] Bloch insists was 'uninventable' and who was the unalienated man and in many ways the humanist ideal *par excellence*. We can concede with Bloch that 'no doubt Jesus is surrounded with myths', but these are as Bloch added, 'merely the frame a man stepped into, the frame a man filled'.[84] It might be suggested that the mystery of Jesus, called the Christ, above all indicated that human possibility is realizable. As [Edward] Schillebeeckx, the Dutch Dominican theologian, puts it, 'the message which Christianity brings to the secular world is this – humanity is possible'.[85] Maybe even to show this is to liberate men from the shackles of meaninglessness and offer the springs of hope.

[Alexander] Solzhenitsyn, in his Nobel Prize acceptance speech, spoke of the artist as a source of unity to this world, capable of breaking down barriers by closeness to humanness. In a sense a doctor is called to be an artist, seeking and expressing the meaning of humanness in our time, in its limitations and its possibilities, both of which are experienced by him not only in his own life but in the lives of those he is permitted to serve. The doctor as artist is not master but servant (though not a slave) and participant in, listener to and explorer of the human mystery, and it is his privilege to etch in his own flesh and to elicit in the lives of others the depths of humanness, becoming aware as he does so, like Rieux (Camus' doctor) at the end of *The Plague* that 'there are more things to admire in man than to despise'.

There is need in our time for a new experience of ecstasy, a new celebration of life in the utter going out from self, a celebration of community, a celebration not only of the past and present but of the open future which it is the task of us all to build. [Friedrich] Nietzsche's Zarathustra challenges us indeed: 'Let the future and the farthest be for you the cause of your today … Walk among men as fragments of the future'.

References

1 Buber, M. *A Believing Humanism*. Gleanings. trans. M. Friedman, Simon & Schuster, New York, 1967, 138.
2 Mill, J.S. 'On Liberty' (1859) in *Utilitarianism, On Liberty, Essay on Bentham*, by J.S. Mill, ed. M. Warnock, Collins 1962.
3 Young, C.M. *Mortality Patterns and Trends in Australia*. National Population Enquiry. Research Report No. 5. Australian Government Publishing Service, Canberra 1976.
4 Hetzel, B.S. *Health and Australian Society*, Penguin Books, Ringwood, Australia 1974 (revised 1976).
5 Furnass, B. 'Changing Patterns of Health and Disease', in *The Magic Bullet*, ed. M. Diesendorf, Society for Social Responsibility in Science, Canberra 1976, 5–32.
6 The Royal Australian College of General Practitioners, 'The Australian General Practice Morbidity and Prescribing Survey 1969 to 1974', *Med. Jnl. Aust.*, ed. C. Bridges-Webb, 2: Special supplement No I, 1976.
7 Roe, M. 'Smallpox in Launceston, 1887 and 1903', *Papers and Proceedings, Tasmanian Historical Research Association, 23.* (1976) 111.
8 Unpublished typescript; some of these studies (e.g. Pridmore) are in preparation for publication.
9 Windschuttle, K. 'Stress and Death amongst Adolescent Males', *New Doctor, 3* (1977) 45–7.
10 Maxwell, R. Health Care. *The Growing Dilemma*, McKinsey and Company, New York 1974.
11 Among the papers of the late Albert Baikie, Foundation Professor of Medicine, University of Tasmania, was found an analysis of Australian data using Maxwell's methodology: the authorship has not yet been established.
12 Heschel, A. *The Insecurity of Freedom*. Essays on Human Existence. Schocken Books, New York 1972, 34. See also Powles, J., 'On the Limitations of Modern Medicine', in *The Challenges of Community Medicine*, R. L. Kane, Springer, New York 1974, 89–122.
13 W.H.O. Expert Committee, *Smoking and its Effect on Health*. Technical Report series No. 568, 1975. See also 'Smoking and Disease: the evidence reviewed'. *W.H.O. Chronicle, 568 (1975)* 26.
14 Doll, R. and Peto R. 'Mortality in Relation to Smoking: 20 years' observations on male British doctors in relation to smoking.' *Br.Med.Jnl., 2*, (1976) 1525.
15 Hedrick, J. L. 'The Economic costs of Cigarette Smoking' in *Drug Use and Social Policy*, ed. Susman, A.M.S. Publication, New York 1972, 180–186.
16 Editorial, *Med.Jnl.Aust., 2* (1976) 775–6. The proceedings of the annual summer schools or seminars on alcoholism and drug dependence,

St. Vincent's Hospital, Melbourne, Departments of Medicine and Community Medicine, offer a wealth of data on the Australian scene over the last decade.
17 Diehm, P. 'Alcohol: What's the Problem?' *New Doctor, 3* (1977) 32–33.
18 Saint, E.G. 'Bacchus Transported, purporting to be an Historical Impression of Alcoholism in Australia.' *Med.Jn.Aust. 2* (1970) 548–551.
19 Notable contributions are those of B. Mitchell and K. Jamrozik (in preparation) 1976.
20 Bolger, P. *Hobart Town*, Australian National Univ. Press, Canberra 1973.
21 Cited by B. Mitchell (1976); the following appeared in the *Tasmanian Colonist*, 2 Nov. 1854, and is taken from a copy in an article by Rod Kilner, 'Temperance and the Liquor Question in Tasmania in the 1850s'. *Papers and Proceedings Tasmanian Historical Research Association*, June 1973, vol. 20, no. 2, and is included by permission of Mary McRae, Principal Archivist, Archives Office of Tasmania.

TEMPERANCE AND THE LIQUOR QUESTION
IN TASMANIA IN THE 1850s
by Rod Kilner
THE TREE OF DISSIPATION
The
sin of
drunkenness
expels reason,
drowns memory,
distempers the body,
defaces beauty, dimin
ishes strength, corrupts
the blood, inflames the liver,
weakens the brain, turns men
into walking hospitals, causes
internal, external and incurable
wounds, is a witch to the senses, a
devil to the soul, a thief to the pocket,
the beggars companion, a wife's woe and
children's sorrow – makes man become
a beast, and a self-murderer, who
drinks to others good health
and robs himself of
his own
THE
ROOT OF
ALL EVIL IS
DRUNKENNESS!!
(*Tasmanian Colonist*, 2 November 1854)

22 Lickiss, J.N. *The Aboriginal People of Sydney with special reference to the Health of their Children. A study in human ecology.* M.D. thesis, University of Sydney 1971.
23 Dax, E.C. 'The Criminal and Social Aspects of Families with a Complexity of Problems.' *Aust. & N.Z. Jnl. of Criminology* (1974) 197–213.
24 Hetzel, B.S. *op. cit.* 127.
25 Criteria Committee, National Council on Alcoholism, 'Criteria for the Diagnosis of Alcoholism.' *Annals of Internal Medicine* 77 (1972) 249–258.
26 Hetzel, B.S. *ibid.* 127.
27 Murray, R.M. 'Characteristics and Prognosis of Alcoholic Doctors.' Br.Med.Joi., 2 (1976) 1537. [Prof. A Conigrave in 2022 has pointed out an error in the numbers quoted which relied on the published Abstract]
28 Arnaldus de Villanova, quoted in B. Roueche, 'Cultural Factors and Drinking Patterns, *Annals New York Academy Sciences, 133* (1966) 849.
29 Baikie, A.G.; Baker, H. Henderson, A.S. and Lewis, I.C. 'Some Aspects of Behaviour in Selected Group of High School Students.' *Proceedings 13th International Congress of Paediatrics 15* (1971) 171.
30 cf. Account of a notable international symposium: Society, Stress and Disease.' *W.H.O. Chronicle 25* (1971) 168.
31 Shaw, G.B. *The Doctor's Dilemma* (1911), Penguin edition 1971, 9.
32 Clendening, L. *Source Book of Medical History* (first publ. 1942), Dover publications, New York 1960, 5.
33 Maxwell, R. *Health Care. The Growing Dilemma.* McKinsey, New York 1974. See also Mahler, H. 'Problems of Medical Affluence.' *W.H.O. Chronicle 31* (1977) 8–13.
34 Terris, M. 'The contributions of Henry E. Sigerist to Health Service organization.' *Milbank Memorial Fund Quarterly 53* (1975) 495. (This article is an invaluable guide to Sigerist's scattered writings).
35 Sigerist, H. *Medicine and Human Welfare*, Yale University Press, New Haven 1941, 114–16.
36 Sigerist, H. *ibid.* 119–24.
37 Sigerist, H. 'The place of the physician in modern society' in *Henry E. Sigerist on the History of Medicine* ed. M.I. Roemer, MD Publications, New York 1960, 69.
38 Gregg, A. 'Henry E. Sigerist: His Impact on American Medicine.' *Bulletin of the History of Medicine 22* (1948) 32–4.
39 Bruhn, J.G. 'Human Ecology: A Unifying Science?' *Human Ecology 2* (1974) 105.
40 Magee, B. *Popper*, Collins, London 1973, 30, 39.
41 Popper, K. *The Logic of Scientific Discovery*, Hutchinson 1968.
42 Popper, K. *The Open Society and its Enemies*, vols *1* and *2*, Routledge, London 1945, revised edition 1966.

43 Camus, A. Notebooks, quoted by A. Alvarez, *The Savage God. A Study of Suicide*, Weidenfeld and Nicolson, London 1971, 217.
44 King, A. *Another Kind of Growth: Industrial Society and the Quality of Life*. David Davies Memorial Institute of International Studies, Annual Memorial Lecture, London 1972.
45 World Health Organization. 'Fifth Report on the World Health Situation, 1969–72.' *WHO Official Records* (1975) *225*. See also 'Mortality and Morbidity Trends 1969–1972', *WHO Chronicle 29* (1975) 377–86.
46 World Health Organization. 'Fifth Report on the World Health Situation, 1969–72.' WHO Official Records (1975) 225. See also 'Mortality and Morbidity Trends 1969–1972', *WHO Chronicle 29* (1975) 377–86.
47 Meadows, D.H.; Meadows, D.L.; Randers, J and Behrens, W.W. *The Limits to Growth*, First Report to the Club of Rome, Earth Island Limited, London 1972.
48 Mesarovic, M. and Pester, E. *Mankind at the Turning Point*, Second Report to the Club of Rome, Hutchinson, London 1975.
49 Hammarskjöld, D. *Markings*, trans. L. Sjoberg and W.H. Auden, Faber, London 1966, 77.
50 Masterman, P. Atheism and Alienation. *A Study of the Philosophical Sources of Contemporary Atheism*. Penguin Books, Harmondsworth 1973, 131.
51 cf. Winter, G. *Elements for a Social Ethic. Scientific Perspectives on Social Process*, MacMillan, New York., chap. 4.
52 Dahrendorf, *Homo sociologicus*, Routledge and Kegan Paul, London 1973, 25.
53 Dahrendorf, R. *op. cit.* 60.
54 Dahrendorf, R. *op. cit.* 69.
55 MacMurray, J. *Persons in Relation*. (Gifford Lectures, University of Glasgow 1954). Faber, London 1961, 150.
56 MacMurray, J. *op. cit.* 211.
57 Frankl, V. *Man's Search for Meaning*. trans. I. Lasch, Beacon Press, Boston 1962, 65.
58 Gibran, K. (1883–1931) *The Prophet*. Heinneman, London 1959, 44.
59 Boros, L. *We are Future*. Herder, New York 1970, 105.
60 de Beauvoir, S. *The Second Sex*. ed. and trans. H.M. Parshley, Jonathan Cape, London 1953, 632.
61 Lawrence, D.H. *Sex versus Loneliness: Selected Essays*, quoted by R. Williams in Culture and Society, Penguin Books, Harmondsworth 1961, 213.
62 Popper, K. *The Open Society and its Enemies: The Spell of Plato*. Routledge and Sons, 1, 1945, 97.

63 Hammurabi in *Growth of Ideas*, ed. J. Huxley, J. Bronowski, G. Barry, and J. Fisher, Macdonald, London 1965, 214.
64 Nathanson, B.N. 'Deeper into Abortion.' *New Eng. Jnl. of Med. 291*, (1974), 1189.
65 *cf* Goodman, E. *A Study of Liberty and Revolution*. Duckworth, London 1975, 67.
66 Bronowski, J. *The Ascent of Man*, BBC, London 1973, 365.
67 Westermann, C. *Creation*. trans. J.J. Scullion, SPCK, London 1971, 92.
68 Bronowski, J. *op. cit.* 144.
69 Benson, H. *The Relaxation Response*, Collins, Glasgow 1976.
70 Beattie, R. Personal communication 1976.
71 Hammarskjöld, D. *op. cit.* 65.
72 Reich, C.A. *The Greening of America*. Bantam Books, New York 1971, 2, 379.
73 Mortimer, K.E. 'The Impossible Profession: The Doctor/ Priest Relationship.' *Proceedings Australian Association Gerontology 2*, 1974, 81.
74 Hammarskjöld, D. *op. cit.* 51.
75 Merleau-Ponty. *Sense and Non-Sense*. trans. by Dreyfus and Dreyfus, North Western University Press, Chicago 1964, 69.
76 Brown, N.O. *Life and Death. The psychoanalytical meaning of History*. Wesleyan University Press, Middleton, Connecticut 1959, 109.
77 Erikson, E. 'Identity and the Life Cycle.' *Psychological Issues. I* 1959, 98.
78 Bloch, E. 'Karl Marx, Death and the Apocalypse' in *Man on His own: Essays in the Philosophy of Religion*. trans. by E.B. Ashton. Herder and Herder, New York 1970, 47.
79 Muller, M. 'Freedom' in *Encyclopedia of Theology: The Concise Sacramentum Mundi*. ed. K. Rabner 1975, 535.
80 Arendt, H. *The Human Condition*, University of Chicago Press, Chicago, 1958, 19.
81 Mills, C.W. 'On Reason and Freedom' in *Identity and Anxiety. Survival of the Person in Mass Society*. Free Press of Glencoe, Illinois 1960, 110.
82 Lickiss, J.N. 'Towards the Human Future. Medical Practice and Human Possibility.' *Med. Jnl. Aust. 2* 1972 896.
83 Westermann, C. *op. cit.* 9–15.
84 Bloch, E. 'Man's Increasing Entry into Religious Mystery' in *Man on His Own. op. cit.* 180.
85 Schillebeeckx, E.H. *God the Future of Man*. Sheed and Ward, London 1968 198. (See also Bloch, E. *Atheism in Christianity*, trans. J.T. Swan, Herder and Herder, New York 1972, 123–4. 'We in our turn have never emerged from ourselves, and we are where we are. But we are still dark in ourselves; and not only because of the nearness, the immediacy of the here and now in which we, as all things, have our

being. No – it is because we tear at each other, as no beasts do: secretly we are dangerous. And because in so many other ways we are hidden: unrealized, unachieved as no other living being, still open to what lies ahead, with a finger even in the yet-tocome, which is coming, far ahead. And at the same time we start, over and over again, at the beginning, ever restless. But with a sign that our plan is good; a sign called Jesus: one that is not yet rid of restlessness and journeying; but one that is bound in unique intimacy to man, and stays by him. As the mildest of signs, it is true; but precisely for that reason as the most fiery, the most disturbing, the most uprooting. If it had not been so, if the hypocrisy had continued, no shoot would ever have blossomed, there would have been no 'I am he'; but just more soothing words. Something else is afoot here, though; for this Jesus calls us by our name and stands by it. The awakening can be a quiet one and yet still be unsettling. It is a renewal.').

5

THE DOCTOR AND EDUCATION

I

A CONSIDERATION OF PERSONAL DEVELOPMENT IN RELATION TO DEAF CHILDREN
1971

Presentation at Triennial Conference,
Australian Association of Teachers of the Deaf, Brisbane, 1971.

Children are 'people beginning to be'[1] Carl Rogers (1902–1987) speaks of 'becoming a person',[2] Carl Jung (1857–1952) wrote of the 'achievement of personality' and stated that 'it is nothing less than the best possible development of all that is a particular, single being'.[3] Human development, indeed all human life, is a process then, the process of becoming what one has the capacity to be. Actualisation of potential occurs throughout life but the transformation wrought in childhood is striking enough and influential enough to deserve close scrutiny, and at least a glimpse of it will be taken today as part of our concern for children who happen to be deaf.

i

'Anything that grows has a ground plan and ... out of this ground plan the parts arise, each part having its time of special ascendancy, until all parts have arisen to form a functioning whole'.[4] So Erikson states the principle (the epigenetic principle) which is basic for a consideration of growth and development. It is essential to stress at the outset, however, that the process through which a fertilised ovum becomes a mature human person depends not only upon the inherent plan (which we might term genetic endowment) but also upon continuing interaction with the environment. The shape of the future is contained in the present but whether this shape is realised, whether potentialities are fully actualised, depends on the quality of the environment – especially that bit of reality in immediate relationship with the developing organism.

Development proceeds, then, in accordance with a ground plan, a complexus of laws inherent in especially the molecular patterns of the genes, and is expressed in ways which we call physical, psychological, social and so on. The organism – or rather, child – develops as a whole. The so-called components of development are merely aspects of the whole isolated for descriptive purposes. Physical expressions of development are very obvious – the embryo becomes a man with increasing size, differentiation, complexity, degree of coordination; and perceptive powers become more attuned to the widening environment as the womb gives way to the cradle, the cradle to the home, neighbourhood, school, city ...

Intellectual development is closely dependent on the level of structural differentiation. Emotional development – the emergence of feelings, and control of them, becomes more and more complex as growth in self-consciousness proceeds parallel with awareness of a widening world. Social development is also clear – from the *in utero* situation where the little human's horizon is the womb, to the years of maturity where there is kinship with the cosmos, there is ideally a steady growth in depth and complexity of interpersonal relationships and sensitivity to their demands. Many factors come into play, including:

 i poor inherent capacity in the organism,
 ii inadequate environment in terms of quantity (of quantifiable things) or quality,
 iii noxious elements in the environment: viruses, drugs, hatred, mistrust …

All this may not only retard development of some aspects of the whole but may lead to such degrees of imbalance and deviant development that wholeness in the future is doubtful.

The personal environment influences to a high degree the interaction of the child with other components of the environment (and it is a personal environment which is the concern of educators). A well-fed child may fail to thrive, may fail in emotional and intellectual as well as physical development and even die if the personal environment is inadequate. Studies in parental deprivation have stressed this point, and no further consideration will be given here.

In the total development of the child the role of the family is paramount. The peculiar dynamics of the little social system (which the family is) provide that personal environment in which the child undergoes the experiences – conflicts, joys, sorrows, hopes, fears – which enable him/her to grow towards full humanness.

The child receives its genetic endowment, in fact, comes to *be* in the roots of the familial life at its dynamic centre: his/her only physical environment is his mother for the first nine months of his existence. He goes through the birth process with his/her mother and for the next half year or so his/her mother is his/her world, gradually becoming differentiated from his/her self. The role of the father and siblings becomes more prominent in the next few years as the child goes through its toilet training period, becomes more aware of self and others, wants to express aggression, yet must learn control, needs to be independent and delights in expressing autonomy in various ways and in all this he is groping for his/her identity including sexual identity.

The resolution of the triangular situation in which the child finds himself/herself, competing with one parent for possession of the parent of the opposite sex, is a very important task of the years from three to six. Resolution of this conflict through identification with the parent of the same sex might usually be the most satisfactory outcome. Maybe the conflict is not universal, nor is it as clearly sexual, as Sigmund Freud (1856–1939) thought, but certainly it is a period of life when instinctual urges come to the fore and anxiety is frequently noted. The child in this period normally internalises the parent figures in some way to lead to the formation of conscience, and he can know guilt when appropriate. It is to be stressed that the first 6 or 7 years of life are critical with regard to future personal happiness, since in those years are laid down the shape of the personality (this may even be well established in the first year of life), and sexual and moral attitudes in the widest sense are firmly fashioned. It is well known that neurosis usually has its roots in dislocation in the interpersonal environment in these early childhood years.

It is noteworthy that 'internalisation of the socio-cultural environment provides the basis, not merely of one specialised component of the human personality, but of what in the human sense is its very core'.[5]

Any discussion of personal development would be incomplete without some mention of the clarifications brought (I think) to a confused field by Erik Erikson (1902–1994)[6] in his writings over the last 20 years. David Rapaport (1950)[7] summed up Erikson's contribution as follows:

> Each phase of the life cycle is characterised by a phase-specific developmental task: which must be solved in it, though this solution is worked out further in subsequent ones. Each phase is described in terms of the extremes of successful and unsuccessful solutions which can be arrived at in it, though in reality the outcome is a balance between these extremes; (1) Basic trust vs mistrust; (2) autonomy vs shame and doubt; (3) initiative vs guilt; (4) industry vs inferiority; (5) identity vs identity diffusion; (6) intimacy vs isolation; (7) generativity vs stagnation; (8) integrity vs despair.

Finally, to sum up the healthy personality we may accept Marie Jahoda's (1907–2001) definition: 'A healthy personality actively masters his environment, shows a certain unity of personality, and is able to perceive the world and himself correctly.'[8]

ii

1. Martin Heidegger (1889–1976) wrote that 'language is the home of being, it is in it that man establishes his abode'.[9] Eduard Bergstein (1850–1932) referred to language as a second womb: 'From the biological womb the child is born into the womb of language in which it develops into a human being'.[10] It is to be expected that a deaf child confronts several hazards to personal growth.

2. Throughout the whole process of development there is reduced environmental interaction: there is reduced impact and reduced capacity for response to stimuli. Reduced

interaction with the material environment is a source of sorrow – but reduced interpersonal interaction caused by impaired communication is a more serious deprivation.

Incomplete and incorrect perception of reality is likely – not merely the inaccurate perception of auditory stimuli in the physical sense but rather the deprivation of language by which reality is codified and is made relevant. Bernstein pointed out that, 'language marks out what is relevant, affectively, cognitively and socially, and experience is transformed by that which is made relevant' (Bernstein, 1961).[11] Anything which leads to inaccurate or incomplete perception not only of oneself but also of the culture in which one lives and the culture of other people and other times is a serious threat to personal development. Margaret Mead wrote strongly on this point:

> Humanity as we know it is not merely a matter of human physique ... but of our capacity to accumulate and build upon the inventions and experiences of previous generations. A child who does not participate in the great body of tradition, whether because of defect, neglect, injury, or disease, never becomes fully human.[12]

3 A deaf child may be in considerable danger of dislocation of family relationships by maternal rejection, heightened sibling rivalry or even early institutionalisation. The last, though occasionally essential, is a grave threat to normal personal development for during the first years of life the family is the required environment for the formation of a secure identity, sound conscience and clear sexual identification.

4 There may be fewer opportunities of choice in a deaf child's everyday world, and decision making with

consciousness of self-directedness is an important aspect of personal growth. The deaf child may be subject to more external control with less opportunity for active exploration of his environment; there may be insufficient outlets for 'the drive for life', and difficulties in achieving control of aggressive and sexual drives. Such restrictions may be aggravated by unenlightened institutionalisation.

5   The deaf child may have to cope with other handicaps, for example, intellectual or visual impairment: this is particularly seen in some rubella affected children.

iii

The approach of the educator to the handicapped child must take into account, among other matters, the basic concepts of personal development and the specific process of personal growth, for education is intently concerned with personal reality. A few brief points are made merely to indicate areas for more profound reflection.

Education goals may be and have been conceptualised in many ways. A useful concept is that education aims to 'awaken awareness'[13] of reality in all its dimensions: of the self, of the other, of the cosmos, of the ultimate. The whole human community is involved in the educational process, intimately concerned with the awakening of a child to himself and to his environment: formal education focuses this communal action.

Through growth in awareness of self, other persons, the non-personal world outside self, and of ultimate realities, a person grows towards increasing richness of life. There have been many attempts to delineate the attributes of a 'rich' human life: self-actualisation, freedom from obstacles to self-directed living, opportunities for choice and creativity, self-giving and receiving the self-gift of another typically in stable marriage, consciousness that the shape of the human condition is dialogue in which one person is open to another as 'thou' not 'it' …[14] Educators need to be mindful of such considerations.

Specifically, the formal educator of a deaf child needs: (a) to recognise the particular difficulties encountered by the deaf child and his/her family; (b) to offer continuous confirmation of the child's being with assistance in his search for identity and encouragement in overcoming obstacles and deviant trends; (c) to provide an atmosphere of respect, affection, and basic trust, where the psychosocial needs are consistently met; (d) to integrate all the educational influences of the child's life, centred clearly on the role of the family. Carl Jung wrote:

> Personality is the highest realisation of the inborn distinctiveness of the particular living being. Personality is an act of the greatest courage in the face of life and means unconditional affirmation of all that constitutes the individual, the most successful adaptation to the universal conditions of human existence, with the greatest possible freedom of personal decision-making.
>
> To educate someone to *this* seems to me to be no small matter. It is surely the heaviest task that the spiritual world of today has set itself. And, indeed, it is a dangerous task, as dangerous as the bold and inconsiderate undertaking of nature to let women bear children.[15]

The Tower of Babel represented the aspirations of men to an impossible goal. Education should lead to the possible. 'Surely there is no greater gift to a man than that which turns all his aims into parching lips and all life into a fountain.'[16]

References

1. Rasey, M, 'Toward the End', in *The Self*, Moustakas (ed), Harper and Row, NY, 1956.
2. Rogers, CR, 'What it Means to Become a Person', in *The Self*, Moustakas (ed), Harper and Row, NY, 1956, and many major books.
3. Jung, CG, 'The Development of Personality', in *The Self*, Moustakas (ed), Harper and Row, NY, 1956.
4. Erikson, EH, *Identity and the Life Cycle*, International Universities Press, NY, 1959, p52.
5. Parsons, T, 'Social Structure and the Development of Personality', in *Studying Personality Crossculturally*, Kaplan, B (ed), Harper and Row, NY, 1961.
6. Erikson, EH, *Identity and the Life Cycle*, (note 4 above); Childhood and Society, 2nd ed, Penguin books, London, 1965; *Identity, Youth and Crisis*, Faber and Faber, London, 1968, etc.
7. Rapaport, D, 'A Historical Survey of Psychoanalytic Ego Psychology', Introduction to *Identity and the Life Cycle*, by Erikson (see note 4 above).
8. Jahoda, M, (1950), cited by Erikson, *Identity and the Life Cycle*, p51.
9. Heidegger, M, *Letter on Humanism*, quoted by Marcel, *Problematic Man*, trans. B Thomson, Herder, NY, p46.
10. Bergstein, T, 'Complementarity and Philosophy', *Nature*, 1929, 222:1033.
11. Berstein, B, 'Aspects of Language and Learning in the Genesis of the Social Process', *J Child Psychology and Psychiatry*, 1961, 1:313.
12. Mead, M, in *Childhood and Contemporary Cultures*, Mead and Wolfenstein (eds), University of Chicago Press, Chicago, 1955, p6.
13. Morris, VC, *Existentialism in Education*, Harper and Row, NY, 1966.
14. Buber, M, *I and Thou*, revised ed, Clarke, Edinburgh, 1958.
15. Jung, CG, ibid, see note 3.
16. Gibran, K, *The Prophet*, Heinemann, London, 1926.

II
ON UNDERGRADUATE MEDICAL EDUCATION
1973

Presentation to Annual Meeting,
Australian College of Education, Hobart 1973.

It is appropriate at a time when all aspects of education are under scrutiny and when the role of the doctor in a changing society is rightly being reconsidered, that a long hard look be taken at undergraduate medical education. It is an axiom that, at the very least, a doctor's education should fit him to meet the real health needs of the society in which he practices as well as to be a leader within society and a contributor to the total store of human knowledge. Further if medical practice is to play an adequate role in the face of increasing awareness of the social dimensions of health problems, the doctor should be competent not only as a clinician in varying contexts but also as an analyst of social change, as a contributor to the shaping of health-related social policies as an informed social critic.

There are conventional problems with regard to medical education and these have been ably and recently considered by many, for example the problems of curriculum design (and the implementation of ideal designs), the matter of inter-relationships between teaching hospital, university and community services, the re-evaluation of teaching techniques, and on the wider issue of the role of medicine in societal change. It may on this occasion be profitable to take up another issue, namely, the conceptual basis and overall goal of undergraduate medical education in the search for a unifying perspective against which one may more fruitfully tackle problems such as those mentioned above.

As a point of departure, the pronouncement of the Royal Commission on Medical Education[1] is apposite:

> We cannot emphasise too strongly that the undergraduate course in medicine should be primarily educational. Its object is to produce not a fully qualified doctor but an educated man who will become fully qualified by postgraduate training.

George Pickering[2] in his discussion of medical education urged in the same vein that, 'whatever else we do, we should be absolutely sure that each of us ... leaves the student with a finer mind than when he started.

What is an educated man? There have been innumerable opinions throughout the ages and some of these are clearly relevant to our present consideration. John Amos Comenius,[3] the seventeenth century follower of Jan Hus [Czech philosopher], considered that the educated man is one whose senses are attuned to the learning possibilities of the world – a notion which is echoed in more existential terms by Van Cleve Morris[4] that an educated man is a man of awakened awareness. Another contemporary writer[5] holds that an educated man is, 'the man capable not of providing specialised answers but of asking the great and liberating questions by which humanity makes its way through time'.

Some of these notions are worthy of further discussion.

First – the educated man, a man of 'awakened awareness'. Awareness may be considered to have four dimensions, each of relevance to the education of a medical student.

Self-awareness

A doctor needs to be comfortable in and with himself – not bereft of the fruitful discontent with self which is part of the thrust of creative living – but marked by a degree of self-understanding, self acceptance, self-direction and clarity of self-identity whilst continuing, like other human beings, to grow as a person throughout life. Is there anything we can add to the processes of time to help our students grow in self-awareness? The answer to that question should seriously influence curriculum design, course content, and teaching methods.

Awareness of other

The personal is constituted by personal relatedness.[6] There is need to listen, need to accept the other as other, need for growth in awareness of common humanness, of communication codes, of understanding and acceptance of sexuality in the perspective of interpersonal communication.

D.H. Lawrence[7] tellingly wrote that:

> [I]f only our civilization had taught us ... how to keep the fire of sex clear and alive, flickering or glowing or blazing in all its varying degrees of strength and communication, we might, all of us, have lived our lives in love, which means that we should be kindled and full of zest in all kinds of ways and for all kinds of things.

There is an urgency in the need to rediscover the human capacity for relationships based on a heightened awareness of common humanness. In the UNESCO sponsored consideration of education there is a warning:[8]

> The great changes of our time are imperilling the unity and the future of the species, and man's own identity as well. What is to be feared is not only the painful prospect of grievous inequalities, privations and suffering, but also that we may be heading for a veritable dichotomy within the human race, which risks being split into superior and inferior groups, into masters and slaves, supermen and submen. Among the risks resulting from this situation would be not only those of conflict and other disasters (for present day means of mass destruction might well

fall into the hands of destitute and rebellious groups) but the fundamental risk of dehumanization, affecting privileged and oppressed alike. For the harm done to man's nature would harm all men.

The doctor, surely a guardian as well as healer of the human needs to understand the risks to dehumanisation as well as the opportunities for the liberation of the human, inherent in our changing world. Social change[9] implies changing relationships, a changing personal field – and only a doctor who understands human togetherness can help persons under the stress of change.

Further, there is need for growth in understanding how the human community is welded together by the interlocking of life cycles in a multitude of ways, such that self and other are seen in the context not merely of immediate relationships but in the context of the human totality. This global consciousness of humankind is an enriching dimension of the pattern of thought and feeling of a truly educated man capable therefore of constructive community-building action.

Awareness of the cosmos – 'at homeness' in the non-personal environment. Harmony and tranquillity with acceptance of one's situation in space and time, capacity to discern (and preserve) what is of value and to shape the earth in accord with its most rich possibilities: all these are hallmarks of an educated mind. This is a sweeping statement but if there is truth in it, there is value in learning about the evolutionary history of mankind and thinking about the inter-relationship of men with the earth. It is true that we have only one earth to live on, to tend, to enjoy, to shape to hand on …

> Alone in space, alone in its life – supporting systems, powered by inconceivable energies, mediating them to us through the most delicate adjustments, wayward,

unlikely, unpredictable, but nourishing, enlivening and enriching in the largest degree – is this not a precious home for all of us earthlings? Is it not worth our love?[10]

It is fitting for an educated man, for a doctor, to ponder on these things, in order to assist truly human development in the context of this earth, recognising clearly the fact and consequence of the limits to growth.[11]

Further, it is our privilege as men not only to live on and care for this earth but 'to discover the latent significance of things'[12] and to give significance where it is not yet. Man is like that ... Margaret Mead[13] when asked what was the most important thing in life for her answered, 'that life should have meaning ... that everything one does should be felt to be in a context which is significant'. Our search for significance and our capacity to join with the whole human community in the quest for meaning and in the task of bestowing significance surely involves the awareness of our place in the total environment, a comprehension of human ecology in all its dimensions.

Awareness of ultimate reality

There need be no apology for placing the awareness of ultimate things as a fourth dimension of awareness of a truly educated man. There are indeed signs that the deeper one penetrates into the fundamentals of the major human disciplines such as physics or sociology one is brought up sharply against the possibility that religious concepts, far from being an illusion or projection of need, may be a reflection in man of his instinctive though fragile grasp of the real.[14]

Each man develops within him a symbol system, a concept of the meaning of life, of goodness, of truth, of evil, of death, of the roots of hope ... A man closed against a consideration of the ultimate may be, to that degree, less a man. As the ageing Marxist Bloch wrote,[15] 'even amid the mythical nonsense that is so easy to note, there ... rises the unfinished question that has been burning only in religions, the question of the sense we cannot make out, of the meaning of life. It is the true realism that will be stirred by this question, one so removed from mythical nonsense so as to be responsible, rather, for every bit of sense'. The days are gone when one man's religious concepts can be dismissed out of hand – for the search now for meaning is too critical. The discernment of what is abiding amid the ephemeral is a life-long task, involving sometimes personal tragedy in which the issues become sharpened. How can we assist future doctors in their growth in this discernment?

Ethical issues in medicine have never been so prominent as they are now in learned medical journals. By what criteria can we judge the value of a man? How can we decide which life should be sacrificed? aborted? not prolonged? 'The momentum of modern medicine has provoked a philosophical dialogue forcing all parties to it to consider certain questions that not too long ago seemed more clear and settled: those questions concerning the value of human life, the basis of human dignity, the goal of human existence and the corollary duties of medicine to be governed by these assumptions'.[16]

Modern medical practice certainly involves confrontation with the ultimate dimensions of human being: how can we help our students learn that which we as teachers struggle through our lives to grasp?

Our young doctors need, then, to have much awareness of self, of others and of this earth and of the learning possibilities of this world, together with a concept of ultimate realities deep enough to provide a frame of reference within which to live and to die and to grow in wisdom that they can, as Tom MacGleish urges, begin to ask the right questions.

What are 'the great and liberating questions' to be asked by men such as doctors in our time?

1. Of the ways in which human beings are adapting to the accelerating change of our period of time which are maladaptations?

   > Man is so adaptable that he could survive and multiply in underground shelters even though this regimented subterranean existence left him unaware of the robin's song in the spring, the whorl of dead leaves in the fall, and the moods of the wind – even though indeed all his ethical and aesthetic values should wither.[17]

   We humans are under stress. We are capable of devising new ways of coping with almost any problem which arises – be it disease, infertility, overpopulation or urban crowding. We can live with war, with hate, with terrorism, with oppression, with poverty. We can – or at least some of us – can adapt to almost anything even if our aesthetic values should whither. A young doctor can, after initial abhorrence, adapt to performing the abortions allotted to his unit. How can we judge maladaptation? When should we protest? – and how?

2. How should human beings respond to the 'loss of the stable state'?

   Donald Schon[18] in the BBC Reith lectures on this subject, after outlining the basis for his claim that our society is beyond stability, warned us of the 'anti-responses' to the situation. He detailed them as either an attempt to return to the last stable state or revolt; the only adequate response is the development of new learning systems in which human beings grow in the capacity to live within a context of change.

What can a doctor, with his experience of persons under stress within our rapidly evolving culture contribute to the search for new learning systems? The widespread anxiety and depression within Western culture (and the extraordinary expenditure on psychotropic drugs) raise these questions very seriously. At the very least, we have the obligation to help our medical students to become aware of the problem with its sharp ethical dimensions and to raise the question of what a doctor can do in the face of the stress and distress of our time in which a crisis of the self does seem to be at least more evident than previously.[19] What are the learning and teaching experiences which will help raise these questions? – and generate some causal hypothesis as a basis for action and prevention.

3   What are the most fruitful possibilities of man? What can man be? What do we want to become?

The fundamental difficulty in formulating a programme for the genetic improvement of man is that we do not know what we want to become or where we want to go.[20]

In our time, what is at issue is the very nature of man, the image we have of his limits and possibilities as man.[21]

We have here a problem of serious consequences.

In a situation of almost limitless possibilities, the burden of choice is increasing. In some ways we are unfree, in others we are frighteningly free. To live a life of indecisiveness is a serious and dangerous possibility. The burden of responsibility for what one becomes is heavy, and the failure to bear the burden may contribute to some of the widespread depression in our culture. Is there any way out? Can we learn ourselves and teach our students that freedom is a precious burden and that the bearing of it needs to be shared at times? We may be on the verge of the rediscovery of a sense of community. Our students may understand this better than their teachers – and there is room for more two-way communication in the learning and teaching situation. Certainly the skill in understanding the burden of freedom may be the prerequisite to sound medical care in our time.

In all this a doctor and therefore a student with his teacher need to be asking as philosophers of our time (such as Ernest Bloch) ask, 'Where are the springs of hope?' Ultimately, surely, hope lies in the intrinsic capacity of man to be open to all that is.

It was the editor of New York Times in 1970 who said that, 'Man persists chiefly because he is endowed with thought and blessed with dreams ... With the dream, there is mankind, capable of what we call compassion and understanding and hope ...' This would seem to be where the doctors come in, capable of embodying compassion, understanding and hope – not mere mockery but real hope that even at midnight we can be confident of the dawn.[22]

4. A final area of questioning raises wide issues, of painful consequence to any doctor with a global sense of mankind. Why is it that there is between nations and within nations such unspeakable maldistribution of medical care resources on the face of this one earth? – and what are the factors which perpetuate the situation and enable us to accept it?

How have we become immune to the impact of the facts which indicate so clearly that a small proportion of the real health needs of a small segment of humankind are being met by escalating use of health resources whilst the majority of men have far from minimal standards of health care?

How can we teach our students to understand the issues when our minds have been clouded? and to act when we have rationalised ourselves and our communities into inertia?

We do have only one earth and we will rightly be held responsible by our descendants for its continuing unspeakable inequalities.

Maybe in all this we need the courage to tap more vigorously the collective wisdom of men. It is consoling that, as the biologist Paul Alfred Weiss[23] wrote, 'human tasks are not punctuated episodes but run on uninterruptedly from the past into the future – each of our contributions but a point on a time line, a thread in an endless fabric being woven.'

It may be that the primary goal of medical education is achieved if a student becomes aware and gladly aware that he, like his teacher, is part of the human fabric, part of the human pattern, and as he becomes creative so awareness grows in unresting/creative/discontent. As William Hobbes[24] wrote three centuries ago, 'There is no such thing as perpetual tranquillity of mind while we live here ... because life itself is but motion and can never be without desire, or without fear, – no more than without sense; there can be no contentment but in proceeding.'

REFERENCES

1 Royal Commission on Medical Education (1968), Report (TODD), H.M.S.O., London.
2 Pickering, G. (1959), quoted by D. Sinclair in *Basic Medical Education*, Oxford University Press, London: 183.
3 Comenius (1592–1670), in *Models of Man*. 'Explorations in the Western Educational Tradition', edited by P. Nash, John Wiley, New York: 203.
4 Morris, V.C. (1966), *Existentialism in Education*, Harper and Row, New York: 103. New York Times, Editorial, July 5, 1970.
5 MacGleish, A. (1968), 'Our Altered Conception of Ourselves', in *Evolution of Man*, (1970) edited by L.B. Young, Oxford University Press, New York: 612.

6. MacMurray, J. (1961), *Persons in Relation*, Faber and Faber London: 61.
7. Lawrence, D.H. (1961), 'Sex versus Loneliness'. Selected Essays, quoted by R. Williams in *Culture and Society*, Penguin Books, Harmondsworth: 213.
8. Faure, E. et al (1972), 'Learning to Be', *The World of Education Today and Tomorrow*, UNESCO, Paris xxi.
9. Dunphy, D. (1972), 'The Challenge of Change', Boyer Lectures Australian Broadcasting Commission, Sydney.
10. Ward, B. and Dubos, R. (1972), *Only One Earth: The Care and Maintenance of a Small Planet*, Penguin Books, Harmondsworth: 298.
11. *Lancet*, (1971), 'The Human Predicament', 2, p. 1015.
12. Dalmais, I.H. (1961), *Introduction to the Liturgy*, translated by R. Capel, Chapman, London: 2.
13. Mead, M. (1973), Interview, Australian Broadcasting Commission, June 16, 1973.
14. Berger, P. (1970), *A Rumour of Angels*, Penguin Books, Harmondsworth.
15. Bloch, E. (1970), *Man on His own, Essays in the Philosophy of Religion*, translated by E.B. Ashton, Herder and Herder, New York: 202.
16. Stumpf, S.E. (1966), 'Some Moral Dimensions of Medicine', *Annals Internal Medicine*, 64: 480.
17. Dubos, R. (1965), *Man Adapting*, Yale University Press, New Haven: 434, 278.
18. Schon, D. (1971), *Beyond the Stable State: Public and Private Leaving in a Changing Society*, Temple Smith, London.
19. Dunphy, D. (1972), 'The Challenge of Change', Boyer Lectures Australian Broadcasting Commission, Sydney.
20. Dubos, R. (1965), *Man Adapting*, Yale University Press, New Haven: 434, 278.
21. Mills, C.W. (1960), *On Reason and Freedom in Identity and Anxiety: Survival of the Person in Mass Society*, edited by M.R. Stein, A.J. Vidich, D.M. White. Free Press of Glencoe, Illinois: 114.
22. Bloch, E. (1970), *Man on His own, Essays in the Philosophy of Religion*, translated by E.B. Ashton, Herder and Herder, New York: 202.
23. Weiss, P.A. (1971), *A Cell is not an Island Entire of Itself: Perspectives in Biology and Medicine*, 14: 183.
24. Hobbes, W. in *Leviathan* quoted by P.F. Medawar, 'The Hope of Progress', Methuen, London, 1972.

III
THE IDEA OF A UNIVERSITY, NOW
1978

Address to Convocation,
University of Tasmania, October 1978.

The asking of such a question implies the existence of a fundamental problem; I believe the time is ripe for a reappraisal of the raison d'etre, the 'idea' of the University of Tasmania – and this paper is merely a small contribution to such an exercise. It appears to me that, having completed a growth period, generated from without, the University is in a state of crisis.

'Let the past illuminate the present' said Mao Tse Tung, and a glance backward may pay dividends.

The prehistory of the founding of the University of Tasmania, as outlined by Maurice French[1] set the stage for a difficult growth period. French delineated three periods:

i the period of sectarian conflict beginning in the 1830s,

ii the period of grand vision beginning in 1855 with a request made to the Legislative Council by Dr. Crooke for a vote of £20,000 per annum for a university described as 'a vision of magnificent buildings, extensive halls, capacious colleges and chambers, and long lines of professors' – a request not acceded to, but which sparked off several moves,

iii the period of personal ambition (often bitter) beginning in the 1870s at a time of political stability and prosperity and concluding with the foundation of the University from 1 January 1890, still amidst controversy.

The University had at its foundation an annual vote of £3000 (£4000 in 1892) and no land, and commenced initially as an examining, not teaching, body; three years later the first lecturers were appointed and lectures commenced 15 March 1893 with a handful of students.

French concludes his account thus, 'Such is the long history of the founding of the University that it cannot be said to have been born – it simply happened; and in the coming decades the University did not thrive – it merely existed.'

Tony Kearney as registrar, in a talk to staff in 1976 outlined the subsequent history of the University and a major work is being prepared by a group of scholars. Kearney noted that, 'the premature and puny institution led a precarious existence for thirty-five years' with parliament several times moving to abolish it as an economy measure.

From a numerical point of view further development was as follows:

	ANNUAL GRANT	STAFF	STUDENTS
1893	£4,000	3 lecturers	33
1917	£8,000	15 including six professors	75
1938	£25,000	20	422
1947	£40,000	40	700
1976	$15 million	300	3,500

Kearney, after giving much useful and interesting detail, summarized the very great changes which occurred between 1945 and 1976, emphasizing the complexity of the University in structure and function, concluding, 'The University is, therefore, no longer just a community of scholars and students'. He noted also the plateau of student numbers in the 70s and could well have added the plateau of financing also reached in the last part of the decade.

It does appear that having completed a quasi-adolescent growth spurt, the University is faced with the challenge of growth in a steady state, growth initiated not from without but from within. Since the core of the University is still, despite its complexity, a community of scholars, it appears essential to look into the core, into the idea of a university, in order to seek how the present task of the University can be understood and achieved. Discussion will be restricted here to an examination of some of Newman's[2] writings relevant to the Tasmanian scene. Leinszer-Mackay (1977) and other writers have discussed the *Idea* of a University more broadly.

At the time the movements towards founding a university in Tasmania were gaining some foothold, and when the Universities of Sydney (1851) and Melbourne (1853) were being founded, John Henry Newman of Oxford was asked by the Irish bishops to found a new university in Dublin. Newman, born in 1804, had been at Oxford since 1822, and for most of this period as an Anglican and, later, Catholic priest. In May 1852 he went to Dublin to deliver the first of a series of lectures or discourses which subsequently were published as *The Idea of a University*; in addition, he wrote a series of articles for the Catholic University Gazette, published subsequently as *University Sketches*.

Newman's efforts in founding the university were marked by controversy, his opposition coming mainly from the bishops whose notions of the idea of a university did not at all coincide with Newman's. In 1860 he wrote sadly in a diary, 'I have no friend in Rome, I have laboured in England, to be misrepresented, back bitten and scorned. I have laboured in Ireland, with a door ever shut in my face.' From Newman's writings several points emerge of relevance to the present consideration.

1 First, he considered the function of a university to establish an intellectual culture, for the cultivation of the mind. This notion comes out in several places in his writings.

I say a university taken in its bare idea ... has this object and this mission; it contemplates neither moral impression nor mechanical production; it professes to exercise the mind neither in art nor in duty; its function is intellectual culture; here it may leave its scholars, and it has done its work when it has done as much as this. It educates the intellect to reason well in all matters, to reach out towards the truth and to grasp it.

Newman in several places made it clear that it is not the university's task to teach the applications of knowledge as required by the professions but to train the mind in preparation for such specific learning:

> ... As health ought to precede labour of the body, and as a man in health can do what an unhealthy man cannot do, and as of this health the properties are strength, energy, agility, graceful carriage and action, manual dexterity, and endurance of fatigue, so in like manner general culture of mind is the best aid to professional and scientific study, and educated man can do what illiterate cannot; and the man who has learned to think and to reason and to compare and to discriminate and to analyse, who has refined his task, and formed his judgement, and sharpened his mental vision, will not indeed at once be a lawyer, or a pleader, or an orator, or a statesman, or a physician, or a good landlord, or a man of business, or a soldier or an engineer, or a chemist, or a geologist, or an antiquarian, but he will be placed in that state of intellect in which he can take up any one of the sciences or callings I have referred to or any other for which he has a taste or special talent, with an ease, a grace, a versatility, and a success, to which another is a stranger.[3]

The Royal Commission on Medical Education in Britain (Todd Commission, 1968) made a point in harmony with Newman's concepts:

> We cannot emphasize too strongly that the undergraduate course in medicine should be primarily educational. Its object is to produce not a fully qualified doctor but an educated man who will become fully qualified by postgraduate training.[4]

However, and here is the problem: society and the professions within it, whilst paying lip service to the cultivation of the mind as being the crucial role of the university, do in fact expect its graduates to be adequately prepared for professional occupations (whilst conceding the need for further education and experience). The medical course, for example, is so structured to almost exclude the quiet reflection and dialogue with other disciplines so essential to the cultivation of the intellect.

2. Newman clearly differentiated teaching (diffusion and extension of knowledge) from 'advancement' of knowledge.

   > To discover and to teach are distinct functions; they are also distinct gifts, and are not commonly found united in the same person. He, too, who spends his day in dispensing his existing knowledge to all comers is unlikely to have either leisure or energy to acquire new. The common sense of mankind has associated the search for truth with seclusion and quiet.[5]

The contemporary University of Tasmania involves both teaching and the advancement of knowledge and there is little opportunity for seclusion and quiet. Certainly promotion can be made on the basis of teaching or research, but the two functions are usually embodied in individual persons.

The argument can be made for removing research from universities into research institutes, and certainly within medical science this trend is clearly perceptible. On the other hand, a mind not seeking to advance knowledge may, in one view, although capable of imparting information, not be the mind to stretch students towards their intellectual capacity.

The dilemma may be approached more surely in the light of Karl Popper's (1902–1994) concepts of World 3, that is, the world of ideas, concepts, problems – which world is man's creation – and his notion of how this World 3 grows.[6]

Popper holds that there exist both matter (World 1) and mind (World 2) and the products of the human mind (problems, theories, critical arguments) as World 3. The university is profoundly concerned with shaping the form and history of World 3. Seclusion from mundane reality may assist us in the generation of solutions but may steer us away from the seminal problems. It may be that in our day we must deliberately choose to be immersed for part of our time in the everyday blood, sweat and tears and, just as deliberately leave it ... in order to be free to generate wise solutions. Mere nostalgia for a former way of life will not solve the problems felt by many academics between the demands of teaching (and worse, administration) and the desire to contribute to the creation of World 3.

There are quite specific points in which, according to Popper's theory of the advancement of science, the community of scholars plays an essential role. Popper points out that in logic, a scientific law is conclusively falsifiable although it is not conclusively verifiable. Popper urges, therefore, that we do not systematically evade refutation but we formulate our theories as unambiguously as possible so that they may be exposed to refutation. Where an observation is made which refutes the theory by methodology which is truly rigorous, then we must search for a new hypothesis which may then be tested by devising confrontations between its consequences and new observable experience.

Criticism, then, is to be prized and the competent criticism of the scientific community is part of the process of growth of science.

The university, in order to assist in the advancement of knowledge, does need to be above all a community of scholars, able and ready for constructive criticism. Those mostly given to teaching rather than research may play, then, an active role in the growth of knowledge.

This function of the university would require rigorous intellectual interaction and a critical mass of those competent to comment. Interaction with scholars in other universities is seen to be also essential in the face of small numbers of competent critics locally.

Relevant to this is Newman's concept of the genesis of the university:[7] A university is a place of concourse the place to which a thousand schools contribute. Newman would not have understood the idea of reserving places for local (in this case, Tasmanian) residents, but would have welcomed scholars from far away – a notion on which to ponder.

3   Newman, in his preface, stated thus:

> The view taken of a university in the Discourses is of the following kind:– that it is a place of *teaching* universal *knowledge*.

In discourse V (Knowledge its own end) in the 1917 edition, Newman expounded the unit of knowledge:

> All branches of knowledge are connected together, because the subject matter of knowledge is intimately united in itself, as being the acts and the work of the Creator. Hence it is that the sciences, into which our knowledge may be said to be cast, have multiplied bearings one upon another, and an internal sympathy, and admit, or rather demand, comparison and adjustment. They complete, correct, balance each other. This

consideration, if well-founded, must be taken into account, not only as regards the attainment of truth, which is their common end, but as regards the influence when they exercise upon those whose education consists in the study of them.[8]

He went on to discuss a consequence of this point, namely, the necessity for a wide range of studies.

It is a great point then to enlarge the range of studies which a university professes, even for the sake of its students and though they cannot pursue every subject which is open to them, they will be the gainers by living among those and under those who represent the whole circle. He (the student) profits by an intellectual tradition, which is independent of particular teachers, which guides him in his choice of subjects and duly interprets for him those which he chooses. He apprehends the great outlines of knowledge, the principles on which is rests, the scale of its parts, its lights and its shades, its great points and its little, as he otherwise cannot apprehend them. Hence it is that his education is called 'liberal'.

A habit of mind is formed which lasts through life, of which the attributes are freedom, equitableness, calmness, moderation, and wisdom.

Here we are at the heart of another tension, the tendency to specialisation almost demanded by the increasing volume of knowledge pulling against the instinctive desire of the academic mind to hold a holistic view of things, in order to maintain perspective in a runaway world.

Maybe this tension is not to be resolved at an institutional level, but at least the present trend to specialisation, even at school, needs to be resisted strongly. Society may now need perspective more than specialisation, if the currents appearing in learned journals are to be noted, as well as the instincts of educated men.

4 In the preface to the Discourses and elsewhere, Newman stressed that the university was primarily a place for teaching knowledge: its object is intellectual not moral.

> To open the mind, to correct it, to refine it, to enable it to know, and to digest, master, rule and use its knowledge, to give it power over its own faculties, application, flexibility, method, critical exactness, sagacity, resource, address, eloquent expression, is an object as intelligible ... as the cultivation of virtue, while, at the same time, it is absolutely distinct from it.

It is probable that this stress was laid down in the face of contrary views of the Irish bishop(s) who may have tended to see moral instruction as central and questioned the value of knowledge for its sake. Newman was obviously very concerned with moral issues and despite the words above, I do not think Newman would other than support the growing consciousness in academic circles, certainly in biomedicine, of the need for examination of ethical and moral issues and values in the face of extraordinary growth of scientific knowledge.[9]

The tension which arises for the academic is that between leaving the student entirely free to grope towards a value system of his own choosing, and the need to reveal one's own moral convictions, and maybe thereby attempt to influence a young mind. The Swedish State Commission on Sex Education In Schools attempted to solve this by dividing values into fundamental values (about which a teacher should be didactic) and controversial values (about which the teacher should seek to inform the student but not influence choice). The problem is that the initial classification of values into 'fundamental' or 'controversial' is itself a most telling expression of values and the system falters on this point.[10]

From Newman's idea of a university emerge, then, four major points, each a source of tension, if not contention:

- *i* that the university is primarily for the cultivation of the mind (not the learning of a profession);
- *ii* that teaching and the advancement of knowledge are distinct functions;
- *iii* that knowledge is one and that the range of studies which a university professes should be broad indeed to reflect the breadth of knowledge;
- *iv* that the object of the university is intellectual not moral.

On these issues Newman serves as a point of departure, but not, I believe of return. He was himself deeply committed to the concept of the evolution of ideas, reflecting probably the Darwinism of his day. We cannot go back to Newman's idea of a university, but it may be possible to incorporate his notions in the new paradigm of the university which is called for and may be emerging in our day.

Thomas Kuhn (in the *Structure of Scientific Revolutions*)[11] has taught that ideas grow, not as it were towards a goal placed from without a teleological view of World 3 – but through debate and intellectual interaction within the scientific community. Out of this interaction new paradigms are born. A new idea of the university is needed:

- *i* in which the university is seen as the place for 'intellectual culture' but also as undertaken more evidently for the human community (including the global community) than for the self,
- *ii* where teaching and the advancement of knowledge may be formally distinct, but where the teacher is perceived by the student as a fellow learner, a questioner after the truth of things, continually open to new questions, to new criticism in order that concepts be refined, rather than as a defender of unquestionable certainties,

iii where knowledge is understood as unity not so much by perceiving the extraordinary scope of human sciences in a splendid mosaic but by penetrating to the depths of disciplines; and finding at the limits of present understanding, analogies which give a sense of the unity of reality: many disciplines forced to their limits begin to ask similar fundamental questions about ultimate issues,

iv accepting that the object of the university teaching is primarily intellectual, not moral growth, but recognizing with the hard light of the crises of the last half of the twentieth century that the search for values is part of the intellectual life of the human community.

The sequence of Reports to the Club of Rome* illustrate clearly that fine scientific minds seeking for solutions to the global problems of our time abut on the world of values and moral issues.

I believe Newman would approve of the evolution of his Idea in these directions.

Finally, one concept of Newman requires no revision, and lays down an unspeakable challenge to every university teacher.

He wrote in the *University Sketches*:

> If learning is to live in us, we may need to place under scrutiny the contributions we make to the birth of ideas. The springs of inventiveness must still dwell within an institution which cost so much and attracted so many fine minds. The blocks to creativity, to the generation of ideas, need to be sought out individually and collectively,

---

* Club of Rome has now published over 45 Reports. They continue to challenge established paradigms and advocate for policies that can practically address the many emergencies facing society and the planet today.

for if we stagnate we have collectively lost our *raison d'être* as a university.

If we are tired, we must seek refreshment; if downhearted or disillusioned, we need, I believe, to be in more contact with the young and seek again for the springs of hope; if cynical of the university because cynical of life, we need to learn to live (even if this means leaving the university for a time). If we have a sense of powerlessness and alienation within the university, then the whole institution needs a review from bottom to top so that the potential of each person should be realized *now*.

If, however, we have truly lost the love of learning, or to cherish knowledge for its own sake, have ceased to reach out towards the truth and to grasp it, and have lost faith even in the road on which we travel, then we are lost indeed, and Newman has something still to say.

REFERENCES

1 French, M., 'The Prehistory of the University of Tasmania', *The Australian University*, 1973, 11, 185–201.
2 Newman, JH., *The idea of a university: discourses on the scope and nature of university education*, Duffy, Dublin, 1852, p203.
3 ibid p255.
4 Royal Commission on Medical Education, 1968, H S London.
5 Newman, op. cit., preface.
6 Popper, K., *Objective knowledge: a revolutionary approach*, Oxford, 1972.
7 Newman, JH., *University Sketches*, Scott, Newcastle on Tyne, 1902, p6.
8 Newman, JH., *The idea of a university: defined and illustrated*, Longmans, 1917, London, pp 99–101. (omitted from Discourse VI in 1952 edition).
9 Kass, LR., *The new biology: what price relieving man's science*, 1971, 174: 779.
10 Swedish State Commission on Sex Education, Stockholm, 1974; Royal Commission on Human Relationships Final Report, Vol. 2, 1978.
11 Kuhn, T., *Structure of Scientific Revolutions*.

IV
Address at a Graduation
2017

*Occasional Address at conferral
of Honorary Doctorate of Medical Science,
University of Sydney, 2017 (Citation p 617)*

I wish to acknowledge again the Aboriginal people of this region, past and present. After all, learning and teaching (the core of a university) has been occurring in this place, not merely for over 150 years, but for maybe 40,000 years!

My first note is that of *gratitude*, on behalf of all Graduates, to those who have contributed to our education and made it possible for us to reach this day. And above all, gratitude to the University of Sydney for enhancing our lives and for placing new trust in us today.

I wish to express also my personal gratitude to my family, to the teachers and colleagues who inspired me, and notably to the University of Sydney, to the Aboriginal people of Sydney who enriched my life, to the thousands of patients who taught me so much, to those students and junior doctors who trusted me to be part of their education and training, to the administrators here and afar who also trusted me, and to the many junior and senior colleagues and friends who walked beside me over many decades. It has all been a rare privilege!

The philosopher Immanuel Kant (1724–1804), in the 18C, famously posed three questions: What can I know? What should I do? and What may I hope? and today I add another one: What is worth saying now, in this hallowed place? I will not dare to comment on the tasks ahead of you – maybe just a few simple thoughts about our own selves. Maybe a few words about mountains ...

We are all standing on top of mountains today, especially all the new graduates. But what does it mean to be on the top of a mountain – apart from the obvious thing that one has done a lot of hard work getting here?

1

First, we may have a sense of exhilaration, of having arrived, a sense of freedom at last!

So, a few remarks about liberty ... There are several old, but ever new, issues for health professionals. Even philosophers notice!

J S Mill in *On Liberty* (1859) famously exalted non-interference by others even for motives of beneficence:

> Each is the proper guardian of his own health, whether bodily, or mental or spiritual. Mankind are greater gainers by suffering each other to live as seems good to themselves, than by compelling each to live as seems good to the rest.

The issue is immediately raised concerning whether or not one's individual actions are truly individual. I would suggest that the nature of persons in the human web, is such that hardly any so-called 'individual' action fails to have social dimensions; indeed, actions sometimes spoken of as 'private' or 'individual' are intrinsically *social* – such as *how* we are born, live, suffer, or *how* we love, hate, or die. This needs much pondering if we are to judge wisely. When should I insist on a so-called 'individual' action which is intrinsically social – with social consequences? And when is it justified to intervene to restrict the freedom, or privacy of an individual for the sake of that individual or of others – or community? Serious questions always.

In fact the freedom which education gives is freedom of thought. Education increases our personal liberty not only by leading us out into a new country but by enhancing our capacity to *think*.

Each of us must form some concept of the good, and accept responsibility for what we do and become, but thoughtfulness should lead to a realisation that *freedom is not merely the right to choose or control* ... There is a mood, at least in the West, for glorifying choice not as a means, but as an end in itself (even in health care), as a central expression of autonomy; and also a tendency, in the name of autonomy, for success to be measured by the pushing away of all obstacles to my individual desires, and frustration in the face of what must be, of what philosophers call 'necessity'. Such notions betray, I think, an inadequate concept of autonomy.

Seventeenth century philosopher Spinoza offered an alternative concept, far richer than that currently prevailing, traceable to Descartes. I quote Sydney philosopher Genevieve Lloyd (UNSW):

> Spinoza offers instead a vision of freedom as the joyful acceptance of what must be ... freedom derives from the active engagement of the mind with necessity, an engagement that flows from the understanding of the truth.

As citizens (anywhere) and especially as medical scientists and health professionals the truth we need especially to understand is the truth about *persons*, about *human life* in all its phases and complexities, about personal development throughout the whole of life – even in the last phase, and what we really mean by personal care and human flourishing in community and the relief of human suffering. For this is our purpose: we are pledged to further the good of persons as our central task.

Freedom understood as the 'joyful acceptance of what must be' is not a recipe for passivity or fatalism! Spinoza is the same philosopher who highlighted the impulse inherent in all living things, what he called *conatus* – a striving to continue in being. Clearly we need freely to accept what must be, whilst at the same time striving to relieve suffering and to enhance human flourishing. This is a far cry from the glorification of 'choice' or misunderstood autonomy. The highest expression of autonomy may indeed be the yielding of control, to surrender in trust to the kindness of strangers. It is hard to learn this!

Another question. Does being professionally bound to the care of others impair our personal freedom?

Why commit to the care of others as our central professional task? Why spend years of arduous study to prepare for it? Why embrace such a life and why continue, hour after hour, day after day, year after year? ... I am (as a citizen but specifically as a health professional) in a relationship of *covenant* with persons in need of my competence: I am bound (and trusted) to be beneficent, to act for good. Being so bound, am I less free? Thought is required.

Desmond Manderson (Formerly Professor of Jurisprudence, University of Sydney) helped me understand that Emmanuel Levinas (1906–1995), a twentieth century philosopher, considered that the *basis of the duty of care* is not law, or contract, (external to my being) but the *call of the other*. But *why* respond? I think now that the same Baruch Spinoza (1632–1677) threw light on this – I respond to the call of the other as an expression of my 'striving to continue in being': something in me would die if I simply pass by someone to whom I am present (Levinas says 'proximate') in need of my competence as a person or as a professional. Such would also apply to a community in need.

Are there limits to the duty of care? I leave that question in the air ... but note that the law does not define morality. The moral requirement to respond to another in need (or a difficult community situation within one's portfolio), cannot merely be defined by law – a sensitive moral compass and an interiorised ethical sense are essential. This issue will cost you in the years ahead ...

Can restrictions on what we can do (fraudulent institutions or even administrators, personal affliction, political pressures, even violence, or torture) *utterly crush freedom*? Not according to psychotherapist Viktor Frankl (1905–1997), who (after the experience of Auschwitz) wrote about 'the last of human freedoms' – 'to take an *attitude* in a given set of circumstances'.

Why does this matter? In fact, the *attitudes* of doctors and other health professionals are critical. Leo Alexander (1905–1985), observer at the Nuremberg trials of Nazi doctors, tried to analyse the roots of the moral collapse of some of the most eminent medical academic leaders, and in a classic paper in NEJM 1949,* pinned the beginning on a 'shift in *attitude* to the non-rehabilitatable sick' – a caution for our own times and forever.

It is a long-standing tradition that doctors are advocates for the weakest in society, those in danger of exploitation or abuse – or suffering it, the wounded, the refugees, the poor, the handicapped, the rejected, the dying. Specifically, we health care professionals need extraordinary sensitivity all our lives to any shift in attitude towards what Alexander called the 'non-rehabilitatable sick'. We need to be alert to what Erich Fromm (1900–1980) called 'evil without horns', evil in the guise of good

---

* Alexander, L., Medical Science under Dictatorship. *NEJM* 241, 39–47, 1949.

emerging among human possibilities. The burden to society of loss of integrity – or soul (if you will) is immeasurable.

Consideration of the nuances of personal freedom has taken us into many difficult territories, but there is more to mountain tops than a sense of liberty at last: we touch now (briefly) on some other ideas.

2

The one thing certain about being on the top of a hill is that we all must have known valleys – times of darkness, even falls, when all seems obscured and even the way out has seemed hard. Such experiences are almost universal. But dark times may be public, when even the truth is obscured and institutions seem to have failed. History teaches us, that even in dark times there are persons who provide flickers of light because they think, judge rightly, and do not conform to the destruction around them.

3

But there is more to being on a mountain top than simply understanding valleys! *We now can see further*, can glimpse new horizons, and new possibilities: we have new perspectives on old realities.

[This may include perspectives about what we mean by 'person'. There is long philosophical tradition about 'person'. My association with the Aboriginal people of Sydney in 1968–70 enriched my ideas about persons and set me thinking about 'person' as fundamentally a relational term. Maybe we need to think of a person truly as a web of relations – with persons, with place, with things, with the past (as memory), with culture and inheritance, with hopes/dreams, with all-that-is (maybe expressed in ritual – which may or may not be deemed religious) – we cannot live without ritual. And unless all of this is taken into account even very briefly, by health professionals, caring is diminished, and suffering may be actually increased. Thinking about persons like this helps to understand suffering (understood best as a sense of impending personal disintegration – after Eric Cassell [1928–]) – which can be triggered by a break in any of these relations: we say the person may be 'broken'. But it also gives a glimpse of the possibilities of healing.]

As we glimpse new possibilities in personal, social and in professional life, *we need to withstand the winds which blow hard* on mountain tops. How? We need to have such deep roots that we can be a source of stability, nourishment, justice, wisdom and renewal in a world in transition, and to stand back appropriately to make careful judgements – and not be overcome by the bombardment of news feeds or the waves of fashion.

And where do we find our roots? Not only in a belief in oneself as radically good, and in conscience as a sure guide, and in our world and the universe as radically good – we need to hold to this – but also in *connectivity* not only with the present (through a sense of embeddedness in all that is, now), but also with the past. We need, in these times more than ever, a deep grasp of the wisdom of the past (to be found in all cultures over thousands of years). Roots firmly placed in the past, and rich connectivity with the real, (not merely virtual) present, and with one's deepest self, give us a sure platform for exploring new perspectives and for shaping the future wisely.

4

There is another truth about being on a mountain top – one cannot stay. One has to go down again (carefully!). One may, having experienced the mountain top, become a leader, both of those on the way up, and then in the valleys, not as one who controls others but as one who can see the way ahead, and whose judgement and integrity can be trusted even in very dark times. And who holds fast to realistic hope.

I recall again Immanuel Kant's questions – What can I know? What should I do? What may I hope? In dark times (and as one grows older) the last question haunts the mind and heart. We need, in hard times, time and space to rethink the springs of our hope. It may be useful to recall the words of a philosopher (Ernst Bloch) who lived most of the twentieth century: 'A leader is one who at midnight is confident of the dawn'. Some of you, my fellow graduates, may have to face extreme difficulties even as national leaders and may find solace in those words.

In conclusion, life begins in wonder – have you looked recently at a new-born baby's eyes? – but it may also end in wonder! I wonder at the potential of you all to shape our future! I have far more questions than answers these days … Even the old (like me) must be explorers – the poets insist on that. Can you think of even those close-to-death as explorers? (Emily Dickenson: *Dying is a wild night and a new road*.) There is always something new to find, and new questions to ask and try to answer. There is in fact always another mountain to climb!

And finally, my fellow citizens (and explorers), two weeks ago I watched, late at night after a concert, the closing stages of the now classic movie, *Schindler's List*: Schindler (a flawed man) saved 1100 people from Auschwitz by employing them in his factory. As he was being honoured by those he had saved, he broke apart and blurted, 'I could have done more', 'I could have done more'. I, in miniature, as I am being honoured this day, share that sentiment …

Congratulations to all new graduates and to your families and friends who have a right to be very proud today! And to the University of Sydney, which has not lost its soul!

6

MEDICINE AND COMMUNITY

A

THE POSSIBILITIES AND LIMITATIONS OF MEDICAL PRACTICE
1981

Essays based on three 1981 presentations:
a) ES Myers Memorial Lecture,
   University of Queensland, Brisbane,
b) Annual Scientific Meeting,
   Royal Australian College of General Practitioners, Newcastle,
c) Clive Hamilton Address, Hobart.

> Men are men before they are lawyers, or physicians, or merchants, or manufacturers; and if you make them capable and sensible men, they will make themselves capable and sensible lawyers or physicians.
> —*John Stuart Mill*

In the closing years of the nineteenth century there appeared consternation at the ills of humanity. Emile Zola (1840–1902) in an address to students in Paris urged men to go on working ('I am convinced that the only faith that can save us is a belief in the efficacy of accomplished toil') but Tolstoy, in commenting on Zola's speech warned of the dangers of mindless labour stopping men from pausing 'to concentrate their thoughts or to consider what they ought to be'[1] and Leo Tolstoy (1828–1910) went on to write: 'If I were called on to give one single piece of advice, the one I considered most useful for men of our century, I should say this to them: For God's sake pause a moment, think of what you are and what you ought to be – think of the ideal.' We live in a world torn apart by talk, in the midst (it well seems) of the death throes of one social structure and the birth struggles of the new (with abundant commentators on the situation[2] of dramatic changes in social consciousness[3] and imperatives for decisions influencing the shape of the future despite our collective weariness of the burden of freedom. The advice of the novelist – 'Only connect – live in fragments no longer' – may appear a mere joke in the midst of such a miscellany of fragmented experiences, drifting we know not where in response to forces from which (or whom) we know less: such is at least one scenario of contemporary life in the West.

In the midst of all this the talk often takes shape (in articles, news and even theatre) around matters which are in some way the responsibility of health care personnel. A catalogue would include the following:

 i ageing of the population – in Australia by the year 2000, we will need twice the resources we have now to care for the aged[4] – and planning appears to be fragmented if existent at all;

ii the shift to chronic disease – over 45% of all Australians have some chronic condition as shown in a recent survey[5] – the shift being largely due to ageing of the population (chronic conditions were noted to increase in number and severity as age advances) and to the life-saving success of acute medicine (some persons who are 'saved' are not cured but are left more or less disabled) ... but the health care system (including the health insurance system) has not adapted to this shift from acute to chronic disease as the major burden of a Western community;

iii continuing social inequalities in health[6,7] with higher overall mortality rates, and higher rates for chronic conditions in lower socio-economic groups: the fact that probably much of the differential may be due 'to life-style induced disease heightens rather than diminishes the fact of the persisting inequality and raises more urgently the issue of individual freedom versus community responsibility in the face of increasing risks of disease or injury and/or early death';[8,9,10]

iv costs of medical care out of control – with increasing evidence of a flat-of-the-curve situation, in which vast increases in expenditure appear to give little improvement in health at an individual and community level;[11]

v increasing manifestations of the inadequacy of hospitals[12] and the health care system as a whole with respect to an understanding of individual human personal needs especially in crisis situations;

vi serious inadequacies with regard to preventing disorders which appear as health casualties but which are manifestations of social malaise: John Knowles, formerly superintendent of Massachusetts General Hospital, edited a telling volume on the US situation under the provocative title *Doing Better and Feeling Worse*;[13]

vii information overload and saturation – with resultant frustration for staff and hazards to patient care, since each patient may have records held by several persons or agencies without linkage;

viii the evidence that technology has outstripped ethical debate.[14,15,16]

In the midst of all this, those of us who are doctors must faithfully carry out our daily tasks, but we also must heed the wise, and (as Tolstoy urged) pause, to look around us, think of what we are and ought to be. Above all to ask the right questions.

It has been well said that the educated man 'is capable not of providing specialised answers but of asking the great and liberating questions by which humanity makes its way through time'.[17]

What is the ideal role of a doctor in relation to the human community – and what are the obstacles to the realization of that role? It may be time for our possibilities to be revealed even to ourselves so that we may apply the words of James Hemming, 1970, to the modern doctor's identity crisis:

> Modern man's identity crisis ... does not hinge upon restoring something that was lost but on his entering into himself fully revealed – a being magnificently endowed with capacities for living that he can bring into fruition by entering, as a person, into relationships with other people and the world.[18]

In this context, I wish to consider in turn the doctor as leader, the doctor as healer and as advocate of the weak: let us review again our own possibilities.

References

1. Tolstoy L. *Non-Acting* (1893): Trans. A. Maude. London: in Recollections and Essays. Oxford University Press, 1937.
2. Toffler A. *The Third Wave*. London: William Collins, 1980.
3. Berger PL, Berger B, Kellner H. *The Homeless Mind*. Harmondsworth: Penguin Books, 1974.
4. Sax S. *The Challenge of post-Clinical Medicine*. The Richard Gibson Medicine. Oration, Australian College of Rehabilitation Sydney, 1981. (See Also: Howe A (editor) *Towards an older Australia*. Readings in Social Gerontology. 1981) St. Lucia: University of Queensland Press.
5. Australian Health Survey 1977–78.Chronic Conditions. Canberra: Australian Bureau of Statistics, 1980.
6. Morris JN. 'Social Inequalities Undiminished'. *Lancet*, 1979; 1: 87–90.
7. Taylor R. 'Health and Class in Australia'. *New Doctor*, 1979; 13: 22–28.
8. Lickiss JN. *On Liberty and the Health of the Community in Community Health in Australia*. R. Walpole, ed. Harmondsworth: Penguin Books, 1978. (See also: *On Limits and Liberty: An Exploration*. University of Tasmania, Occasional Paper, 1978 – inaugural address by J.N. Lickiss as Professor of Community Health).
9. Beard T. *Promoting Health Prospects for Better Health Throughout Australia*. Canberra: Australian Government Printing Service, 1979.
10. Beauchamp DE. 'Public Health and Individual Liberty'. *Am Rev Public Health*, 1980; 1: 121–36.
11. Enthoven AC. *Cutting Cost without Cutting the Quality of Care* – Shuttock Lecture. N Engl J Med, 1978; 298: 1229–1238.
12. Roberts SL. *Behavioural Concepts and Nursing Throughout the Lifespan*. New York: Prentice Hall, 1978.
13. Knowles JH (ed.) *Doing Better and Feeling Worse: Health in the United States*. New York: Norton, 1977, p2.
14. Kass L. 'The New Biology: What Price Man's Estate'. *Nature*, 1971; 174: 779–788.
15. Kirby M. 'Test Tube man'. *Med J Aust*, 1981; 2 pp1–2.
16. Kennedy I. *Unmasking Medicine*. (Reith Lectures) London: George Allen & Unwin, 1981.
17. MacGleish A. *Our Altered Perception of Ourselves in Evolution of Man*, Young LB, ed. New York: Oxford University Press, 1968.
18. Hemming J. *Individual Morality*. London: Panther Books, 1970; p.102.

I
DOCTOR AS LEADER

> Every epoch has its character determined by the
> way its population reacts to the natural events they
> encounter. This reaction is determined by their basic
> beliefs – by their hopes, their fears, their judgements
> of what is worthwhile. They may rise to the greatness
> of an opportunity, seizing its drama, perfecting its art,
> exploiting its adventure. On the other hand they may
> collapse before the perplexities confronting them.[1]

When the philosopher Alfred Whitehead (1861–1947) wrote these words in 1933 he considered that humanity was 'shifting its ground'. How much greater are the perplexities now, some fifty years later and who can have wisdom enough to offer leadership now?

Doctors have a potential and even responsibility, based on their gifts of intelligence and education, which compels them even when young to encounter the limits of the human, and thus to have precious and privileged experience of human affairs.

Can one be more specific with respect to concepts relevant to the human condition which should be appreciated by doctors, if their grasp of humanness is to be deep enough to justify a leadership role within the human community?

Doctors should first of all be more aware than most of the rhythms of the phases of personal development and of the role of crisis. William Shakespeare, in his talk of the 'seven ages of man' (*As you like it*, Act II, Scene vii), recognised the biological fact of the stages of human development – and such is familiar indeed to the practising doctor – but personal development of a human being throughout life is complex, and over the last few decades there has been increasing clarification of the processes involved.

Erik Erikson (1902–1994) has given much food for thought in his writings.[2] He presented human growth from the point of view of the conflicts, inner and outer, which the healthy person weathers, emerging and re-emerging with, among other things, an increased sense of inner unity. He held that there are inner laws of development, laws which create a succession of potentialities for significant interaction with others. While such interaction may vary from culture to culture, it must remain within the proper rate and the proper sequence which govern the growth of a personality as well as that of an organism.

Erikson saw human growth as taking place by negotiation of developmental tasks through the resolution of crisis. The growing human being is continually faced by options, each life stage being characterised by its own options which, while they confront a person throughout life, do come to a point of ascendancy in a given stage. For example, the favourable outcome of infancy is an attitude of basic trust, rather than one of basic distrust, and on this basis the child goes on to be faced with the choice of autonomy or fear of decision-making. Where the life process is characterised by the embracing of favourable options, the personality becomes characterised by trust, reasonable autonomy, initiative, capacity for effort, sense of identity (to be oneself and to share being oneself) rather than confusion, capacity for intimate personal relationships (to lose and find oneself in another) instead of isolation, fruitfulness rather than stagnation, and finally (in the elderly) a sense of integrity or wholeness of life rather than despair.

Erikson's analysis of personal growth is sensitive indeed in its consideration of the developmental task of all phases of life: details may be useful of this exposition of the situation of the elderly in this perspective:[3]

> Only he who in some way has taken care of things and people and has adapted himself to the triumphs and

disappointments of being, by necessity, the originator of others and the generator of things and ideas – only he may gradually grow the fruit of the seven stages. I know no better word for it than integrity ... It is the acceptance of one's own and only life cycle and of the other people who have become significant to it as something that had to be an acceptance of the fact that one's life is one's own responsibility. It is a sense of comradeship with men and women of distant times and of different pursuits, who have created orders and objects and sayings conveying human dignity and love.

On the other hand, Erikson noted further:

... the lack or loss of this accrued ego integration is signified by despair and an often unconscious fear of death: the one and only life cycle is not accepted as the ultimate of life. Despair expresses the fear that the time is short, too short for the attempt to start another life and to try out alternate roads to integrity. Such a despair is often hidden behind a show of disgust, a misanthropy, or a chronic contemptuous displeasure with particular people – a disgust and a displeasure which (where not allied with constructive ideas and a life of co-operation) only signify the individual's contempt of himself.

The work of Erikson with regard to each phase of the life cycle has clear relevance to judgements concerning desirable or undesirable lifestyle features in persons of all ages. Lifestyle at all ages should offer opportunities for facing and fulfilling the current developmental tasks and should foster the negotiation of developmental tasks by those with whom one's life is interlocked. His understanding of the elderly is highly relevant to the increased concern with the quality of life of the elderly in Australia: is the spotlight sufficiently focussed on the developmental needs of the elderly?

Daniel Levinson (1920–1994) has more recently offered an arresting account of processes of adult male development based on the detailed study of a group of 40 men in four occupational subgroups over five years, the emphasis being on the middle adult years.[4] The subjects varied widely in social class, racial, ethnic and religious origins, and educational status. Levinson identified four overlapping eras in the life cycle, each lasting some twenty-five years (childhood and adolescence, early adult era, middle adult era, late adult era), the eras together forming the skeletal structure of the life cycle. Within each era he identified specific developmental periods:

> The life structure evolves through a sequence of alternating periods. A relatively stable, structure-building period is followed by a transitional, structure-changing period. The major developmental tasks of a structure-building period are to make crucial choices, to create a structure around them, to enrich the structure and pursue one's goals within it. These periods ordinarily last six to eight years. In a transitional period the major tasks are to reappraise the existing structure, explore new possibilities in self and world, and work towards choices that provide a basis for a new structure. The transitional periods generally last four or five years.

With Erikson, Levinson recognised the sequential rather than hierarchical nature of development.

> Each season plays its essential part in the unfolding of the life cycle, and the sequence follows a prescribed course. Winter is fallow, quiet time in which the previous growth comes to an end and the possibility of new growth is created. It is the ultimate transitional period. Unless the creative work of winter is done and the seeds take root, nothing further can grow. Spring is a time of blossoming, when the fruits of the winter's labour begin to be

realised. The blossoms will not appear unless the seeds have been nourished, and the blossoms in turn, make way for the blooming, fully grown flowers.

So too with our developmental periods. The Early Adult Transition provides the cross-era shift into early adulthood. The next three periods ... permit a man to build a first adult life structure. At about forty he enters the Mid-Life Transition. Now he must terminate the early adult era and plant the seeds for middle adulthood when he will go through a similar sequence of building, modifying and rebuilding the life structure. The tasks of one period are not better or more advanced than those of another, except in the general sense that each period builds upon the work of earlier ones and represents a later phase in the cycle.

The negotiation of developmental phases (or tasks) involves inevitably close personal relationships and the whole spectrum of human communication, both within the non-verbal and between the past and present (verbal and non-verbal) and between the past and present.[5]

In the course of such communication, life cycles, as Erikson called them, are interlocked cogwheeled, as it were, welding together the human community into a matrix in continuous process or movement.

The doctor as leader must have a dynamic view then of human life both individual and communal, with a commitment to assisting authentic human development.

Social dimensions also need appreciation.

It has long been appreciated that the integration of the individual into a human network by social bonds appeared to be necessary for health but over the last decade there have been several significant conceptual advances. This dimension needs to be understood by doctors. There has been clarification of the role of stressors in health (physical and mental), and the emphasis in research of the recent past on analysis of the adverse effects of certain life events appears to be giving way to a focus on the means by which the person copes with stressors of varying types and especially with the significance of social networks: L. Levi,[6] B.A. Hamburg and M. Killilea[7] and S. Henderson[8] all offer valuable reviews relevant to this field.

The study by S.L. Berkman-Syme[9] in Almeda county (USA) offers an example of the association between social networks and mortality. In a nine year follow-up of approximately 7000 adults, it was found that people who lack social and community ties appear more likely to die when compared with those with more extensive contacts: the effect appeared to be independent of the so-called 'health habits'. Henderson's group in Canberra demonstrated the association between non-psychotic mental illness and a lack of social bonds. A recent study by medical students in Hobart, Tasmania using Henderson's methodology demonstrated a paucity of social bonds in young alcoholics (Tilsley, Loughnan and Gibson, unpublished).

In such studies the question of the direction of causality has yet to be defined and Henderson's group has contributed richly to this debate. In the perspective of the present consideration of interpersonal interaction as a component of lifestyle it is sufficient to note that if the lifestyle does not include evidence of a good range or depth of social bonds, health is likely to be at risk. From the point of view of research into lifestyle as related to health it is obvious in this type of problem, that sound longitudinal studies, short and long term, are important in facilitating the understanding of the antecedents of human distress and indeed premature death, as well as the effectiveness (or not) of interventions.

The concept of social networks may be usefully related to the concept of 'a sense of coherence' as put forward in Israel by Aaron Antonovsky.[10] He defines a sense of coherence as:

> [A] global orientation that expresses the extent to which one has a pervasive, enduring though dynamic feeling of confidence that one's internal and external environments are predictable and that there is a high probability that things will work out as well as can reasonably be expected.
>
> The sense of coherence explicitly and unequivocally is a generalized, long-lasting way of seeing the world and one's life in it. It is perceptual, with both cognitive and affective components. Its referent is not this or that area of life, this or that problem or situation, this or that time, or in our terms, this or that stressor. It is, I suggest, a crucial element in the basic personality structure of an individual and in the ambiance of a subculture, culture or historical period.

Antonovsky developed a model of those factors which assisted in the maintenance of (or resisting the loss of) a sense of coherence. He described a 'general resistance resource' as a characteristic (e.g. cognitive, emotional, attitudinal) of an individual, primary group, subculture or society that provides extended and continued experience in making sense of the countless stimuli with which one is constantly bombarded and facilitates the perception that the stimuli one transmits are being received by the intended recipients without distortion. After discussing the social support literature Antonovsky stated his view that, 'social supports enhance the ability to obtain meaningful information, or in my terms, enhance the sense of coherence.'

And what of global dimensions?

In addition to the appreciation of the patterns of personal development and the role of social bonding in the nurturing of this development and to the maintenance of health (and vice versa), a doctor today needs to have a global vision of human welfare. There is a real danger that by immersion in a busy round of problem solving in the immediate vicinity, global perspectives can be lost.

The situation has been well documented by the World Health Organisation, but the message is clear that the health problems are part of a total problem set. Alexander King, Director-General of Scientific Affairs, O.E.C.D., Paris, and Founder Member of the Club of Rome outlined the problem thus:

> The problems themselves in their wide spectrum which ranges through disparities between developed and under-developed countries, inflation, unemployment, race, environmental deterioration, individual alienation, crime and violence, have a number of features in common. They seem to appear in all countries at a certain level of development irrespective of the political system. They are extremely multi-variant in their elements and they all seem to interact in ways that are only dimly understood. There is a tendency to refer to this cluster of problems as 'the problematique', a series of difficulties so intimately interrelated that it is increasingly difficult to identify discrete problems and apply discrete solutions. To tackle elements of the problematique appears increasingly to be an attempt to remove symptoms of a disease which has not been fully diagnosed with the consequences that interactions within the system may lead to further difficulties in other parts which are not obviously recognised as being due to the initial remedial action.[11]

The Club of Rome [The Club of Rome is a nonprofit, informal organization of intellectuals and business leaders whose goal is a critical discussion of pressing global issues.] has made available several major studies undertaken of the total global situation, the first *The Limits to Growth*, under the leadership of Professor Dennis Meadows.[12]

The computerized model projected into the future current trends in a limited number of quantifiable elements of the 'problematique' – population growth with the consequent demands for food and agriculture, capital and industrial growth, raw material depletion and pollution, taking account of their cross impacts, and predicted virtual collapse of world population and society within the next one hundred years. It was asserted that dramatic changes in such variables as population growth and resource usages are essential NOW to alter these disastrous trends. It is widely accepted that, despite criticisms of methodology and estimates, the portrait drawn in *The Limits to Growth* must be taken seriously.

The second Report to the Club of Rome, entitled *Mankind at the Turning Point* (and dedicated to 'future generations') was prepared under the direction of Mihajlo Mesarovic and Eduard Pester.[13] This study set out to look at five major regions of the world and the interactions between them and significantly includes a telling chapter on 'Limits to Independence': the chapter concludes that we must acknowledge 'the dawn of an era of limits to independence even for the strongest and biggest nations of the world.' In the epilogue the Report notes:

> If the human species is to survive, man must develop a sense of identification with future generations and be ready to trade benefits to the next generation for the benefits to himself. If each generation aims at maximum good for itself, Homo Sapiens is as good as extinct.

In the last few years, the Club of Rome Reports have included a study of the various world regions under the title *The Goals of Mankind*, and of education and its inequalities and inadequacies (*No Limits to Learning*). It has become clear that the debate of the 80s is centering on values and the elucidation of the psychological blocks that can prevent human beings from making rational decisions in the face of gross degrees of inequality on the face of the globe, trends in population growth and the hazards of nuclear catastrophe.

There are indeed 'inner limits' to Mankind. Those prominent in Club of Rome have been most concerned with this issue of late, and Ervin Laszlo, in a book titled *The Limits of Mankind*, has written:

> The root causes even of physical and ecological problems are the inner constraints on our vision and values. We suffer from a serious case of 'culture lag'. Living on the threshold of a new age, we squabble among ourselves to acquire or retain the privileges of bygone times. We cast about for innovating ways to satisfy obsolete values. We manage individual crises while heading toward collective catastrophes. We contemplate changing almost anything on this earth but ourselves.
>
> People still prefer the acrobatic feat of reading the handwriting on the wall while their backs are up against it, to concerns and concentrated forward planning to attain the things and conditions they desire.[14]

Doctors are becoming more involved in such issues, but the vast majority of doctors are quite uninvolved and appear to welcome leadership from elsewhere (except in the domestic affairs of doctors): one can wonder whether the cluttering of the mind with information or a passive mode of learning encourages these tendencies.

One is reminded of Bertrand Russell's warning of 1916, 'The habit of passive acceptance is a disastrous one in later life. It causes men to seek as a leader whoever is established in that position'.[15]

What is the essence of leadership? Kenneth Galbraith, in *The Age of Uncertainty* alleged: 'All the great leaders have had one characteristic in common: it was their willingness to confront the major anxiety of their people in their time.'[16]

In the contemporary Australian community it may be possible to discuss the lineaments of the major anxieties. There are data, disturbing data, concerning the levels of personal anxiety in our people – for example the recent study in Sydney of several thousand persons going to a health screening agency (persons who might be expected to be rather more financially secure, health motivated, future orientated, than the 'average' Australian).[17] Over one quarter of these subjects had very significant emotional problems related to marriage, work, etc. At a less personal scale there is frequently expressed anxiety that the Australian community is drifting, moving in response to this or that stimulus, with no clear goals of what we wish to become: the lack of goals is a fundamental and major anxiety for any person or group since if the goals be unclear, anxiety concerning processes or means being adopted (and in which one is immersed) can become intolerable of community goals. Some focus may be justified therefore on the issue.

Much has been written about the need for goals (social and personal). What Allen Wheelis wrote concerning the individual can certainly be applied to a group or community, and even a nation:

> Without meaningful goals modern man has understandably no source of direction; for he does not look where he is going. Like an anxious soldier on a drill field he covertly watches those around him to make sure he stays in step. He sticks to the group, and where the group will go next nobody knows. He despairs of its zigzag course, but hesitates to strike out on his own in any direction because of the likelihood that no one direction can be long maintained. He adjusts to the group

and executes increasingly frequent manoeuvres with increasing alacrity.'[18]

René Dubos, the Nobel prize winning microbiologist, once wrote: 'Man is so adaptable that he could survive and multiply in underground shelters, even though his regimented subterranean existence left him unaware of the robin's song in the spring, the whirl of dead leaves in the fall, and the moods of the wind – even though all his ethical values should whither ...'[19]

It is not merely adaptation which is needed to the rapidly occurring new technological revolution already begun in the 80s or to the violent international tensions – or to the continuing inequalities within as well as between nations with reference to basic lifestyle necessities: conflicts and inequalities which manifest themselves in ways relevant to doctors. There is a future to create. Aurelio Peccei, founder of the Club of Rome, in an address at a Club of Rome conference in Berlin in 1979 outlined first some signs of a deteriorating global situation and then indicated the directions in which we need to think and move.

> The key can indeed be only a profound conceptual and behavioural renewal of the human protagonist himself ... A philosophical and cultural effort of major magnitude is required to update and mend, if not reverse, our concept of ourselves, of our world, and our place in it.[20]

Thus far, we have noted a lack of clear goals – and have remarked that mere adjustment to change is an inadequate way to proceed, as an individual or as a society.

How can a community with the assistance of leaders, including its doctors, shape its own social goals?

Leaders and would-be leaders of thought and action from Plato onwards have offered blueprints of an ideal society. The United Nations Bill of Rights has codified the rights of each citizen (including the disabled citizens). In addition to what is due by right (and expected of as responsibility) in regard to each person, other features of life become desirable: human dignity and value is at stake. Much political debate (in the broad sense) centres on which order of priority should be observed and which means should be adopted in seeking to achieve a social system in which all rights are freely recognized. Debate concerning processes by which goals are to be achieved must take into account ethical issues.

Both the debate concerning social goals and the means by which they are to be achieved requires input by persons such as doctors, in close contact with not only the strong but also the weaker members of society. The role of the doctor as advocate of the weak is taken up elsewhere: suffice to say here that the development of social goals and social policy must deliberately take into account the interests and needs, priorities and values of the least powerful members of the human community, and an advocate for the weakest of the weak should be an active participant in all relevant decision making.

How can the doctor-as-leader confront anxieties like these in self and the community? Where does the doctor (who belongs to a profession with a high suicide rate) look for the springs of hope?

It may be no accident that it is an Australian, Ross Fitzgerald, who has edited recently an invaluable book entitled *The Sources of Hope*.[21] In his preface and in his own essay which concludes the book, Fitzgerald laments that universities and scholars ('The Academy') neglect the issue of hope ('and what medical courses mention it?'). He concludes that, 'it is only beyond the 'self' that hope lies and despair ends'. With regard to obsessive self-absorption, Victor Frankl in the year of his death employed an extremely appropriate metaphor:

> As the boomerang returns to the hunter who has thrown it only when it has missed its target, so Man returns

to himself, reflect upon himself and becomes overly concerned with self-interpretation only when he has, as it were, missed his mission, having been frustrated in his search for meaning.

> Unless we transcend to future self, the ultimate in meaninglessness and despair will compound and overtake us in the face of death ... For if there is nothing beyond the isolated self to give life meaning, this death is utter annihilation and life is absurd. If a person has not contributed to or served something other than the 'self', then instead of accepting death and dying (like suffering) as a natural and meaningful process, one can do little else but fight one's extinction with resentful and impotent fury ...[22]

How can the doctor lead him or herself in the journey beyond the self? – for the journey must be made if the doctor is to lead (*educate*) other persons out of despair and towards hope. The doctor is often tired, weary, lonely even, in times of difficult decisions but the doctor who does not share the darkness as well as the light of the human condition cannot truly be a leader. A certain solitariness is in fact essential for adequate reflection – Carl Jung's words of 50 years ago are more relevant than ever:

> I must say that the man we call modern, the man who is aware of the immediate present, is by no means the average man. He is rather the man who stands upon a peak, or at the very edge of the world, the abyss of the future before him, above him the heavens, and below him the whole of mankind with a history that disappears in primeval mists ... Since to be wholly of the present means to be fully conscious of one's existence as a man, it requires the most intensive and extensive consciousness, with a minimum of unconsciousness ... He alone is modern who is fully conscious of the present.

The man whom we can with justice call 'modern' is solitary.[23]

The leading (education) of other persons towards hope may be seen as a form of 'liberation' – the doctor having the privilege of assisting in the removal of obstacles to human growth towards hope and towards the good both within and beyond the self. This role of the doctor in relation to the removal of obstacles to growth has been explored elsewhere in respect to the care of the dying[24] but in its essence the notion is very old and one can recall Plato's image of the cave follows:

Plato has Socrates describing an image of human life as:

Behold! Human beings living in an underground den, which has a mouth open towards the light ... Here they have been from the childhood, and have their legs and necks chained so that they cannot move and can only see before them, being prevented by the chains from turning round their heads. Above and behind them a fire is blazing at a distance and between the fire and the prisoners there is a raised way ... and a low wall built along the way, with men passing along the wall.

Plato goes on in the dialogue to explain that since the prisoners are chained and can only look ahead, they see only shadows of the things on the wall and of themselves, but because there is no chance of seeing anything else than shadows, the human beings consider the shadows as real. He goes on to describe what happens if one of the prisoners is freed and turned around towards the light: how the glare will distress him and how the sight of the real things will confuse him since he has been so used to mere shadows. Then Plato describes the painful process of learning to gaze even at the light of the sun outside the den and so come to a grasp of the good. It is a privilege indeed to help another human turn to the Real.

So, in sum, if the doctor is to be a real leader within the contemporary human community, then he or she needs to be capable of confronting anxieties (and sustaining contradictions) concerned with lack of clear goals, uncertainties of the road, a sense of meaninglessness, and a loss of hope, and capable above all of moving out from the self towards the source of hope (however conceived) beyond the self and thereby coming to terms with the reality and mystery of human death.

Then and only then, one can 'at midnight be confident of the dawn' (Ernest Bloch), as a leader must be.

Ernst Bloch, a Marxist philosopher, who died in 1977 in his nineties, having had significant influence on philosophy and theology in Continental Europe, concluded his *magnum opus* (*Das Prinzip Hoffnung*) with these words:

> Man still lives everywhere in pre-history, everything is still before the creation of the world – as a right world. The real genesis is not at the beginning, but at the end. And it only starts to begin when society and existence become radical, that is, when they comprehend their own roots. But the root of history is the creative working man, who rebuilds and transforms the given. Once man has comprehended himself and established in real democracy existence without externalization and alteration, something arises in the world which all men have glimpsed in childhood, but where no one has yet been: homeland.[25]

The role of the doctor-as-leader may seem to be summarized in the concept that the doctor has the privilege of assisting other persons to be at home on this earth and the earth to be a homeland for all. No matter how weary of work and even of life the task is there – and the words of Dag

Hammarskjöld, written when Secretary-General of the United Nations, may be both consolation and inspiration to the real doctors among us:

> Tired
> And lonely
> So tired
> The heart aches.
> Meltwater trickles
> Down the socks
> The fingers are numb,
> The knees tremble.
> It is now,
> Now, that you must not give in.
>
> On the path of the others
> Are resting places,
> Places in the sun
> Where they can meet.
> But this
> Is your path,
> And it is now,
> Now, that you must not fail.
>
> Weep
> If you can,
> But do not complain.
> The way chose you –
> And you must be thankful.[26]

References

1. Whitehead AN. *Adventures of Ideas*, 1933. Reprinted 1947. Cambridge University Press.
2. Erikson EH. *Childhood and Society*. 2nd ed. Penguin Books, 1965. Harmondsworth
3. Erikson EH. *Identity and the Life Cycle*. Universities Press, 1959.
4. Levinson DJ. *The Seasons of a Man's Life*. New York: International New York: Knopf, 1978.
5. Lickiss JN. *Speech and Community*, Proceedings Annual Convention of Australian Association of Speech and Hearing. 1978, pp4–12. (Keynote address).
6. Levi L. 'Psychosocial Factors in Preventive Medicine, in Healthy People: The Surgeon General's Report on Health Promotion and Disease Prevention'. *Background Papers*. U.S. Department of Health, Education and Welfare, 1979.
7. Hamburg BA, Killilea M. *Relation of Social Support, Stress Illness and Use of Health Services in Healthy People*: The Surgeon General's Report on Health Promotion and Disease Prevention. Background Papers. Washington, D.C.: U.S. Government Printing Office, 1979.
8. Henderson S. 'A Development in social psychiatry: The systematic study of social bonds'. *J Nerv Ment Dis*, 1980; 168: 63–69. (See also for development of the subject, Henderson AS, Byrne DG, Duncan-Jones P. Neurosis and the Social Environment. Sydney: Academic Press, 1981).
9. Berkman-Syme SL. 'Social Networks: Host resistance and mortality', *Am J Epidem*, 1979; 109: 186–204.
10. Antonovsky A. *Health, Stress and Coping*. Jossey, Bass, 1979. San Francisco.
11. King A. *Another Kind of Growth: Industrial Society and the Quality of Life*. David Davies Memorial Institute of International Studies, Annual Memorial Lecture. London, 1972.
12. Meadows DH, Meadows DL, Randers J, Behrens WW. *The Limits to Growth*. First Report to the Club of Rome. London: Earth Island Limited, 1972.
13. Mesarovic M, Pester E. *Mankind at the Turning Point*, to the Club of Rome. London: Hutchinson, 1975. Second Report.
14. Laszlo E. *The Inner Limits of Mankind*. 1978. Oxford: Pergamon Press.
15. Russell B. *The Principles of Social Reconstruction*. Allen and Unwin, 1916. London.
16. Galbraith JK. *The Age of Uncertainty*. London: B.B.C., 1977; p.330.
17. Reynolds I, Rizzo E, Gallagher H, Speedy B. *Psychosocial Problems of Sydney Adults*. Health Commission of N.S.W., 1979.
18. Wheelis A. *The Quest for Identity*. New York: Norton, 1958; p.87.

19 Dubos R. *Man Adapting.* New Haven: Yale University Press, 1965; p.278.
20 Peccei A. 1979 'Whither Humankind'? Opening address to the coming decade of Danger and Opportunity, Club of Rome Conference. Berlin, 1979.
21 Fitzgerald R. *The Sources of Hope.* Oxford: Pergamon Press, 1979.
22 Frankl V. Postscript 1975: 'The Unconscious God', revised and enlarged 1977; p.97. New Research in Logotherapy: Hodder & Stoughton, London.
23 Jung CG. *Modern Man in Search of a Soul.* Paul, 1933; p.226. London: Routledge & Kegan.
24 Bloch E. *The Sources of Hope*, Fitzgerald R (ed.). Rushcutters Bay: Pergamon Press, 1979; p.161.
25 Hammarskjöld D. Markings. Trans. Sjöberg and Auden. London: Faber, 1966.
26 Erling B. *A Reader's Guide to Dag Hammarskjöld's* Waymarks, Minnesota, 2010, p.273

II
The Doctor as Healer

> You can hold yourself back from the sufferings of the world, this is something you are free to do and is in accord with your nature but precisely the holding back is the only suffering that you might be able to avoid.
> —*Franz Kafka*

The doctor as a healer, within the human community, has the responsibility to comfort, from a privileged experience of humanness, the central anxieties of our times and to seek to assist other persons to be at home on this earth, and the earth to be a homeland for all. It is in his or her role as healer that the doctor is unequivocally on the side of and at the service of mankind. The doctor – as a healer is the central relationship of the doctor with the human community, the cornerstone indeed – and as such, is worthy of scrutiny.

As a point of departure, let us take academic lawyer, Professor Sir Ian Kennedy in the 1980 BBC Reith lectures:

> Science has destroyed our faith in religion. Reason has challenged our trust in magic. What more appropriate result could there be than the appearance of new magicians and priests wrapped in the cloak of science and reason? Please understand that it is we, all of us, who have hitched our wagon to the wrong star, scientific medicine, as our guiding light.[1]

The thesis I wish to propound is that medicine needs to be more, not less, scientific. Such a thesis will concern some who would to recognise that science is an art and indeed a humanistic discipline. Alvin Feinstein (1925–2001), who offered what the editor of a prominent medical journal called a 'cogent analysis of scientific methodology in clinical medicine',[2,3,4,5] might allay the fears of some:

> As humanist and artist, the clinician need not fear that medicine will be dehumanised by improved scientific methods for observing and analysing the intact body, mind, existence, and clinical treatment of men. The traditional human values of clinical medicine may seem threatened today, but not by a technology or science that draws the clinician closer to human beings. The threat comes from beliefs that give the label of 'science' to a dissection of a patient's protoplasm but not to a description of his pain; from the concept that a 'disease' is the derangement of a molecule or the dysfunction of a cell, but not the illness of a person; from devices that perceive man as a reduced fragment but not as an intact whole; and from the false scientific dogmas, intolerant of the dignity of the past, that have distracted clinicians from their ancient domain: the care of the sick.[6]

It can be argued that, in the Reith lectures, Kennedy expresses an inadequate view of science. 'Science' is defined by the Oxford dictionary as 'systematic and formulated knowledge' ... and 'scientific' as 'according to rules laid down in science for testing soundness of conclusions, systematic, accurate ...'. It is my view that medical practice needs to be more not less scientific, with pressing needs for clear articulation of goals and objectives, more appropriate processes of diagnosis and interventions in achieving these goals, less archaic methods for the management of information and clearer recognition of limits.

First, let us consider the *goals and objectives of medicine* (without getting bogged down or befogged by an excess of management terminology).

The ancient Greeks had a clear idea of the goal of medical endeavour: witness the words of Hippocrates:

> I will define what I conceive medicine to be. In general terms, it is to do away with the sufferings of the sick, to lessen the violence of their diseases, and to refuse to treat those who are overmastered by their diseases, realizing that in such cases medicine is powerless.
>
> For if a man demand from an art a power over what does not belong, to the art, or from nature a power over what does not belong to nature, his ignorance is more allied to madness than to lack of knowledge. For, in cases where we may have to master through the means afforded by a natural constitution or by an art, there we may be craftsmen, but nowhere else. Whenever, therefore, a man suffers from an ill which is too strong for the means at the disposal of medicine, he surely must not even expect that it can be overcome by medicine.[7]

Many centuries later, Francis Bacon (1561–1626) assured us that 'the office of medicine is but to tune this curious harp of Man's body and to reduce it to harmony.'[8] He also wrote that: 'There is another powerful and great cause of the little advancement of the sciences, which is this: it is impossible to advance properly in the course when the goal is not properly fixed. But the real legitimate goal of the sciences is the endowment of human life with new inventions and riches.'[9]

In our own times, men are no less articulate concerning the goals of medicine, although we see diversity of emphasis. Feinstein (with specific reference to clinical medicine):

> The care of a sick person is the ultimate, specific act that characterizes a clinician. It is the reason for his existence, and its function differentiates him from all other biologists and students of human disease. Its responsibility is transmitted as the heritage of his

profession, and its performance is his unique contribution to the multifarious services exchanged by mankind to sustain human civilization and life.[6]

Thus far, there is no real controversy. However, in the everyday practice of medicine today, the debate can arise with respect to what we mean by care. In the face of a far wider range of options, it has become essential to specify far more precisely what is the primary goal of medical endeavour: cure of a disease process? control of a disease process although not cure? control of symptoms even though the disease process itself can neither be controlled nor cured? Surely these three identifiable and distinct particularized goals need to be articulated within a more general framework – namely, that the goal of any medical intervention at the individual level should be improved quality and, if possible, length of life of the individual at a price (in monetary terms, in convenience, effort, time spent by both patient and staff) proportionate to the gain achieved, and within the community's resources in the face of competing priorities. It is to be noted that such a concept of goals can of course embrace interventions directed towards prevention of ill health and health promotion.

These conclusions seem obvious, but the consequences, if taken seriously, will revolutionize clinical medicine.

Let us take, for example, the problems posed by an elderly woman with considerable cardiac failure caused by long-standing hypertension causing tiredness, some exertional dyspnoea and swelling of the ankles at the end of the day. The goal of treatment will not be eradication of the cardiac disease (for it may not be reversible) nor even control of the disease process (her vascular problem will slowly progress), nor even removal of all signs of cardiac failure, but improvement in the quality of life. Relief of her symptoms (not her signs) must be the goal of treatment. To eliminate all signs of cardiac failure at a dose of drugs which leads to cramps at night, biochemical problems (needing visits to the doctor and blood tests, both of which use up time and risk further misadventures) or even falling (with its attendant dangers) due to postural hypotension is inappropriate, unscientific and misguided medical practice. Yet we have become, since student days, mesmerized by disease processes and clinical signs – and we have magnificent technology now to assist in giving additional information concerning signs (be they lumps, abnormal heart sounds, or disturbance in muscle power or nerve conduction, etc.). Yet the subjective rather than the objective aspect of illness – namely, *symptoms* rather than *signs* must be the real focus of our endeavour. In centuries past symptoms formed almost all the data base upon which a doctor had to make decisions; now signs and extensions of signs by means of investigations predominate. Symptoms used to be written down by patients in long letters to doctors ... but now the weight given to symptoms has shrunk – for the 'harder' information objectivized in signs and investigations impresses more the doctor of the later Twentieth Century, working in a milieu in which addiction to information is in danger of usurping judgement – including clinical judgement,

Precision of diagnosis by application of the technologies available is in no way justified where inconvenience or hazard is involved, unless the increased precision will reasonably be expected to influence intervention decisions for the benefit of that patient.

Precision of diagnosis by autopsy is, of course, quite another matter and certainly may be justified in the interests of others. Another special circumstance may prevail if the patient is, with his or her consent, involved in a scientific investigation, such as a correctly conducted clinical trial – but even in that circumstance 'scientific reasons' cannot justify unnecessary morbidity, cost and major inconvenience, for example, removal of the patient from their home town or inability to work.

There is a strong case for reflection at the point where the data base consists of symptoms and signs – and a working diagnosis is suggested.

Before any attempt is undertaken to go further along the road towards precision of diagnosis, it is necessary to ask these questions: 1) What is the most probable diagnosis? 2) What reasonable alternative diagnoses can be listed? 3) Of all the reasonably possible diagnoses, which are the most treatable? 4) What steps can be taken to exclude or confirm the most treatable diagnosis? (These should be undertaken.) 5) Of the other alternatives, what interventions are available? If the interventions (treatments) available, for say, 3 of 5 possible diagnoses are all the same, then there is a case for seeking no further specification within that trio.

Such an approach requires very precise knowledge of clinical medicine and needs a more intelligent and demanding form of clinical practice. To make correct decisions, the doctor needs to know not only a great deal about the natural history of disease processes in persons of varying age, ethnic group, genetic characteristics, immune status, and so on, and the interaction of one disease process with another and of treatment of one with the treatment of another, but also he or she must understand the sensitivity and specificity of all investigations being considered as well as the hazards they pose to the patient. We do not escape the flat-of-the-curve medicine by a retreat from technology – but rather by more intelligent applications of sound technology, with a minimum of delay. A large literature is arising on decision analysis in clinical medicine and its rational basis,[10,11,12,13] and gradually our thought processes are being refined in this new phase of clinical science, but most of the discussion hitherto has not included the issue of quality of life as being a well-articulated goal, and such is essential if medicine is to be adequately scientific and true to its meaning.*

We can be consoled in one sense that the present debate concerning the appropriateness of investigations is not a development of the 1980s, 70s or even 60s, for Wilmot Herringham, in the British Medical Journal of 1920, wrote as follows:

> It cannot be denied that our present system or want of system wasted the patient's money, and puts him to the utmost inconvenience, and sometimes to great distress. It also wastes everyone's time. Every special test that has to be made, every special examination, every special opinion that has to be asked, means that if the patient is up and about, he has to trot round to a different door, and sit about in a different waiting room, or else send various emanations from his person to another laboratory. Or if the patient is in bed, each of these various authorities has to come to him and carry out the necessary details under the worst possible conditions.[14]

A further dimension needs at least to be mentioned in any consideration of goals. The goal of medicine is not adequately articulated merely in terms even of the quality of function of the patient-as-individual, even though this is a far more accurate formulation of the goal than any definition concerned with diagnosis or labelling of dysfunction. The quality of a person's life is dependent not only on individual function but on whether or not the various components of the environment, personal and impersonal, are such as to permit and indeed facilitate the exercise of individual capacities and to make good

---

* This was true in 1981 but is no longer true in 2023.

deficiencies in those capacities. The goal of clinical practice involves focus on the unique ecosystem of the individual patient; the diagnosis needed is a system-diagnosis, precise identification of a fault in the system, an idea of its etiology and a correct appraisal of the most appropriate processes to be instituted to heal the ecosystem. Medical practice is essentially concerned with human ecology: the human person-in-relationship, the human person-in-community.

In the foregoing clarification of the goals of medical practice, mention has already been made of judicious use of some of the processes to achieve these goals – including the use of investigations in diagnosis and in monitoring treatment. The *healing process* in its totality requires now to be brought into sharper focus – seen first of all as situated within an interpersonal network, the bonds being created by perceived need and presumed skills, and as Eric Cassell (1928–)[15] has stressed, by the capacity of the doctor to connect the unknown and apparently uncontrolled phenomena the patient feels with the remainder of the patient's experience.

Reference has already been made to the need to recognise more adequately the significance of symptoms. Feinstein stressed that the object of clinical science is not disease but disease-in-persons. The person-with-symptoms (or with a disease detected which requires intervention to *prevent* symptoms) is one partner in the healing process – the other partner is the collective comprised of the doctor and his or her colleagues in the health care system, and in a wider sense each person concerned with correcting deficiencies in any part of the patient's ecosystem – whether by, for example, correcting hypotension, making splints, assisting with dressing or with recovery of speech, and the myriad of other ways human beings (with more or less special skills) help one another. The doctor is no more, no less, than an often crucial cog in a healing system.

There is increasing stress on the role of the patient in the healing process. Some approaches to medical practice stress above all else the need to assist the patient to counter the disease: such an approach is inherently logical as long as recognition is made of the limits of this approach. More problematic are the interventions the doctor may seek to implement to attack the disease process directly. Of these, one appropriate for discussion here is the medical use of drugs.

In Australia, the medical use of drugs appears nearly out of control – the findings of the Senate Select Committee concerning this matter are quite horrifying: we appear to be a grossly over-medicalized society.[16] In particular, it appears futile to seek to solve social ills by sedating, tranquillizing or seeking to elevate the mood of a large minority of the population – and, of course alcohol is abused by a larger number of us. Such drug-induced pseudo-tranquillity augers poorly for the future. Debate along these lines could be fruitful but will not be pursued here.

Of particular concern is that a budget spent on unfruitful or unwise prescription of drugs represents siphoning off of funds which need to be applied to other health needs – notably in upgrading the care of the aged and the chronically ill. Also the very significant morbidity (with detraction from the quality of life) due to drug side effects represents a deviation from the optimum scientific application of medical technology. Side effects can occur in the best regulated therapy but it is frequently found that serious side effects are being caused by quite inappropriate use of drugs, for example, overzealous treatment of hypertension in the very elderly.[17]*

---

* The improved quality of antihypertensives and the reductions in cost that have occurred in the last 40 years would appear to have overcome this concern.

In any debate concerned with drug use, due proportion must be maintained. Oliver Wendell-Holmes Sr, in his essay in 1860 *Currents and Countercurrents in Medicine*, probably overstated the point when he wrote as follows:

> Throw out opium which the Creator himself seems to prescribe, for we often see the scarlet poppy growing in the cornfields as if it were foreseen that whenever there is hunger to be fed there must also be pain to be soothed: throw out a few specifics which our doctor's art did not discover: throw out wine which is a food and the vapours which produce the miracle of anaesthesia and I firmly believe that if the whole materia medica as now used could be sunk to the bottom of the sea, it would be all the better for mankind – and all the worse for the fishes.

No specific mention has been made of processes involved in healing psychological symptoms. Suffice to say that within the interpersonal relationships which are at the core of the practice of medicine in whatever context there are countless opportunities for the doctor to assist in the growth of another person through resolution of crises. Occasionally the context will be identifiable counselling sessions or psychiatric practice – more often it is in the day-to-day consultation or therapeutic situation where the opportunities – and challenges occur. There is risk involved in being a doctor: unless one holds oneself back from the suffering of others one is in danger of being exposed in one's humanness, and from time to time being found wanting.

The management of medical information looms large as one of the most pressing tasks of the 80s. The technology is with us and needs urgent application.

There are three major areas of information requiring better management: information concerning basic medical sciences in general, information concerning the problem under consideration, and information held in whatever place concerning this patient. Jean Hamburger (1909–1992) (Professor of Medicine, Paris) pointed out the futility of using the brain to store information – growth in wisdom can be inhibited: 'Heads that are full are not necessarily useful'.[18]

It is worth reflecting that medical literature may contain an over-representation of the writings of relatively inexperienced young medical/clinical scientists on the way up the promotion ladder. The distillation of perspectives in the face of a mass of information (e.g. concerning new tests, new manifestations, new treatments for this and that condition) comes more often with advancing years, and such perspectives are frequently *not* written but embodied in the clinician: not all that is known in medicine is written and in particular much less is written in the area of clinical judgement (where information from several sources is being applied to decide on either a diagnosis, a prognosis or an intervention). Such is a cautionary note for those who would frenetically seek a fast route to wisdom or experience via an on-line literature search.

These observations are not at all novel; John Shaw Billings (1838–1913), the editor of the first *Index Medicus* (1881), wrote:

> There is a vast amount of this effete and worthless material in the literature of medicine, and this is increasing rapidly ... (It is) characterized as 'superlatively middling, the quintessential extract of mediocrity'. Nine tenths at least of it becomes worthless, and of no interest within ten years after the date of publication, and much of it is so when it first appears.[19]

It would certainly appear that information concerning specific problems, for example, concerning the side effects of drugs, could be far more adequately managed so that doctors could retrieve information relevant to a problem on hand by use of a terminal in a practice office rather more efficiently than by thumbing through the index of the right book or journal in a library. A computer-based data bank relevant to various branches of practice should be readily constructible and available for questioning by telephone-linked terminals concerning relevant information, leaving the questioner with a less cluttered mind and with time and space for reflective judgement.*

With reference to information concerning individual patients, record linkage systems appear imperative. Lawrence Weed[20] has recently stressed that since the patient is now the point of continuity in a changing scenario of health professionals, the patient should be responsible, at least in part, for the preservation of information concerning him or her. The day may come when the patient carries a cassette with a computer tape of updated medical information to be given to the doctor at each clinical encounter, for scrutiny and updating (copying maybe), before being handed back. Why not indeed?

So communications technology does offer solutions to the problems of information management, but it is essential for the clinician to recognise that, as stressed above, information is an aid to, not a substitute for, clinical judgement in a highly personalized context. Stanley J Reiser concludes his book *Medicine and the Reign of Technology* (1978) as follows:

> To be free to develop his medical skills to their highest point ... today's physician must rebel. He can use his strongest weapon – a refusal to accept bondage to any one technique, no matter how useful it may be in a particular instance. He must regard them all with detachment, as mere tools, to be chosen as necessary

---

* This is now a reality e.g., with MIMS On-Line.

for a particular task. He must accept the patient as a human being, and regain and reassess his faith in his own medical judgement.[21]

So the healer-doctor is servant but not slave, growing in wisdom, free to reflect, confident in considered decision-making and a true scientist.

The contribution of the doctor as healer inevitably leads to *a recognition of limits*. The recognition of its limits is a sign of a mature intellectual discipline. There are indeed limits to the application of medical science, limits to its power, limits to its appropriateness. If the goal is adequately perceived, these limits will be readily recognised. If medical science is clearly directed toward improved quality (and, where appropriate, increased length) of life, then, provided there is adequate grasp of the notion of quality, medicine will not (as the public fears) overstep its mark, especially in those who are (as Hippocrates puts it) overmastered by diseases and irretrievably so.

There is increasing literature in this area, much of it influenced by St. Christopher's Hospice.[22,23,24] The application of first class clinical medicine in the care of the dying is just as much a moral imperative as is the care of those deemed 'curable' – and is indeed intellectually (as well as emotionally) more demanding because of the complexity of the total situation.

I leave to others to discuss psychological, psychiatric and spiritual concepts of the care of the dying, and the opportunities for preventive medicine (especially with regard to those to be bereaved) inherent in the situation. Neither can the issue of euthanasia be discussed here. The debate was sharpened in the 70s and some of the issues are well discussed in a document (*On Dying Well*) prepared for the Lambeth conference of bishops of the Anglican Church. This document stresses that the call for euthanasia reflects poor application of contemporary clinical science to the care of the dying, especially with reference to the management of pain. Attention might be drawn also to the most recent major Catholic statement on the issue and the useful clarifications contained herein [25] with respect to the need for 'due proportion in the case of remedies':

> In any case, it will be possible to make correct judgement as to the means by studying the type of treatment to be used, its degree of complexity or risk, its cost and the possibilities of using it and comparing these elements with the results that can be expected, taking into account the state of the sick person and his or her moral resources.

The document went on to offer further useful clarifications worthy of restating:

> In order to facilitate the application of these general principles, the following clarifications can be added:
>
> - If there are no other sufficient remedies, it is permitted, with the patient's consent, to have recourse to the means provided by the most advanced medical techniques, even if these means are still at the experimental stage and are not without a certain risk. By accepting them, the patient can even show generosity in the service of humanity.
>
> - It is also permitted, with the patient's consent, to interrupt these means, where the results fall short of expectations. But for such a decision to be made, account will have to be taken of the reasonable wishes of the patient and the patient's family, as also of the advice of the doctors who are specially competent in the matter. The latter may in particular judge that the investment in instruments and personnel is disproportionate to the results foreseen; they may also judge that the techniques applied impose on the patient strain or suffering out of

proportion with the benefits which he or she may gain from such techniques.

- It is also permissible to make do with the normal means that medicine can offer. Therefore, one cannot impose on anyone the obligation to have recourse to a technique which is already in use but which carries a risk or is burdensome. Such a refusal is not equivalent of suicide; on the contrary, it should be considered as an acceptance of the human condition, or a wish to avoid the application of a medical procedure disproportionate to the results that can be expected, or a desire not to impose excessive expense on the family or the community.
- When inevitable death is imminent in spite of the means used, it is permitted in conscience to take the decision to refuse forms of treatment that would only secure a precarious and burdensome prolongation of life, so long as the normal care due to the sick person in similar cases is not interrupted. In such circumstances the doctor has no reason to reproach himself with failing to help the person in danger.'

The clinical and ethical issues involved in the care of the dying in whatever situations are becoming clearer – but the challenge and privilege of a doctor involved needs restating in different terms.

Dying *is* part of living and care of the dying is care of living persons in the last phase of human growth. If we return to Erikson's schema of the developmental tasks to be negotiated in the course of human personal growth – we note that the favourable end point in the resolution of the developmental tasks of the later years is the development of a sense of wholeness (which Erikson called 'integrity') rather than a sense of despair. Just as, in Erikson's schema, the emergence in adolescence of a strong sense of identity (rather than identity diffusion) prepares one for the gift of the self to another in intimacy (rather than the isolation of the self), so the attainment of integrity (in old age or at a younger age when relevant and one sees this telescoping of stages occur in those dying young) may be the optimum preparation for the surrender of the self in death which appears to be the 'normal' human end point after the shock, aggression and depression are (if they occur) worked through.

'Death' wrote the aged philosopher, Ernest Bloch (1880–1959), 'serves as the master test of our journeyman years.'[26] As a person is dying, it is the privilege of doctors to help create the conditions where, as free of pain and other symptoms as possible, and with opportunities for choice, for privacy, for solitude and for intimacy, a person may reveal to himself/herself, if not to others, what he/she has become. Above all, the precious time he/she has left must be at their disposal, to express their own unique priorities – not spent in quite inappropriate medical procedures or investigations. It is not inappropriate to offer a coeliac axis block to a man with severe upper abdominal pain as his/her major (though not only) symptom – even if he/she is likely to live only a week or two. It *is* inappropriate to waste a few half days having chest x-rays, blood counts or even medical consultations which could be conducted by telephone if he/she would prefer to be out on his/her farm ... or in their suburban home – or even on the hospital balcony with a partner during those precious hours.

It has been said that, 'It is the task of medicine to emancipate man's interior splendour'[27] and this task reaches its height in the case of the dying.

There are limits to the appropriateness of medicine, especially in the situation of the dying – but these are readily embraced by sound clinical medicine. The general principle always is that decisions taken must be for the good of the individual; with the individual as the end not the means.

Immanuel Kant, the philosopher, urged us 'So act as to treat humanity, whether in your own person or in that of another, in every case as an end, never as a means only.' In this, the situation of the gravely ill is no different from any other situation in clinical medicine, but because the patient is even more powerless than the average patient, the point needs stressing that no investigation should be done nor treatment given primarily that the doctor may learn more which might be of benefit to others without the patient's informed consent and after the doctor has carefully considered the price the patient will pay in time and inconvenience if consent is given. Such concepts are quite crucial especially in teaching hospitals; in general, in Australia, such concepts are understood and acted upon.

There are serious and pressing problems in other aspects of medical practice but these cannot be further considered here. There are limits also in the area of medical research with respect to the limits of appropriateness and these must be mentioned briefly. Leon Kass (1971), in a thoughtful article suitably entitled *The New Biology: What Price Man's Estate?*, alleged that: 'Our value and our very concept of Man is at stake'.[28]

In some forms of research, the application of biomedical technology is wholly inappropriate. The problem may be illustrated by the sadness of Ian Donald, Emeritus Professor of Midwifery, University of Glasgow. His name was a byword for generations of students of obstetrics and yet the last section of his short work (*Life, Death, and Modern Medicine*) is entitled *Was my life worthwhile?*[29]

In his booklet, he talks of what he calls 'God-baiting research' and refers to work he saw going on in Sweden:

> The procedure is to put live babies aborted by abdominal hysterectomy late in the middle trimester into tanks of artificial liquor and then maintain them alive on cardiopulmonary bypass. These babies could be seen

making crying grimaces and gestures as the effect of various drugs was noted in their circulation.

Finally, as he questions the possible misuse of his own researches into early intra-uterine life, he ends with the words of GK Chesterton:

> I tell you nought for your comfort,
> Yea, naught for your desire
> Save that the sky grows darker yet
> And the sea rises higher.

In sum, a radical reappraisal of clinical practice as a truly scientific activity necessitates reflection on Man, his excellence, his meaning, the process of his development throughout life, his fulfilment, his values and, above all, his mystery. Only in this way will there be true reappraisal of both the goals and the processes of clinical practice. If clinicians are not prepared to reflect and to recognise the crucial relevance of philosophic and religious reflection on Man throughout the ages, there is a very great danger that clinical science will continue to fail to contribute optimally fashion to the quality of life of men and the effort will have missed its mark entirely.

The doctor is at core and above all else a healer – embedded within the community, and through the exercise of this privileged role he or she can be a spark of light in dark times, for as Hannah Arendt reminded us:

> Even in the darkest of times we have the right to expect some illumination and such illumination may well come less from theories and concepts than from the uncertain, flickering and often weak light that some men and women, in their lives and their works, will kindle under almost all circumstances and shed over the time span that was given them.[30]

References

1. Kennedy I. *Unmasking Medicine*. London: George Allen & Unwin, 1981. (Reith Lectures).
2. Feinstein AR. 'Scientific Methodology in Clinical Medicine', I: Introduction, Principles, and Concepts. *Ann Intern Med*, 1964; 6: 564–579.
3. Feinstein AR. Scientific Methodology in Clinical Medicine, II. *Classification of Human Disease by Clinical Behaviour*. ibid. p.757–781.
4. Feinstein AR. Scientific Methodology in Clinical Medicine, Ill. *The Evaluation of Therapeutic Response*. ibid. p.944–965.
5. Feinstein AR. Scientific Methodology in Clinical Medicine, IV. *Acquisition of Clinical Data*. ibid. p.1162–1193.
6. Feinstein AR. *Clinical Judgement Baltimore*, Williams &. Wilkins, 1967; p.363.
7. Hippocrates (W.H. Jones, ed.). *Hippocrates 2*. Cambridge, Massachussetts, 1923.
8. Bacon F. quoted in 'Medicine and the Quality of Life'. *Ann Intern Med*, 1966; 64: 711–713.
9. Bacon F. Novum Organon 1:80, quoted in *Great Treasury of Western Thought* (M.J. Adler and C. Van Doran, eds.). Nevi York: Bowker Company, 1977; p.1110.
10. Hodkinson M. *Biochemical Diagnosis of the Elderly*. New York: Wylie, 1977.
11. Clarke RM, Mason B, Leeder SR. *Cost and effectiveness of Clinical Investigation: the state of the art*, Aust NZ, J Med, 1980 10: 572–580.
12. Schwartz WB, Garry GA, Kassirer JP, Essig A. 'Decision analysis and clinical judgement'. *Am J Med*, 1973; 55 459–471.
13. Pauker SG, Kassirer JP. 'Decision making: The threshhold approach to clinical', *N Eng J Med*, 1980; 302: 1109–17.
14. Herringham W. 'The Consultant'. *Br Med J*, 1920; 2 36–40.
15. Cassell EJ. *The Healer's Art: A new approach to the Doctor-Patient Relationship*. Harmondsworth: Penguin Books, 1978.
16. *Senate Standing Committee on Social Welfare*. Another side to the Drug Debate. A Medicated Society? Canberra: A.G.P.S., 1981.
17. Isaacs B. 'Should we treat hypertension in the elderly?', *Ageing*, 1979; 8: 115–120.
18. Hamburger J. *The Power and the Frailty*: 'The Future of Medicine and the Future of Man'. Trans. J. Neucroschel. New York: Macmillan, 1973.
19. Billings JS, International Medical Congress, Seventh Session, 'An Address on Our Medical Literature', London, August 1881.
20. Weed L. 'Physicians of the Future'. *N Engl J Med*, 1981; 304 903–907.

21 Reiser SJ. *Medicine and the Reign of Technology*. Cambridge: Cambridge University Press, 1978.
22 Saunders CM. *The Management of Terminal Disease*. London: Edwin Arnold, 1978.
23 Lamerton L. *Care of the Dying*. Harmondsworth: Penguin, 1980.
24 Lickiss JN. 'Dying from Cancer: What are the questions?' *Aust Fam Physician*; 1979; 8: 991–1003.
25 Sacred Congregation for the Doctrine of the Faith. *Declaration on Euthanasia*. Rome, 1980.
26 Bloch E. *Man on His Own*. Trans. E.B. Ashton. New York: Herder & Herder, 1970; p.47.
27 Mortimer K.E. 'The Impossible Profession: the doctor-priest relationship', Proceedings. p. 81., *Aust Assoc Gerontology*, 2 (2), 1974.
28 Kass L. 'The New Biology: What Price Man's Estate'. *Nature*, 1971; 174 779–788.
29 Donald I. 'Life, Death and Modern Medicine'. Social Responsibility Series, Order of Christian Unity. London, 1974.
30 Arendt H. *Men in Dark Times*. New York: Harcourt, Brace and World, 1955. Extract is taken from preface to 1968 printing.

III
The Doctor as Advocate of the Weak

> Doctors are the natural attorneys of the poor.
> —*Rudolf Virchow* (1821–1902)

> Three passions, simple but overwhelmingly strong, have governed my life: the longing for love, the search for knowledge, and unbearable pity for Mankind.
> —*Bertrand Russell* (1872–1970)

These words could have been written of all those committed to the care of the sick, of humankind, as doctors radically are. One of the features of the relationship between doctors and the human community of which they form part is the note of advocacy for the weak. Doctors are, as it were, at the interface of the weak and the strong: there appears need to explore this notion anew from the vantage point of the late twentieth century.

In the human community, there have always been the weak – those who through lack of physical or mental stamina or social status lack the power to share significantly in decisions made concerning themselves and to control actions stemming from these decisions.

Social history from the earliest recorded times up to the present bears eloquent testimony to the possibilities and actualities of the crushing of the relatively weak: the conquered, the alien, the maimed, the unwanted (whether infant or aged) the mentally ill, the poor, unskilled labourers, members of a particular race or creed.

As we race towards the close of the twentieth century, we need to remind ourselves of the unspeakable exploitation of the labourers and little children even in England in the eighteenth and nineteenth centuries. Friedrich Engels (1820–1895), the son of a wealthy German textile worker whose father owned a factory in Manchester, wrote in his now classic work in the mid-nineteenth century[1] of the almost unspeakable conditions of life and work of the labourers and their families: it is not necessary to espouse the philosophy which Engels with Karl Marx (1818–1883) developed on the basis of their observations in order to recognise with them the horror of the situation which prevailed. Those children who survived (and Engels reports that in Carlisle, Preston and Leeds more than 40% of children under 5 years of age died) had a life of almost unbelievable harshness. Stone[2] gives some details concerning treatment of children in England in the eighteenth and nineteenth centuries:

> For the few who survived (in workhouses), the prospect was a grim one. The older females were frequently handed over to a master who is either vicious or cruel: in the one case they fall victim to his irregular passions; and in the other are subjected with unreasonable severity, to tasks too hard to be performed. These were the lucky ones, others being virtually enslaved by criminals and trained for a life of prostitution if female or robbery and pick-pocketing if male.
>
> Some had their teeth torn out to serve as artificial teeth for the rich; others were deliberately maimed by beggars to arouse compassion and extract alms. Even this latter crime was one upon which the law looked with a remarkably tolerant eye. In 1761 a beggar woman, convicted of deliberately 'putting out the eyes of children with whom she went about the country' in order to attract pity and alms was sentenced to no more than 2 years' imprisonment.

There have always been the weak because men, members of one species – Homo Sapiens – are, from an empirical point of view, unequal.

Vast tracts have been written by wise (and unwise) men down the centuries on the issue of the equality – and of the natural inequality – of men, and debate has waxed strong with varying positions forming the basis of various political ideologies.

Friedrich Nietzsche (1844–1900) (*Twilight of the Idols*) wrote of the doctrine of equality, 'There exists no more poisonous poison.' Richard Henry Tawney (1880–1962), who in 1903 as a young student, was sent by Edward Caird (1835–1908), the Master of Balliol College, to visit the poor of London ('to discover why with so much wealth, there was so much poverty in London') clarified the debate in his writings by accepting empirical differences among men whilst stressing society's responsibility to respect all and facilitate the development of all:

> It is obvious ... that the word 'Equality' possesses more than one meaning, and that the controversies surrounding it arise partly, at least, because the same term is employed with different connotations. Thus it may either purport to state a fact, or convey the expression of an ethical judgement. On the one hand, it may affirm that men are, on the whole, very similar in their natural endowments of character and intelligence. On the other hand, it may assert that, while they differ profoundly as individuals in capacity and character they are equally entitled as human beings to consideration and respect, and that the well-being of a society is likely to be increased if it so plans its organisation that, whether their powers are great or small, all its members may be equally enabled to make the best of such powers as they possess.[3]

Jacques Maritain (1882–1973), the Thomist philosopher, writing in war-torn Europe amidst the brutalizing of *Man by Man* (1943), articulated the reality of the true equality of men, prescinding from the extremes of nominalism and idealism:

> The equality in nature among men consists of their concrete communion in the mystery of the human species; it does not lie in an idea, it is hidden in the heart of the individual and of the concrete, in the roots of the substance of each man. Obscure because residing on the level of substance and its root energies, primordial because it is bound up with the very sources of being, human equality reveals itself, like the nearness of our neighbour, to everyone who practices it; indeed, it is identical with that proximity of all to each, and of each to all. If you treat a man as a man, that is to say, if you respect and love the secret he carries within him and the good of which he is capable, to that extent do you make effective in yourself his closeness in nature to and his equality or unity in nature with yourself. It is the natural love of the human being for his own kind which reveals and makes real the unity of species among men. As long as love does not call it forth, that unity slumbers in a metaphysical retreat where we can perceive it only as an abstraction.
>
> In the common experience of misery, in the common sorrow of great catastrophes, in humiliation and distress, under the blows of the executioner or the bombs of total war, in concentration camps, in the hovels of starving people in great cities, in any common necessity, the doors of solitude open and Man recognises Man.[4]

There have always been the weak and men have exploited the weak. Bertrand Russell deplored that 'throughout past history power has been used to give to the strong an undue share of good things and to leave to the weak a life of toil and misery.'[5] And yet there have been voices speaking out against the exploitation of the weak by the strong, voices raised as advocates of the weak, calling on the strong to recognise the rights and the value even of the weak within Society.

Man recognises Man even in weakness ...

In the early Hebrew scriptures there is repeated testimony to fundamental features of the human condition. In the early chapters of Genesis, we see a glimpse of human possibility – unalienated Man.

In the following books, we see injunctions for the man of power to recognise the rights and needs of the poor, the oppressed, the alien ... and there is a thread running through the Hebrew scriptures of the special value and significance of persons in these categories, the *anawim*, the little ones. The poor man has a special claim on God – and on Man.

Millennia later, in the nineteenth century, Charles Darwin (1809–1882), in the *Descent of Man*, wrote:

> The aid which we feel impelled to give to the helpless is mainly an incidental result of the instinct of sympathy, which was originally acquired as part of the social instincts, but subsequently rendered ... more tender and more widely diffused. Nor could we check our sympathy, if so urged by hard reason, without deterioration in the noblest part of our nature. The surgeon may harden himself whilst performing an operation, for he knows he is acting for the good of his patient; but if we were intentionally to neglect the weak and the helpless, it could only be for a contingent benefit, with a certain and great present evil ...

Not all agreed with this point of view. Nietzsche, in Germany in the nineteenth century, propounded the need for men to be strong, and the writings of this fiery genius influenced many, including the poet, Rainer Maria Rilke (1875–1926), who as a young man, after reading some of Nietzsche, wrote in 1896 as follows:

> He whom men worship as the Messiah turns the whole world into an infirmary. He calls the weak, the unfortunate, the disabled His children and His loved ones. What about the strong? How are we ourselves to climb if we lend strength to the unfortunate and the oppressed, to idle rogues with no wits and no energy? Let them fall, let them die, alone and wretched. Be hard, be terrible, be pitiless! You must thrust yourselves forward, forward! A few men, but great ones, will build a world with their strong, muscular, masterful arms on the corpses of the weak, the sick and the infirm.[6]

It is consoling that this youthful piece of work is not considered to represent Rilke's mature thought[7] – but the ideas embodied in it continued to be nurtured in fertile ground. This stream of thinking glorifying, in some measure, the powerful may have been significantly complemented by ideas emanating in the nineteenth century from August Comte (1798–1857) and his followers.[8]

In 1847, Comte gave a series of lectures and one of his hearers, Dr. Robinet, wrote: 'In those hallowed hours that heralded such great destinies, we felt the breath of Humanity, we caught a glimpse of its reality, its greatness, we bowed before it.' The glorification of Humanity as such – not the sheer celebration of Man as had been seen in some features of the Renaissance – but a triumphalism concerning Humanity, continued palpably in the positivist tradition. In the following generation another fervent positivist (addressing Catholics) said: 'We shall convince the men, we shall persuade the women, and the day is not far off when we shall enter your forsaken temples as masters, bearing above our heads the banner of triumphant Humanity.'

A further nuance was expressed by Contrat, another positivist, in the 1930s: 'Objectively, the only individual being that surpasses the individual is his species, carrying in it ... that extraordinary additive faculty which enables Man to outclass the animals. This suggests an inspiring extension of the humanist attitude. We seek to divert religious feeling towards the species, as the Marxians tried to divert it towards class warfare, the dictatorship of the proletariat or the organisation of industrial production.'

Once the good of the species moves to the centre of the stage then the context is ripe for the upsurge of ideas that the Well-being of individuals – especially the weak and apparently unprofitable – can be logically sacrificed as a manifestation of concern for the species.

In this context came Adolf Hitler. In *Mein Kampf* (1925), he wrote:

> Defective people (must) be prevented from propagating equally defective offspring ... For, if necessary, the incurably sick will be piteously segregated – a barbaric measure for this unfortunate who is struck by it but a blessing for his fellow men and posterity.[9]

As we know, this logic was mercilessly put into effect, and although there have been further brutal and brutalising cruelties inflicted on a large scale by *Man on Man* since the Hitlerian programmes, concern and speculation continue to be focused on that phenomenon – because of the grave questions it poses and the assumptions it challenges.

Mr. Justice Kirby, Chairman of the Law Reform Commission of Australia, recently noted (when discussing experimental therapies) that the Nazi euthanasia programme began as a means of 'relieving' the severely and chronically sick, with the medical profession advancing the programme. It seems that many of the doctors who presided over the killings saw themselves as idealists – parties in a 'vast revolutionary biological therapy'. Recently Kirby quoted Leo Alexander (1905–1985), observer at Nuremburg Trials:

> It started with the acceptance of the attitude, basic in the euthanasia movement, that there is such a thing as life not worthy to be lived. This attitude in its early stages concerned itself merely with the severely and chronically sick. Gradually, the sphere of those to be included in this category was enlarged to encompass the socially unproductive, the ideologically unwanted, the racially unwanted and finally all non-Germans. But it is important to realise the infinitely small wedged-in lever from which this entire trend of mind received its impetus was the attitude towards the non-rehabilitatable sick.[10]

It will already be apparent that some of these issues are (unfortunately) relevant now forty years later. It is instructive, therefore, to look more closely at the involvement of the medical profession (and others equally informed) in such manifest evil.

Erik Fromm (1900–1980), in his work *The Anatomy of Human Destructiveness*, discussed the phenomenon of Hitler and the involvement of good men in evil, and offered a significant analysis 'of the main fallacy which prevents people from recognising potential Hitlers before they have shown their true faces.':

> This fallacy lies in the belief that a thoroughly destructive and evil man must be a devil – and look his part; that he must be devoid of any positive quality; that he must bear the sign of Cain so visibly that everyone can recognise his destructiveness from afar ... more often the intensely destructive person will show a front of kindliness;

courtesy; love of family, of children, of animals; he will speak of his ideals and good intentions. But not only this. There is hardly a man who is utterly devoid of any kindness; of any good intention ... Hence, as long as one believes that the evil man wears horns, one will not discover an evil man.

The naive assumption that an evil man is essentially recognisable results in a great danger; one fails to recognise evil men before they have begun their work of destruction.[11]

Is it possible that there is unrecognised actual or potential evil – not only within us (the great playwrights, novelists assure us of that possibility if we needed any confirmation) but also within our society? Remembering that, as Fromm stressed, evil does not wear horns, but can appear even under the guise of the good, is there evidence of our society falling into the trap of justifying exploitation or even destruction of the 'weak' – or at least inadequate care of the weak for the good of the strong? If so, we are in extreme moral danger as a society and already bear within us the seeds of our destruction. The question is hard to face, but needs to be faced – and in those terms, not as a political but as a moral question.

Violence, cruelty – for example, attacks on defenceless elderly – all these are recognised as evil, and we have a criminal code to deal with them. It is the 'evil without horns' which is the danger and it could be that evil may be present wherever and whenever a decision made by the powerful concerning the relatively powerless (the aged, the frail, the chronically ill, the dying – or the very young or unborn) benefits the powerful ... and certainly any such decision must be highly suspect.

Can we be more specific in our reflection? It is surely the ideal of every true doctor to be an advocate of the weak, and not to be involved albeit unknowingly in evil. What can this mean now in practice?

We do not have to consider only the pressures for active euthanasia for the unfit or unwanted; there is serious imbalance in our system for caring for people in need – with waiting lists of frail elderly and non-rehabilitatable sick for places in nursing homes, seriously inadequate resources for the care (at home where possible) of the chronically ill and the very elderly. Yet the trend to chronic disease will gather momentum with increasingly aged population, as well as the continuing relative success of 'acute' medicine leaving some with lives saved but residual disability. However, neither the health care systems nor the insurance systems have reflected the increasing ratio of chronic to acute disease in our community. The poor elderly have the greatest need of medical care but available information suggests that they do not have a proportionate share of the health bill (whether private or public).

It is clear that care of our frail elderly cannot be based on concepts of economic return to the community. William Farr (1807–1883), the British Statistician in his nineteenth century work, *Vital Statistics*, progressed to calculating the value to the state of a life according to future accrued income; that is, setting off investment in early nurture and sanitation against late wages and taxes. He estimated that a Norfolk agricultural labourer was worth five pounds at birth, fifty-six pounds at 5, one hundred and seventeen pounds at 10, one hundred and ninety-two pounds at 15, two hundred and thirty-four pounds at 20, a peak of two hundred and forty-six pounds at 25, two hundred and forty-one pounds at 30 and thereafter declining to one hundred and thirty-eight pounds at 55 and one pound at 70, and thereafter at a rising cost to the community, until at 80 the old man was costing forty-one pounds a year. Smith, after discussing Farr, notes, 'This investment-oriented approach positively discourages expenditure in areas that will not yield a higher return.'[12]

There are pressures for more resources to be allocated in several areas of the health care system. What shall be the principles which should guide decision-making in the face of competing needs? The principle of economic worth just will not do in the face of all the foregoing discussion.

Contributions from three sources appear relevant: the Maxwell Enquiry, the recent major contribution by social philosopher, John Rawls (1921–2002), and concepts of contemporary philosopher, Karl Popper (1902–1994).

RJ Maxwell, in 1974, undertook a detailed study of the health care systems of over twenty Western nations – with Australian statistics incorporated in a second edition in 1975, and the points he made are still valid.[13]

By way of preamble, Maxwell outlined the paradox of health needs:

> The fundamental paradox of health care is that medical advances so often breed further needs and increase future requirements for care ... In short, every inch of ground gained is won with greater difficulty and at higher cost than the last. It is the familiar phenomenon of diminishing returns, with one vital difference: no new gain, however costly, can ever be dismissed as marginal if it promises some real reduction of human suffering. There is, in the nature of things, no possibility of saturating 'demand' for the reduction of mortality and the relief of pain. In every nation, the demand for health care is growing and the balance of needs is changing towards less tractable problems associated with handicap, affluence and age.

It was clear that 'in every country studied health expenditure has been rising faster than the Gross National Product, no matter how fast the latter has risen.'

The Maxwell enquiry considered many other facets of the health care delivery system: patterns of supply of health professionals, their geographical distribution, patterns of use of hospitals and the cost effectiveness of the systems prevailing in the various countries. It was clear that each country requires a means of confronting and resolving the question of priorities.

In every health care system there are organisational problems which the Maxwell enquiry lists as: (1) barriers to patient access (simple non-availability, financial problems, the complexity of the system); (2) inflexibility of resource use (e.g. by boundaries between hospital services and services outside hospital, professional demarcation); (3) ill-defined responsibilities with inadequate planning; (4) excessive complexity and cost.

The Maxwell enquiry concludes that 'four kinds of shifts in strategy will be widely called for', and details these as:

1 Greater attention to, and expenditure on, prevention and health education.
2 Building and maintaining stronger systems of primary care.

> 'Specialization has been the foundation stone for skilled care of specific, acute illnesses. But such conditions, though intensely important, represent only a small fraction of the total incidence of disease. Something like nine of ten cases can be dealt with quite satisfactorily by a well-trained general practitioner or specialist in primary care. In the absence of such a practitioner, what happens to these nine cases? The patient has to decide to which specialist to turn, many cases are seen by specialists that do not require their skill and are outside their main field of competence, and there is

> little continuity in the doctor/patient relationship. In consequence, the quality of care suffers, and resources are wasted. The greater the proliferation of medical specialities, the more doctors will be needed to deal with a fluctuating caseload.
>
> Only when the specialized skills are really required is this an acceptable price to pay for higher quality care.'

3. Upgrading the treatment of long-term illness and handicap.
4. Streamlining the acute hospitals as an integral part of the total pattern of provision.

> 'The first step, which depends on strengthening the primary and long-term care services, is to relieve the pressure of inappropriate admissions and to allow earlier discharge of patients who no longer require acute medical care. The right use of a major acute hospital's skills is possible only when the acute hospital no longer has to make good the deficiencies of other parts of the health system.'
>
> The Maxwell report has been discussed at some length, not because the points it makes are new nor unexpected but because it represents, from an international perspective, a useful discussion of the health care.
>
> John Rawls of Harvard, in his seminal work, 'A Theory of Justice'[14] in merely ten years has evoked so much interest, discussion and debate[15] that the contribution has been styled the most significant since the nineteenth century utilitarians represented by J.S. Mill. His central idea is a revised version of a contract approach to the distribution of resources, with the principles being worked out by a consensus of persons who do not know their own social status, age, needs, etc. – under the so-called 'veil of ignorance'.

Rawls believes that under such circumstances principles will emerge which ensure the fair distribution of resources:

> We are to imagine that those who engage in social cooperation choose together, in one joint act, the principles which are to assign basic rights and duties and to determine the division of social benefits.
>
> Men are to decide in advance how they are to regulate their claims against one another and what is to be the foundation charter of their society.
>
> Among the essential features of this situation is that no one knows his place in society, his class position or social status, nor does anyone know his fortune in the distribution of natural assets and abilities, his intelligence, strength, and the like. I shall even assume that the parties do not know their conceptions of the good or their special psychological propensities. The principles of justice are chosen behind a veil of ignorance.
>
> This ensures that no one is advantaged or disadvantaged in the choice of principles by the outcome of natural chance or the contingency of social circumstances. Since all are similarly situated and no one is able to design principles to favor his particular condition, the principles of justice are the result of a fair agreement or bargain. For, given the circumstances of the original position, the symmetry of everyone's relations to each other, this initial situation is fair between individuals as moral persons, that is, as rational beings with their own ends and capable, I shall assume, of a sense of justice. The original position is, one might say, the appropriate initial status quo, and thus the fundamental agreements reached in it are fair.

> This explains the propriety of the name· 'justice as fairness': it conveys the idea that the principles of justice are agreed to in an initial situation that is fair.

A basic concept in Rawls' work is that, 'all social primary goods – liberty and opportunity, income and wealth, and the bases for self-respect – are to be distributed equally unless an unequal distribution of any or all of these goods is to the advantage of the least favoured'.

We can reasonably ask what principles for allocation of health resources would emerge if the parties charged with reaching consensus did not know their age, economic status, health status, ethnicity nor their place in the health system – whether acutely ill patient or chronically ill patient, cook, nurse, general practitioner, hospital specialist, health administrator, and so on. Some discussion of applications of Rawls' ideas to the health system is beginning elsewhere (for example, in U.S.A.[16]) and debate is essential in Australia.

If a sign of significance of a philosopher is the seminal nature of his ideas, in that his concepts stimulate progress in thought in a broad range of other disciplines, then Karl Popper, currently in retirement in England and maybe with some of his finest work still to be published, is a highly significant philosopher in our times. His thought is rich and out of this richness may be distilled many lines of enquiry of relevance to medical practice.[17,18]

Popper pointed out that logically a scientific law is conclusively falsifiable although it is not conclusively verifiable. Popper therefore urges that we do not systematically evade refutation but we formulate our theories as unambiguously as possible so that they may be exposed to refutation. Where an observation is made which refutes the theory by methodology which is truly rigorous then we must search for a new hypothesis which may then be tested by devising confrontations between its consequences and new observable experience. It is a liberating thing to turn the mind not to defending (even irrationally) what one holds to be correct but to devising means whereby it could be shown to be false or inadequate. He wrote that: 'The man who welcomes and acts on criticism will prize it almost above friendship: the man who fights it out of concern to maintain his position is clinging to non-growth'.

A proposed medical care system is (if planned at all) basically an hypothesis generated in the face of data concerning needs, resources and foreseeable trends. It could be fruitful to seek deliberately for additional data which would demonstrate that the proposed plan (hypothesis) is inadequate, incorrect, 'false' rather than approaching the 'truth' in relation to the context within which it has been generated. A policy, then, according to Popper is an hypothesis which has to be tested against reality and corrected in the light of experience. Once again, the search for multiple pieces of evidence which would confirm the policy may be far less valuable (even though emotionally more comfortable) than the search for one soundly produced piece of evidence which would refute it.

There is a further area of Popper's thought put forward in *The Open Society and its Enemies* as the general guiding principle for public policy, namely, minimize avoidable suffering'. Popper bases this on his observation of, as it were, a logical asymmetry: we do not know how to make people happy (as the policy 'maximize happiness' demands) but we do know ways of lessening their unhappiness ('minimize unhappiness'). 'Instead of the greatest happiness for the greatest number, one should demand, more modestly, the least amount of avoidable suffering for all; and further, that unavoidable suffering, such as hunger in times of unavoidable shortage of food, should be distributed as equally as possible.' The relevance of this concept of health planning at the national, regional or local level is singularly obvious, and liberating indeed, capable of giving impetus to the creative spirit of health professionals.

The issue of the chronically ill and the elderly and indeed the dying is one focus of what we may call the weak/strong dilemma.

We cannot pass over the issues at the other extreme of life, where weakness is even more manifest. Once again, we must be aware of any decision concerning the weak which favours the powerful – for such is the stuff of evil as seen above. Mention has been made elsewhere[19] of the consternation of Professor Ian Donald (1910–1987) of Glasgow at the inappropriate foetal research he had observed making him question whether his own life had been worthwhile. Also noteworthy is the dismay of Bernard Nathanson (1926–2011) (himself instrumental in founding abortion clinics in New York where the safety of the mothers was assured) in the face of the current escalation of abortion – death in utero is now so common even in Australia that the uterus seems not safe for the human unborn. In a thoughtful paper which shocked his colleagues, Nathanson urgently bade all (as Leo Tolstoy (1828–1910) did) to reflect, for, as he commented, 'The issue is human life and deserves the reverent stillness and ineffably grave thought appropriate to it'.[20]

What can we say in the face of the weak/strong dilemma, the dimensions of which are very grave? It is not possible and maybe not even wise wholly to remove power from the powerful – nor to remove weakness from the weak, however much we try by health measures, income supplementation, social legislation or by resolutions, and so on – and nor can we move backwards into an extended family system where the weak can be cared for within a family network and thereby possibly though not necessarily be protected from exploitation.

There will always in human societies be disparities of power whatever the prevailing ideology. We may wish to return to (or move towards) a situation devoid of serious personal choice – what Karl Popper calls the 'closed society' rather than progress towards the 'open society' in which individuals are confronted with personal decisions. It is not surprising that after insisting that to remain human 'there is only one way, the way into the open society', Popper discusses the issue of the weak, and he needs to be quoted in full:

> According to a modern writer (G.H. Eastbrooks [1895–1973]), Man made the decisive mistake when he became civilized, and especially when he began to help the weak; before this, he was an almost perfect man-beast; but civilization, with its artificial methods of protection, must ultimately destroy itself. In reply to these arguments ... the theory that the human race might have lived a little longer if it had not made the fatal mistake of helping the weak is most questionable; but even if it were true, is mere length of survival of the race really all we want? Or is the almost perfect man-beast so eminently valuable that we should prefer a prolongation of his existence (he did exist for quite a long time anyway) to our experiment of helping the weak?
>
> ... There have been some amazing successes. Many of the weak have been helped, and for a hundred years, slavery has been practically abolished ... (even) if we had to return to the almost perfect man-beast, all this would not alter the fact that slavery once, for a short time, disappeared from the face of the earth. This fact, I believe, may comfort some of us for all our misfits, mechanised and otherwise; and to some of us, it may even atone for the fatal mistake our forefathers made when they missed the golden opportunity of arresting all change – of returning to the cage of the closed society

and of establishing, for ever and ever, a huge zoo of almost perfect monkeys.[21]

The spectre of a zoo of almost perfect monkeys is in harmony with the wholly regulated society of *Brave New World* where no weakness is tolerated. A hardening of society in which no defect and no weakness is tolerated is a society which has lost one of the most essential features of fully developed humanness – namely mercy. Mercy is a feature of highly evolved Man. Sir Charles Sherrington (1857–1952), in his celebrated Gifford lectures of 1937–38 (*Man on His Nature*), pointed to the dilemma which the man who would be truly altruistic faces:

> We think back with repugnance to that ancient biological pre-human scene whence, so we have learned, we came; there no life was a sacred thing. There millions of years of pain went by without one moment of pity, not to speak of mercy. Its life innately gifted with 'zest-to-live' was yet so conditioned that it must kill or die. For man, largely emancipated from those conditions, the situation has changed ... The change is in himself. Where have his 'values' come from?
>
> Those other creatures than himself, even the likest to himself, would seem without the values. There arises for him a dilemma and a contradiction. The contradiction is that he is slowly drawing from life the inference that altruism, charity, is a duty incumbent upon thinking life. That an aim of conscious conduct must be the unselfish life. But that is to disapprove the very means which brought him hither, and maintains him. Of all his new found values perhaps altruism will be the most hard to grow. The 'self' has been so long devoted to itself as end ... Man is grappling with its newly found 'values', yet with no experience except its own, no counsel but its own.[22]

Sherrington comments on the mysterious nature of morality in a scenario of Mother Nature addressing Man:

> You thought me moral, you now know me without moral. How can I be moral being, you say, blind necessity, being mechanism. Yet at length I brought you forth, who are moral. Yes, you are the only moral thing in all your world, and therefore the only immoral. You thought me intelligent, even wise. You now know me devoid of reason, most of me even of sense. How can I have reason or purpose being pure mechanism? Yet at length I made you, you with your reason. If you think a little you with your reason can know that; you, the only reasoning thing in all your world, are therefore the only mad one, ... You are my child.
>
> Do not expect me to love you. How can I love – I who am blind necessity? I cannot love, neither can I hate. But now that I have brought forth you and your kind, remember you are a new world unto yourselves, a world which contains in virtue of you, love and hate, and reason and madness, the moral and immoral, and good and evil. It is for you to love where love can be felt. That is, to love one another.
>
> Bethink you too that perhaps in knowing me you do but know the instrument of a Purpose, the tool of a Hand too large for your sight as now to compass. Try then to teach your sight to grow.

Maybe four decades later we may need to realise that the profound ethical problems of medicine are embodied in these issues: medical practice is for the good of Man, an embodiment of true altruism, expressed ultimately as mercy. We need not belittle the differences men have in naming 'the compass by which we steer our ship if we are to set a true course through life.' But we can go on to agree that 'all such formulations try to express Man's relatedness to a central order.'[23]

Medical practice so deeply immersed in the suffering, joy and mystery of the human is surely called to manifest however weakly 'the central order' of things ... it is concerned with the healing of the wounds of Man, the reintegration of Man, even as he dies.

The quality of mercy is the quality of the truly strong, the truly complete man. What may face us in the West is the need to make, as it were, a quantum leap into a new order of mercy, not as a manifestation of maudlin sentimentality but as the recognition by the strong that the rediscovery of mercy in the face of weakness may be the breath of life for our civilization – and for our health system. The inspiration and model for that mercy may after all need to be sought beyond ourselves.[24]

What can be said in the way of conclusion?

Tolstoy urged us to stop and reflect, and this we have done. For my part in it, I align myself with the comment of Carl Jung (1857–1952):

> I do not forget that my voice is but one voice, my experience a mere drop in the sea, my knowledge no greater than the visual field in a microscope, my mind's eye a mirror that reflects a small corner of the world, and my ideas – a subjective confession.[25]

In which direction shall we go? – 'it is open to every man to choose the direction of his striving',[26] as Albert Einstein (1879–1955) reminded us.

The resolution of the weak/strong dilemma appears to involve the recovery of mercy as a voluntary limit to power. The radical rethinking of the goals and processes of clinical practice needs to be undertaken in the light of reflection on the dignity and meaning of Man. The construction of a dream, the rebirth of a vision requires not only the inventiveness of Man but the tapping of the springs of hope.

MEDICINE AND COMMUNITY PART A SECTION III

Medical science is no 'Deus ex machina' – science is in the minds of men, practice is done by men and the direction must be set from within – by men filled with mercy, hope, inventiveness and a sense of servanthood. Let us above all, in the face of our failures, not be consumed by cynicism – an ever present danger as pointed out by Isaiah Berlin (1909–1997) of Oxford: 'No body of men which has tasted power, or is within a short distance of doing so, can avoid a certain degree of that cynicism which, like a chemical reaction, is generated by the sharp contact between the pure ideal, nurtured in the wilderness, and its realisation in some unpredicted form which seldom conforms to the hopes or fears of earlier times.'[27] Instead of cynicism, we may in our efforts to express mercy need to be merciful to ourselves in our own weakness – whilst still nurturing our ideals in a new wilderness.

Humanity is shifting its ground. The social context is dramatically changing, with, in many ways, a turn full circle as with microcomputer technology increasingly available as means of communication and action the focus can turn again on man-at-home, on individual initiative, on small-scale operation within networks, on life within a web of life, not beneath an umbrella of authority or of power. And yet all is like the spider's web, so delicate, so fragile. The whole web of global life may depend now on the integrity of leadership, as if the leaders were the meeting points or nodes of silken strands – and if these points yield, the results may be catastrophic.

It seems that there is a pressing and urgent need for doctors, who are by vocation on the side of Man, and by tradition embody something of the Good, to go out into the wilderness and rediscover the capacity and responsibility to lead, to heal, to protect – and because of all of this, to be springs of hope, and so to rediscover our real significance, our true power, and our participation in the mystery of mercy.

Victor Frankl (1905–1997) reminded us that: 'our generation is realistic for we have come to know Man as he really is. After all, Man is that being who has invented the gas chambers of Auschwitz: however, he is also that being who has entered those gas chambers upright, with the Lord's Prayer or the Shema Yisrael on his lips.'[28]

It may be fitting, then, that the poet, James McAuley (1917–1976), who died in Tasmania in 1976, has the last word:

> Incarnate word in whom all nature lives
> cast flame upon the earth; raise up contemplatives
> among us, men who walk within the fire
> of ceaseless prayer, impetuous desire.
> Set pools of silence in this thirsty land.

REFERENCES

1 Engels F., *The Condition of the Working Class in England* (1892), London, Granada Publishing, 1969.
2 Stone L., *The family, sex and Marriage in England* (abridged edition), Harmondsworth: Penguin, 1979.
3 Tawney R.H., *Equality*, London, Barnes and Noble, 1931.
4 Maritain J., *Redeeming the Time*. Trans. H.L. Binsse. London, Geoffrey Bles: The Centenary Press, 1953.
5 Russell B., 'Human Society in Ethics and Politics II'. Quoted M. Adler & C. van Doren (eds.) – *Great Treasury of Western Thought*, New York, Bowker, 1977.
6 Rilke RM., *Der Apostel* 1896, Quoted in *The Drama of Atheistic Humanism*, New York, World Publishing, 1963, in Translation in H. de Lubac, Trans. E.M. Riley, (First English Edition, 1950).
7 de Lubac H., op. cit.
8 Comte A., (in de Lubac op. cit.)
9 Hitler A., *Mein Kampf* (1925). Trans. R. Manheim, 1943, in Fromm E, *The Anatomy of Human Destructiveness*, 1973.
10 Kirby M., Chairman of the Reform Commission of Australia.
11 Fromm E., *The Anatomy of Human Destructiveness*, Holt, Rinehart and Winston, 1973.
12 Farr W., 'Vital Statistics', in F.B. Smith, *The People's Health 1830–1910*, Canberra, A.N.U. Press, 1979.

13 Maxwell R., *Health Care: The Growing Dilemma* (2nd ed.), New York, McKinsey and Co., 1975, p 2.
14 Rawls J., *A Theory of Justice*, Oxford, Oxford University Press, 1971.
15 Daniels N. (ed.), Reading Rawls, *Critical Studies of a Theory of Justice*, Oxford, Blackwell, 1975.
16 Beauchamp DE,. 'Public Health and Individual Liberty', *Health*, 1980; 1: 121–136, Ann Rev Public.
17 Popper K., *The Open Society and Its Enemies, Vols. 1 and 2*, London, Routledge, 1945, revised edit. 1966.
18 Popper K., *The Logic of Scientific Discovery*, London, Hutch Jon, 1959. (see also Magee B., Popper K., London, Collins, 1973).
19 Donald I., Life, Death and Modern Medicine. Social Responsibility Series, Order of Christian Unity. London, 1974.
20 Nathanson BN., 'Deeper into Abortion', N Engl *J Med*, 1974; 291:1180 (see also Nathanson B., *Aborting America*, Garden City, NY, Doubleday, 1979).
21 Popper K., *The Open Society and Its Enemies, Vol.2, The Spell of Plato*, London, Routledge, 1945, p268.
22 Sherrington CS., *Man on His Nature*, London, Cambridge University Press, 1940.
23 Eccles JC., 'The Human Psyche', *The Gifford Lectures*, University of Edinburgh, 1978–1980, Berlin: Springer International, 1980.
24 John Paul II., *Dives in Misericordia (On the Mercy of God)*, Encyclical Letter, 1980.
25 Jung C.G., *Modern Man in Search of a Soul*, and Kegan Paul, 1933, London, Routledge.
26 Einstein A., 'Considerations concerning the fundaments of theoretical physics', *Science* 1940 XCI: 487–92. (Reprinted in *Science, Faith and Man*, Wagar WW ed. London, Macmillan, 1968, p22).
27 Berlin I. *Four Essays on Liberty*, Oxford University Press, 1969.
28 Frankl V., *Man's Search for Meaning*, Beacon Press, 1962, p136. Oxford, Oxford University Press, 1969, Trans. I. Lasch. Boston.

B
OTHER PSYCHOLOGICAL AND SOCIAL DIMENSIONS OF MEDICINE

I
SPEECH AND COMMUNITY
1979

Edited version of presentation, in
Proceedings of Voice and Communication Disorders Convention,
The Australian Association of Speech and Hearing,
Annual Convention, Tasmania, 1979.

The momentum of modern medicine has provoked a philosophical dialogue forcing all parties to it to consider certain questions that long ago seemed more clear and settled: those questions concerning the value of human life, the basis of human dignity, the goal of human existence and the corollary duties of medicine to be governed by these assumptions.[1]

The earliest human records – art forms before words – bear testimony to the awareness of man of the mystery of himself, and history is strewn with attempts to formulate concepts concerning matters such as those raised by Stumpf: the value of human life, the basis of human dignity and the goal of human existence. Indeed, as Karl Popper stressed in a recent paper on his own work: 'All men are philosophers, because in one way or another all take up an attitude towards life and death'.[2]

In order to approach the mystery of humanness, many models, as it were, of man have been proposed through the ages.[3,4] Plato and Aristotle stressed the fundamental need for intellectual understanding. In more modern times the voluntarists tend to treat freedom and autonomy as ends rather than means, seeing autonomy as the final realisation of man's nature. Determinist views of man reject the concept of freedom and choice entirely, and attribute all thinking, acting, and making to the interplay between basic drives and environmental influences. Sigmund Freud saw man as 'driven' whilst modern behaviourists such as Skinner see man as wholly 'malleable'. Karl Marx in his early writings conceived of man as primarily a productive animal: 'We can distinguish men from animals as soon as they begin to produce the means of life ...'[5]

More recently man is seen more clearly as 'inventor', and some writers see this as a unifying focus for the consideration of man in the face of many other models reflecting particular perspectives or capacities. Philip Rhinelander of Stanford university wrote (1974):

> It is my belief that a unifying focus may be found if we stress man's capacity for inventiveness, recognizing that such inventiveness is displayed not merely in man's arts and crafts, but in his ability to establish complex symbol systems to make and modify social systems and to build elaborate normative system to guide his own behaviour. The root of man's inventiveness seems to lie in his capacity – evidently correlated with his highly developed brain – to envisage *possibilities* beyond the actualities of immediate experience.[6]

Man's capacity for symbol making finds one of its highest expressions in language, one of the most important and remarkable of human inventions. If we consider the model of man as inventive symbol maker as probably the richest model we have, and accept that language is the most remarkable symbol system invented by man, it is clear that language (written or spoken) is close to the core of what is human.

Speech therapists are involved in alleviating difficulties in a specifically human activity. Language, and therefore speech, is not only a specifically human activity (like laughter) but is crucial in personal development (which laughter may not be). Some discussion of the processes of personal development may indicate some reasons for such significance.

A Schema of Personal Development

Being human means being in process, on the way, in becoming, not a static entity. We are not yet what we fully are to be. What I am includes what I may become, just as it includes what I have been (and what my biological and cultural ancestors have been). My present incorporates my past but also enfolds (without determining) my future.

The process of human becoming is life-long from conception to death. From the mother's womb the babe is born into the womb of language,[7] of personal relationships, and other experiences within which slowly the personal lineaments become more clearly etched, or better, generated. We are continually becoming persons, being continually defined in relationship, for 'the personal is constituted by personal relatedness'.[8]

The environment is critical for optimum personal development and in one writer's words, 'the environment must provide that *outer wholeness and continuity* which, like a second womb, permits the child to develop his capacities in distinct steps.[9] The non-personal aspects of the environment – poverty, physical surroundings – may exert their most profound effects by any influence they have on the personal growth of the significant figures in a child's milieu. [The analogy here between the child and a hospitalised adult (still in the process of personal growth) should be obvious: the quality of persons interacting with the patient influences his or her human potential far more than the physical surroundings – though one must not decry the value of comfortable pillows and adequate pain killing drugs and other essential skills and technological hardware.]

William Shakespeare, in his talk of the seven ages of man, recognised the biological facts of stages of human development. Carl Rogers has written much on what it means to become a person, expressing in psychological terms the notions of the existentialist philosophers who would see man spending a life time shaping his own essence.[10] Erik Erikson has given much food for thought in his analysis.[11] He presented human growth from the point of view of the conflicts, inner and outer, which the healthy personality weathers, emerging and re-emerging with, among other things, an increased sense of inner unity. He held that there are inner laws of development, laws which create a succession of potentialities for significant interaction with others. While such interaction may vary from culture to culture, it must remain within the proper rate and the proper sequence which govern the growth of a personality as well as that of an organism.

Personality can be said to develop according to steps predetermined in the human organism's readiness to be driven toward, to be aware of, and to interact with, a widening social radius, beginning with the dim image of a mother and ending with mankind, or at any rate that segment of mankind which counts in the particular individual's life.[12]

Erikson saw, then, human growth as taking place by negotiation of developmental tasks through the resolution of crisis. The growing human being is continually faced by options, each life stage being characterised by its own options which, while they confront man throughout life, do come to a point of ascendency in a given stage. For example the favourable outcome of infancy is an attitude of basic trust, rather than one of basic distrust, and on this basis the child goes on to be faced with the choice of autonomy or fear of decision. Where the life process is characterised by the embracing of favourable options, the personality becomes characterised by trust, reasonable autonomy, initiative, capacity for effort, a sense of identity (to be oneself and share oneself) rather than confusion, capacity for intimate personal relationships (to lose and find oneself in another) instead of isolation, fruitfulness rather than stagnation, and finally a sense of integrity or wholeness of life rather than despair.

The negotiation of these developmental tasks involves inevitably personal relationships and the whole spectrum of human communication both within the present (verbal and non-verbal) and between past and present. In the course of such communication, life cycles, as Erikson called them, are interlocked, cog-wheeled as it were, welding together the human community into a matrix in continuous process or movement.

Language and the Life Stages

We are not involved here in a consideration of how language is acquired or used: that is fortunate and it is consoling that Noam Chomsky noted, 'Honesty forces us to admit that we are as far today as Descartes was three centuries ago from understanding just what enables a human to speak in a way that is innovative, free from stimulus control, and also appropriate and coherent.'[13] Nor will attention be paid to the way the form of social relationships acts selectively on the speech possibilities of the individual, with subsequent influence on behaviour: a field extensively researched by Bernstein and others and more familiar to this expert audience than to me, and usefully summarised for speech pathologists by Orlando Taylor in 1973.[14]

Rather, it might be useful to reiterate some points of particular relevance to the life stages outlined by Erikson in relation to certain other seminal and relevant concepts.

Personal development occurs through social interaction; growth in solitude is in a sense through interaction with the self. Weber defined social action: 'Action is social in so far as, by virtue of the subjective meaning attached to it by the acting individual (or individuals), it takes account of the behaviour of others and as is thereby oriented on its course.'[15] The essential note of meaning implies that social action is symbolic – and the most important symbolic action is language, spoken or written. As Robert Nisbet wrote in his analysis *The Social Bond*:

> It is language alone that makes possible the development of the human mind, the sense of self, the consciousness of personal identity, and that very fundamental capacity, unique in mankind, of being to adopt one or more of the social roles that confront each newborn infant in human society.[16]

It is clear that in the early stages of childhood when the lineaments of the self are being constructed, language is crucial. Nonverbal communication is seriously limited by the lack of what is one of the characteristics of language as a means of communication: namely, the capacity for displacement in time and space, so that the past and the faraway (or the future) are made present. The wider the spectrum of language to which a child is exposed or learns, the richer may be his awareness of self and the world. It is fair to assume that growth in basic trust will (if the personal environment is trustworthy) be facilitated by language not only as a means by which the perception of trustworthiness is reinforced but also as the means by which the child can concentrate the trust growing within him. It appears to be the same for the other developmental options of childhood, with the child needing not only to perceive but somehow externalise, by a symbol relating past and present and here and there, his emerging autonomy, initiative, industry, and sense of self identity. A question asked by my small nephew at 2½ years, 'Mummy, who are I?' embodied the questioning which language permits the emerging self to ask of the environment as part of the beginnings of the search for ego identity. Clarification of ego identity in adolescence by means of self-questioning, together with the search for the reflections of the self in the other, is surely the reason for the telephone blockade which occurs in homes of adolescents in middle class suburbia. It may be worth noting that in subcultures where the 'restricted code' of Bernstein is evident, non-verbal sexual exploration may form a more prominent part of a similar identity search. A sensitive remark of Kenneth Clark quoted by Erik Erikson may not be out of place:

> Illegitimacy in the ghetto cannot be understood or dealt with in terms of punitive hostility, as in the suggestion that unwed mothers be denied welfare if illegitimacy is repeated. Such approaches obscure, with empty and at times hypocritical moralizing, the desperate yearning of the young for acceptance and identity, the need to be meaningful to someone else even for a moment without implication of a pledge of undying fealty and foreverness.[17]

Speech therapists involved with children and adolescents would need to be mindful of the developmental tasks being negotiated to understand the significance of language, and its deficit. Each of the childhood stages has its favourable outcome outlined above and well detailed by Erikson, but at each stage the child is especially vulnerable to the possibility of the unfavourable option of each pair; for example, in the early years at school when the favourable option is development of a sense of industry, that effort is worthwhile. The ever present danger is the appearance of a sense of inferiority. A speech therapist would need exquisite sensitivity to avoid reinforcement of embryonic feelings of inferiority in a speech deficient child of such an age. Similarly, the adolescent has the ever present danger of moving in the direction of identity diffusion instead of that of a deepening ego synthesis. The speech therapist must not be surprised at the variability and unpredictability of the adolescent in this phase – rather she or he may be a point of continuity assisting the adolescent's movement towards constancy – or so it seems to a non-speech therapist.

The phases of adulthood are first the growth in the capacity to go out from self, to lose the self, finding the self again indeed but not continually searching for the reflection of the self as in adolescence, but rather the giving and the finding of the self already known. It is the time for profound partnership in friendship, genital sexuality, cooperative ventures of moment, as well as competition. It is the time of commitment, of marriage, of the taking on of responsibility. The risk is that of opting instead for isolation, withdrawal from intimacy and solidarity, of retreat into the often confused self. The stage merges into the phase characterised by Erikson as that of generativity, either expressed in the establishment of the next generation or in contributions to the human community in other forms of creativity, notably in the world of ideas (which Karl Popper calls 'World 3').[18]

Language (notably speech) is crucial in these adult stages. Stable intimacy implies breadth and depth and continuity of interpersonal communication by several forms of symbolic interaction, both verbal and non-verbal. Animal pairs may fondly caress, though not often apart from a sexual context, but as far as we know they cannot remind each other of a sunset a year ago or even of what was eaten the day before, for that matter. The capacity of language to bring past and future and the spatially distinct into the recent context is highly significant in relationships of intimacy and generativity. But language has limits even as a means of communication. Ivan Illich, in

The Celebration of Awareness, noted the eloquence of silence: 'The man who shows that he knows the rhythm of our silence is much closer to us than one who thinks he knows how to speak'.[19]

The generativity of human persons has implications in the realm of language: two perspectives, both maybe a little oblique but precious, may be introduced.

James McAuley who died in Tasmania in 1976 wrote:

> CREDO
> That each thing is a word
> Requiring us to speak it
> From the ant to the quasar,
> From clouds to ocean floor –
> The meaning not ours, but found
> In the mind deeply submissive
> To the grammar of existence,
> The syntax of the real.[20]

Here is a concept that man responds to what is, discerning its meaning, required somehow to speak the word which each thing is.

There is another concept – long ago articulated by the author (individual or collective) of Genesis. Adam, the first man, is pictured as *naming* the animals: a semitic way of indicating his power and capacity to be a source of meaning. It may be that man is not only a searcher after meaning (and we cannot live with utter meaninglessness), but also has the capacity to be a giver of meaning, a source of significance, and a role therefore in the construction of reality. Peter Berger and Thomas Luckmann in *The Social Construction of Reality*[21] give a glimpse of the role of the community, of humans bonded together in this activity, and in the reinforcement and maintenance of the reality so constructed. Karl Popper's exposé of the growth of human knowledge by observing the objectivising of ideas enabling criticism has affinity with the same concepts.

What relevance has this for the speech therapist? Maybe it is essential to recognise the creativity of man by means of language: to assist a person with a speech deficit not merely to communicate need and emotion, but also to be creative, to invent, to construct, even within the therapeutic relationship, new reality.

Erikson's analysis of personal growth is sensitive indeed in its consideration of the task of the elderly. He conceives the task as the development of a sense of wholeness, of *integrity*:

> Only he who in some way has taken care of things and people and adapted himself to the triumphs and disappointments of being, by necessity the originator of others and the generator of things and ideas – only he may gradually grow the fruit of the seven stages. I know no better word for it than integrity. It is the acceptance of one's own and only life cycle and of the people who have become significant to it as something that had to be … an acceptance of the fact that one's life is one's own responsibility. It is a sense of comradeship with men and woman of distant times and of different pursuits, who have created orders and objects and sayings conveying human dignity and love.

On the other hand, Erikson noted further:

> [T]he lack or loss of this accrued ego integration is signified by despair and an often unconscious fear of death: the one and only life cycle is not accepted as the ultimate of life. Despair expresses the fear that the time is short, too short for the attempt to start another life and to try out other roads to integrity. Such a despair is often hidden behind a show of disgust, a misanthropy or

a chronic contemptuous displeasure which (where not allied with constructive ideas and a life of cooperation) only signify the individual's contempt of himself.[22]

Erikson has been quoted at length not only because the source is relatively inaccessible but also because a large number of speech therapy patients are elderly, and are in a crucial developmental phase. The shape of the task needs to be understood by those in contact with the elderly. They may well vacillate between wholeness and despair and need to be supported gently. They may long for and need to recover the language whereby they can express their internal states, explore the threat of despair, and through dialogue with significant others, reach out again towards the wholeness which is possible. It is surely the task of each man to explore his own possibilities. To express what one has become requires symbols – normally the symbol system of language. So language deficit in the elderly is a grave deprivation and therapeutic skills must be a privilege to possess.

Quite apart from the normal developmental crises, the client of the speech therapist is in what is sometimes called a situation of accidental crisis. Certainly sudden language loss is a crisis situation of the first order. It may be useful to recall that a crisis represents a growth opportunity and the speech therapist in touch with what is most human in the stricken has the opportunity to be a source of hope. If there is a comprehension deficit, the threat of meaninglessness is even worse than in solely expressive dysphasia, and the threat strikes at the human core.

In the end, when no remedy is possible, there may have to be reverence for that in man which is beyond human language; for not only are we called to speak the words which things are, but we ourselves are words spoken. As Martin Buber, the Jewish philosopher, wrote: 'Our being spoken is our existence ... In the measure that each of us reveals himself to the others, fulfilling the speech that he is, we allow the Coming One to come ...'[23]

So beyond speech, finally there is only the listening to the words things are, to the words others are, to the word enfleshed in the self and in openness to the source.

REFERENCES

1. Stumpf SE., 'Some moral dimensions of medicine'. *Annals Internal Medicine*, 1966, 64, 460.
2. Popper KR., 'How I see philosophy', in *Philosophers on Their Own Work*, Vol 3, edited by Andre Mercier and Maja Svilar, Peter Lane, Berne, Frankfurt am Main, Las Vegas, 1977, 147.
3. Nash P., *Models of Man*, Wiley, NY, 1968.
4. Rhinelander PH., *Is Man Comprehensible to Man?* Freeman, San Francisco, 1974.
5. Marx K., *Capital and Other Writings*, ed Eastman, Modern library, 1932, 1 (Quoted in Rhinelander op cit, p71).
6. Rhinelander, op. cit., p 97.
7. Bernstein T., 'Complementarity and philosophy', *Nature* 222 1969 1033–35.
8. MacMurray J., *Persons in Relation*, Gifford Lectures, University of Glasgow, 1954, Faber and Faber, London 1961, p 61.
9. Erikson EH., 'The roots of virtue', in *The Humanist Frame*, ed by JS Huxley, Allen and Unwin, 1962, p 151.
10. Rogers C., 'What it means to become a person', in *The Self*. ed by C Moustakis, Harper and Row, New York, 1956, p 211.
11. Erikson EH., *Childhood and Society*, 2nd Edit. Penguin, London, 1965 (and other writings).
12. Erikson EH., *Identity and the Life Cycle*, Psychological Issues Monograph, International Universities Press, New York, 1968, p52.
13. Chomsky, N. *Language and Mind*, Hardcourt, Brace and World, New York, 1968, p11.
14. Taylor OL., 'Sociolinguistics and the Practice of Speech Pathology', *Rehabilitation Record* 14 1973 pp14–17.
15. Weber M., *The Theory of Social and Economic Organization*, trans by AM Henderson and Talcott Parsons, Oxford University Press, New York, 88 (quoted in Nisbet, vide infra).
16. Nisbet RA., *The Social Bond*. Knopf, New York, 1970, p58.

17 Clark K., *Dark Ghetto*, Harper and Row New York, 1965, p73, quoted by EH Erikson in *Identity: Youth and Crisis*, Faber, London, 1968, p307.
18 Popper KR., *How I see philosophy*, op. cit. 142 'I follow common sense in holding that there exists both matter (World 1) and mind (World 2), and I suggest that there exist also other things, especially the products of the human mind, which include our scientific conjectures, theories and problems (World 3)'.
19 Illich ID., *Celebration of Awareness: A Call for Institutional Revolution*, Doubleday, New York, p47.
20 McAuley J, *Collected Poems 1936–70*, Angus and Robertson, Sydney, 1971, p92.
21 Berger PL and Luckmann T., *The Social Construction of Reality: A Treatise on the Sociology of Knowledge*, Penguin, Harmondsworth, 1967.
22 Erikson EH., *Identity and the Life Cycle*, op. cit., p98.
23 Buber M., 'Since we have been a dialogue', in *A Believing Humanism: Gleanings*, Trans M Friedman, Sinn and Schuster, New York, 1969, p85.

II
Psychological Aspects of Cancer
1980

*Edited version of keynote address at the
New South Wales Cancer Council Workshop on Psychological
and Biochemical Determinants of Cancer, Sydney, 1979.
In The Medical Journal of Australia, April 6 1980 1: 297–302).*

Richard Doll, considering the prospects for prevention of cancer, outlined four recent developments giving grounds for cautious optimism: the recognition that the incidence of cancer varies from place to place and from time to time associated with environmental and behavioural changes; the appreciation that cancer is preceded by detectable and possibly treatable pre-cancerous tissue lesions; recognition of those people prone to cancer; and the notable development in virology.[1] With respect to the third of these developments, Doll wrote:

> Knowledge of factors that affect individual susceptibility – genetic, constitutional and psychological – is beginning to accumulate so that prophylactic efforts may possibly be concentrated where they will be most rewarding.

Discussion for present purposes will be limited to those aspects which assist in providing perspective in a rather confused field, in the interests of avoiding waste of research effort in the future. [Walter] Walshe, in 1846,[2] may have considered that questioning of the reality of the connection between psychological factors and carcinogenesis was 'a struggle against reason'; it may, however, be rational to scrutinize the supposed connection with great care, not only to confirm its reality (if it can sustain the scrutiny), but also to discern fruitful ways to make conceptual advances as to its nature.

A Short History

[Aelius] Galen, in the sixth century AD is said to have alleged that cancer is more common in 'melancholic' than in 'sanguine' women. This idea was taken up again by clinicians many centuries later.

[SJ] Kowal, in a review of the attitudes of eighteenth and nineteenth century physicians towards cancer,[3] noted that they were impressed by the frequency with which adverse life situations seemed to occur before the diagnosis of cancer. A common denominator which they noted was a reaction of despair and hopelessness following various personal stresses.

The excellent reviews of cancer research in the nineteenth century provided by [VA] Triolo[4,5] indicate clearly that experimental pathology was the dominant influence, but it is important to note the scientists recognized that, while tissue and cellular changes were the characteristic phenomena of cancer, both inherent susceptibility and extrinsic influences played a part in genesis of these phenomena – by mechanisms unclear.

Triolo noted that 'hereditary aberrations and physical and chemical disturbances within the tissue environment, as internal seats of disordered growth, become pivotal issues in oncology after 1850'. Some eminent nineteenth century clinicians were adamant that psychological factors contributed in some way to this intrinsic predisposition to cancer.

Willard Parker, who operated on breast cancer patients in New York from 1830 to 1883, wrote up a study of 93 cases and noted:

> There are the strongest physiological reasons for believing that great mental depression, particularly grief, induces a predisposition to such disease as cancer, or becomes an exciting cause under circumstances where

the predisposition has already been acquired.[6]

James Paget wrote in the second edition of his text, *Surgical Pathology*:

> The cases are so frequent in which deep anxiety, deferred hope and disappointment are quickly followed by the growth and increase of cancer, that we can hardly doubt that mental depression is a weighty addition to the other influences favouring the development of the cancerous constitution.[7]

Herbert Snow, in 1893, went further. [Laurence] LeShan and [Richard] Worthington[8] outlined a statistical study undertaken by Snow. In 156 of 250 patients of the Cancer Hospital (London), '... there had been immediately antecedent trouble, often in very poignant form as the loss of a near relative ...', and Snow wrote:

> We find that the number of instances in which malignant disease of the breast and uterus follows immediately antecedent emotion of a depressing character is too large to be set down to chance, or to that general liability to the buffets of ill fortune which the cancer patients in their passage through life share with most other people not so affected.

Snow, in relation to cancers in general, considered that 'lowered vitality, in other words, prostration of the nervous system, might fairly be termed a cause of all cases'.

It is not surprising that, in the early decades of the twentieth century, as Sigmund Freud and his school drew the attention of scientists to the complexities of the human mind and the influence of psychological factors in the genesis of physical conditions, the interest in the possible role of psychological factors in the genesis of cancer waxed rather than waned. An editorial in the *British Medical Journal* in

1925, after discussing some recent work, stated that 'indirectly nervous influence must be regarded as of great importance in the production of cancer'.[9]

In the next decade, further papers appeared. In 1926, [Elida] Evans considered that in persons with cancer, detached energy, upon experiencing the stress of some intense renunciation in adulthood, had turned inward and expressed itself through a primitive erotic outlet.[10] The influence of psychoanalytic concepts is clear.

Studies Since 1945

In the period after World War 11, there was a resurgence of research interest. Excellent reviews of these studies are available.[11,12,13,14,15,16]

Since 1945, studies of psychological factors in neoplastic development appear to have, in the main, fallen into one of six groups: (i) animal studies; (ii) descriptive human studies; (iii) human studies involving a control group; (iv) studies concerning possible mechanisms; (v) studies concerning further neoplastic progression (including metastases); and (vi) studies concerning patient response to diagnosis and to treatment. Obviously, any attempt to categorize the vast numbers of papers on rather broader but related issues (such as social change in relation to cancer) is quite beyond the scope of this paper.

Animal Studies

RC LaBarba,[17] in reviewing studies in animals, noted in passing that methodology in human studies left much to be desired.

His detailed review of the animal work led him to similar conclusions and he urged more concerted efforts towards a systematic standardized research programme. In his review, he did note with some interest the efforts of some researchers to introduce stressors rather nearer to life's realities (for animals) than, say, repeated electric shocks. [RC] LaBarba related that one worker, Matthes, even exposed mice, rats, rabbits and chickens to hungry ferrets to see the effect of such stress on their tumours.

[MM] Jensen,[18] in reporting a study of the influence of stress on murine leukaemia virus infection, outlined several stressing procedures, and a brief description of one of them may assist in preparing for a point to be made below. Jensen described an 'avoidance-learning stress' which involved a shuttle box apparatus automatically programmed to require the mice to jump a barrier to the opposite side of a compartment once every five minutes on the presentation of a warning buzzer and a light. Mice soon learned to avoid the electric shock, and were thus exposed primarily to the stress (Jensen notes) of anticipation of pain and fear.

The problem here is that other factors which are possibly of relevance to tumour development may well be induced by such a 'stress' mechanism. It is known, for example, that exercise has influence on tumour development[19] and so a confounding variable may well be introduced into the system outlined by Jensen. It is a nice point to design a stressor which cannot influence movement, nutrition, mating patterns, exposure to possibly carcinogenic chemicals and so on.

This problem is illustrated by a recent study by [V] Riley[20] who placed some mice in a special type of housing designed to be protective against infections, cross-contamination, aerosols and chemicals, and was thus considered to reduce stress. In addition, unnecessary handling was reduced. Such mice were compared with other mice housed in standard steel shoe-box style cages. There were other groups within the experimental design but the point at issue is that 'stress' was considered to be the difference between the two forms of housing, and the reduction of tumour incidence observed in the animals in the plastic boxes was attributed to a reduction in stress. It appears, however, that many other variables could have influenced the experiment, and that an experiment needs to be devised to control for some of these variables (if this has not already been done by Riley's group).

Descriptive Studies

Descriptive human studies were frequently reported in the post-war years; despite their limitations, they are of considerable interest. At least careful descriptive studies can provide the seeds of hypotheses worthy of rigorous testing. For convenience, the main features of some of these descriptive studies are brought together in the Appendix.[21,22,23,24,25,26,27,28,29]

The concept of loss of an important relationship had arisen in the studies of Snow in 1893, Evans in 1926, and Foque in 1931,[30] all of whom were reviewed by LeShan and Worthington in 1956.[8] More recent studies generated the same concept. Greene, after summarizing his careful studies for the New York Academy of Science meeting in 1966, concluded as follows:

> The study of these three series of patients, which now include over 100 in number, show that the manifest leukaemia or lymphoma developed in a setting in which the patient was also dealing with a number of losses or separations with understandable feelings of sadness. anxiety, anger or hopelessness.
>
> To the extent that psychological factors may prove to be relevant to the pathogenesis of leukaemias and lymphomas, it is my impression that it is not so much a matter of the individual running into psychological conflicts engendering guilt or boomeranging aggression. but rather his running out of psychological resources engendering shame and hopelessness.[28]

In a review at the same meeting, LeShan gave a vivid description of the patterns he had perceived, and is worth quoting at length:

> In this description of the life history pattern which was found so typically in the cancer patients, reference has been made to a quality which we have called 'despair' ... The depth and intensity of this orientation is so great that it is difficult to describe. Basically, it is a bleak hopelessness about ever achieving any real feelings of meaning or enjoyment in life. The person feels condemned to make tremendous efforts to find meaningful relationships and roles which will enable him to share the zest, the enthusiasm and the feeling of belonging that he senses in others, but deeply believes that these efforts will ultimately fail. There will be only the struggle without the rewards. There is a complete loss of faith in the ability of outside objects to bring any meaningful rewards and loss of faith in his own development ever bringing him to a stage where he will feel less cut off. In the patient with a psychotic depression, there is still somehow, somewhere a ray of hope. The orientation that emerged in the cancer patients is bleaker than that. They have utterly despaired of being themselves ... Most of them had repressed the emotions connected with this despair and accepted their lives as they saw them with a stoic lack of bitterness or resentment.[31]

The inability to express hostile feelings successfully was noted by [C] Bacon *et alii* in 1952[24] on the basis of interviews, by [BA] Cobb in 1952[23] on the basis of interviews, questionnaires and projective tests, by [B] Butler in 1954[32] on the basis of psychiatric interviews, and by [L] LeShan and Worthington in 1955[33] using the above-mentioned personal history test.

LeShan and Worthington also confirmed findings of strong unresolved tensions concerning a parental figure. Similar concepts emerged in the work of Evans[10] using a Jungian psychoanalysis, [M] Tarlau and [L] Smalheiser[22] using Rorschach tests, drawings of human figures and interviews, and that of Bacon and colleagues[24] using interviews.

[M] Cutler and colleagues[34] studied 50 patients with cancer. They made observations on the first 18 cases, and, on the basis of these, developed predictive tests which were applied to the next 32 cases. They were able to predict, on the basis of MMPI, Wechsler-Bellevue and Rorschach tests, which patients would have fast-growing tumours and which would have slow-growing tumours. The patients with rapidly growing tumours had more defensiveness, a higher anxiety level, and less ability to reduce tension through motor discharge.

The problem with the descriptive studies (of which researchers are well aware) is the perennial problem of uncontrolled studies: are the trends observed more than would be expected? [WA] Greene rightly points out the problems of a choice of controls for the leukaemia/lymphoma patients reported so carefully. Advances in investigative and clinical medicine have frequently been made on the meticulous observations of astute clinicians. The problems, however, remain. The patients may not in reality be different from the population from which they arose if a valid control group can be examined. Further, the long latent period of human tumours is such that personality traits observed before the diagnosis may be reflections, not causes, of the neoplastic condition – neuropsychiatric sequelae of tumours are well recognized. Kerr, Schapira and Roth[35] concluded from a prospective study of males with affective disorders that:

'Our own findings support the view that a depressive illness developing in men of late middle age without previous psychiatric illness, occurring without apparent cause and characterized by features of both reactive and endogenous depression, may be an early and direct manifestation of malignant disease'.

Some descriptive studies had a comparative element. LeShan and Worthington[33] compared 150 patients with unspecified malignant tumours with patients with non-malignant conditions or no disease. Using their personal history test, they considered and demonstrated three factors which differentiated the patients with malignancy:

i loss of a major cathexis within 10 years before diagnosis;

ii less ability to express hostility; and

iii more tension over the death of a parent, often long before diagnosis.

However, some methodological problems occurred in this study and David Kissen, one of the eminent workers in this field, wrote in 1960:

> What is important is that too many deep studies, involving two few patients and without controls or objectivity, are used as the basis for too many profound conclusions.[36]

His own meticulous studies of psychological factors in lung cancer attempted to overcome these objections and his contribution (with a bibliography of his studies) is summarized in a dedication to his memory by the 1969 conference of the New York Academy of Sciences.[37] His studies, those of [AH] Schmale and [HP] lker,[38,39] and those of [S] Greer and colleagues[40,41] sought to assess patients with a high probability of a particular malignant condition before the diagnosis was known to patient, medical staff members or researchers, and, where possible, these studies tested hypotheses. All these studies sought to avoid sampling errors and investigators' knowledge of the diagnosis, and to give precision with respect to the site and extent of the cancer. The main features of the studies merit some discussion.

[DM] Kissen studied chest patients in chest units before a diagnosis of lung cancer had been made in some of them. In a conference of the New York Academy of Science on the theme of psychophysiological aspects of cancer in 1966, Kissen reviewed his earlier studies.[42] He had demonstrated with a high level of consistency and predictability that lung cancer patients have a diminished outlet for emotional discharge compared with non-cancer chest patients. He also compared lung cancer patients with non-chest unit non-cancer patients as representative of the general population. It was noted in the latter study that those with a poor outlet for emotional discharge appeared to have over four times the risk of lung cancer by comparison with those with good outlets, and the differences were present at all levels of smoking. There appeared to be evidence that the poorer the outlet for emotional discharge, the less exposure to cigarette smoke was required to induce lung cancer. Thus, the distribution of lung cancer patients among heavy smokers did not appear to be random. Kissen also studied the pattern of so-called adverse life events in lung cancer patients, but emphasized the part played by the personality in determining the significance of a life situation to an individual; he foreshadowed here the more recent emphasis on the 'social meaning' to the individual of 'adverse' events.

Schmale and Iker of Rochester, in a series of studies, demonstrated with remarkable consistency that in women with atypical cervical cytology being subjected to biopsy, high levels of hopelessness with awareness of inability to cope with certain life crises ('giving up hopelessness'); are predictive of cancer. In 1971, they summarized their ideas:

> We speculate that such characteristics as low social and economic status, early coitus, promiscuity, early and unhappy marriage, divorce, early pregnancy, etc., are all factors associated with cervical dysplasia but not directly with carcinoma ... We conceive of the cellular dysplasia as the initiator and the psychological experience of hopelessness as a promoter agent. We continue to subscribe to the theory which states that a high hopelessness potential provides a special somatic vulnerability through a loss of ego control for women who are already biologically predisposed to cancer of the cervix.[43]

In the 1979 Kissen Memorial Lecture,[41] Greer summarized the studies which he and his colleagues had done in relation to breast cancer. They tested systematically certain hypotheses which had been advanced previously about the psychological correlates of breast cancer: a history of stressful life events (particularly the loss of a loved person); antecedent depression; the use of denial as a characteristic defence; difficulty in expressing emotions (particularly hostile feelings); and extraversion. They studied a consecutive series of 160 women admitted for breast tumour biopsy, 69 of whom were subsequently found to have breast cancer. No significant associations were found between breast cancer and extraversion, denial as the characteristic response to life stresses, depression during the previous five years or the occurrence of stressful life events (including loss of a loved person) during the previous 20 years. The main positive correlation was with a tendency to extreme suppression of anger throughout adult life: patients were classed as suppressors if they had never or not more than twice during their adult lives openly shown anger and had always or nearly always concealed other feelings. It was found that diagnostic prediction made solely with the psychological variables proved to be as accurate (72%) as one based on the standard clinical variables (size and outline of tumour, superficial or deep tethering, nipple discharge or in version and palpability of ipsilateral lymph nodes). The consistency is impressive of the studies such as those of Kissen, Schmale and Greer and their colleagues. The predictive capacity of their hypothesis is powerful. These studies cannot be dismissed on the evidence available, but the questions they raise are almost innumerable.

Recently, a group at Buffalo reported comparative studies with respect to antecedent social trauma in 358 breast cancer patients compared with 670 patients with other types of cancer;[44] no difference was found between these groups concerning the extent to which the subjects or their families had experienced in the five years before onset of symptoms: death; divorce; illness; economic want; residential mobility; or feeling of being upset. A study was also undertaken, using similar methodology, of social trauma in relation to carcinoma of the cervix.[45] Although the patients with cervical cancer differed from patients with other cancers in certain respects (lower socioeconomic status, earlier marriage, more pregnancies), there was no difference with respect to experience of death, divorce, illness, economic want, residential mobility or upset feelings in patients or their families within five years of diagnosis.

A small group of prospective cohort studies merits discussion.

[O] Hagnell[46] interviewed all 2550 persons in a Swedish population and classified personality according to the method of Sjöbring of Lund in terms of four independent, continuously varying dimensions of personality function: 'capacity factor', 'stability factor', 'solidity factor' and 'validity factor'.

Hagnell located the cancer cases 12 years later, and no associations were observed between cancer incidence and rated levels of validity, solidity or capacity; however, sub-stability was significantly correlated with cancer in women, but not in men. The mechanisms operating were unclear, but it was considered that substability was, in a sense, a measure of the degree of emotional control: sub-stable persons are warm and sociable, but, when depressed, exhibit inertia and inhibition.

[RJ] Keehn and colleagues[47] reported a study of nearly 10 000 World War II United States Army veterans discharged for psychoneurosis in 1944. They did not demonstrate any increased risk of cancer by comparison with a control group matched for age, race, sex, mode of entry into service, and length of service.

[CS] Thomas has reported[48,49,50] the outcomes in terms of various forms of illness of a cohort of Johns Hopkins medical students in 17 successive classes (graduating between 1943 and 1964). The suicide, mental illness and malignant tumour groups had low mean scores for closeness to parents. The mental illness group showed the most nervous tension, depression, and anger under stress, and the malignant group the least. These findings are consistent with the findings of Kissen.

One other prospective study has some relevance. [R] Paffenbarger and colleagues[51] reported the preliminary results of a study of 50 000 former students of Harvard University and the University of Pennsylvania with respect to later development of Hodgkin's disease by 45 of them. It was found that the risk of Hodgkin's disease was lower in men who had experienced common contagious diseases in childhood, and higher for students who had reported early death of a parent (especially from cancer) and for students who were obese, heavy cigarette smokers and coffee drinkers. There was no comment made concerning personality measures.

It is hard not to surmise that there are indeed some interrelationships of 'mind and cancer', despite the extraordinary complexity and heterogeneity of the studies reported. The problems remain of possible mechanisms and of creation of a conceptual framework which can hold observed facts together.

Possible Mechanisms

Several authors, especially Fox[15] and Greer,[41] summarize possible mechanisms whereby psychological factors could work in influencing carcinogenesis, the most obvious pathways being via the immune or endocrine systems. Greer's brief summary of the situation may be usefully quoted (omitting documentation):

> What of the effects of psychological stimuli on endocrine and immune functions? There is firm evidence that emotional arousal leads to changes in circulatory levels of catecholamines, corticosteroids, growth hormone and prolactin ... Emotional arousal may also affect androgens and oestrogens ... as well as thyroid function ... but the evidence for the last-mentioned remains inconclusive ... Of particular interest and importance are a number of studies which have demonstrated that effectiveness of psychological defences is associated with corticosteroid production. The endocrine system can now be reasonably described as a third effector system of the brain, together with the musculoskeletal and autonomic nervous systems.
>
> Less is known about the effects of psychological stimuli on the immune system. It is considered likely that such effects are mediated principally through neuroendocrine pathways; one example is the release in response to stress of corticosteroids which have an immunosuppressive action ... The evidence that psychological factors can alter immune function is mainly indirect, being based either on animal studies, or on

reports of immunological abnormalities in psychotically disturbed patients, or on studies linking stress with the onset and course of diseases associated with dysfunction of the immune system ... Direct evidence is rare: hypnotic suggestion was shown to alter immediate and delayed hypersensitivity responses in an early series of experiments ... Severe psychological stress was reported to produce rises in 48 and 198 class serum proteins in one study and depression of T-cell function in another ...

The mechanisms of neoplastic development were reviewed in the last decade in a masterly two volume study by Leslie Foulds.[52,53] It is clear that the processes leading to clinically evident cancer as an outcome are complex. We are not concerned here with the fundamental nature of neoplasia, and can accept that what is at stake is, as Foulds put it, 'a stable, probably irreversible, replicable intracellular change'. It is essential that all considerations of the possible role of psychological (including behavioural) factors on the genesis of cancer in humans recognize that there is no real doubt that intracellular change is the final common path of these factors. Observed psychological phenomena (such as sadness and hopelessness) must affect subcellular elements by some intermediary mechanism. It is crucial that, in the laudable recognition that a person is one whole with functions that can be considered at several levels (total person, organ, tissue, cellular, subcellular, and so on) and is part of a larger whole, recognition of basic chemicophysical mechanisms be not obscured. A human person is indeed one whole, but the mechanisms are still unclear by which functional relationships within that whole are sustained, such that phenomena at one level of organization do affect and reflect phenomena at another level.

There are even simpler traps to be avoided. The person with feelings of hopelessness may have altered nutrition, interference with sleep patterns, altered exercise patterns, exposure to known environmental carcinogens, and so on. These behavioural changes must be considered without forging an immediate link between mental state and a cellular change, even via the immune or endocrine systems.

Further, it needs to be recognized that, whereas the role of immune factors in neoplasia is evident in animals, the situation in man is both complex and unsure. Immunosuppression has not been shown to predispose to the common tumours and particularly not to the tumours studied by Kissen (lung), Schmale (cervix) and Greer (breast). D. W. Weiss has said:

> It must be emphasized, nonetheless, that there is still no proof for a pathway leading from emotional state via immunological mechanisms to an effect on neoplasia, and even much stronger evidence that is currently available on the impairment of immune function under certain psychodynamic conditions that also favor neoplasia would still not prove categorically that the relationship is causal and not coincidental.[54]

Studies Concerning Further Neoplastic Progression

The metastatic process has been studied from many points of view and there has been considerable discussion of the influence of host factors. Of particular relevance to the present discussion are two Australian observations that smoking may facilitate the formation of metastases in melanoma,[55] and the influence of intensive meditation on regression of metastases.[56,57]

Studies Concerning Patient Response to Diagnosis and Treatment

Greer[41] listed some recent studies relevant to psychological aspects of the clinical situation of the patient with cancer – for example, communication between doctors and patients, causes of delay in medical consultation among cancer patients, and progress of cancer patients after treatment in terms of their psychological and social adjustment. A paper of considerable interest with regard to the last point, but not mentioned by Greer, is that of Weisman and Worden of Harvard[58] concerning what they term the 'existential plight' of the patient with cancer during the phase after diagnosis and definitive treatment. The present paper does not focus on these issues despite their crucial importance concerning quality of life, but the possibility appears credible that psychological factors operating after the diagnosis of cancer has been made may well influence the continuing neoplastic process: the work of Cutler,[34] may be relevant. Any aspect of the clinical management of cancer patients which raises the anxiety level, adds to defensiveness and interferes with tension discharge may well accelerate neoplastic progression. Oncologists will never agree upon which measures do these things; patients may, however, prove to be good guides and research is needed with respect to this matter.

Conclusions and Questions

What are pointers to the way ahead in seeking to unravel what appear to be unspeakably complex constellations of psychological phenomena which may well be causally related to carcinogenesis by routes other than mere behavioural change leading to exposure to known carcinogenic agents? It appears that development is needed of both conceptual models and hypotheses as well as methodology if knowledge and understanding are to be advanced.

[PS] Todd and [CJ] Magarey[59] offer a significant contribution to methodology by developing operational definitions and valid measures of ego defences using a system of explicit behavioural criteria.

Crisp[12] offered a complex model emphasizing the multifactorial aetiology of cancer with what he called the 'mind-body apparatus' in close interrelationship with the 'social-natural' environment.

[J] Cassel,[60] among others, offers probably the simplest model (and possibly the most useful) lending itself to detailed development. In his discussion of psychosocial factors in disease aetiology (he did not deal with cancer specifically, but rather with disease in general), he reviewed 'the clues from animal studies indicating that changes in the social milieu (particularly changes in group membership and the quality of group relationships) could, through demonstrable neuroendocrine mechanisms, markedly alter the responses of the body to a wide variety of stimuli'. Cassel went on to discuss general principles or hypotheses applicable to human studies relating to social disorganization, dominance and subordination, and social buffers. Cassel concluded that certain conditions of social change and disorganization, rather than having a specific aetiological role, would enhance susceptibility to disease in general: 'The specific manifestations of disease would be a function of the genetic predisposition of the individuals and the nature of the physio-chemical or neurobiological insults they encounter'. Cassel's model needs to be complemented by the concept of neoplastic development occurring in definable stages over time, as outlined especially by Foulds: it is distinctly possible that immunoendocrine mechanisms may be concerned with one phase of this process rather than with another – for example, with enhancement of progression of the process rather than with initiation.

With these and other reservations, such a model does offer the opportunities to dissect out some elements in a possible chain of causality, and to design studies either to obtain necessary descriptive data or to test out reasonable hypotheses. Investigation appears to be warranted: (a) in seeking correlation between 'giving up hopelessness' and immunological/endocrine status in cross-sectional and longitudinal studies; (b) in assessing predictability on psychological grounds (at time of initial treatment) of relapse in persons with neoplasms highly likely to relapse within five years (for colon cancer at Dukes stage B and C, certain categories of melanoma); and (c) in 'bereaved' persons, after [RW] Bartrop,[61] to seek correlation between the type of response to bereavement and immunological competence.

[I] Berenblum, after nearly 50 years' work as a scientist seeking to unravel the problems of cancer biology, wrote:

> We find ourselves at the present time in the era of molecular biology, and we are perhaps unduly influenced by the genetic code as the dominant principle in biology. Perhaps, in a decade or two from now, the dominant principle may shift to another plane, which in turn will influence our speculations about tumour causation. A chapter on 'Theories of Tumour Causation' might then relegate those based on genetic principles to the category of 'outmoded theories', with a very different set of 'contemporary' theories presented for serious consideration ...[62]

Medical science demonstrates its creativity in the questions which it frames, and it is inevitable that questions must be raised at ever deeper levels of inquiry. We have barely begun to see even the shape of the questions which will finally need to be asked concerning the interrelationship of the mind and neoplasia since we are involved in reflecting upon the self and, in this, we are, by nature, limited.

Appendix

Some studies which described psychological factors in cancer patients are noted.

1. **Miller, and Jones**, 1948.[21]
   Tumour: Chronic granulocytic leukaemia. The authors reported that 'frequent occurrence of emotional difficulties in patients with leukaemia may be more than a coincidental finding' and described six cases showing marked emotional stress before the leukaemia was diagnosed.

2. **Tarlau, and Smalheiser**, 1951.[22]
   Tumour: Breast cancer. The authors noted that the patients were more likely to have sexual maladjustment, negative attitudes towards sexuality, no premarital experience, late age of marriage and a stable marriage.
   Tumour: Cancer of the cervix. With these patients, the authors noted sexual maladjustment with disturbance more overt than in breast cancer patients, a higher rate of premarital sexual activity, a younger age at marriage and a high incidence of overt marital discord.

3. **Cobb**, 1952.[23]
   Tumour: Not specified, though the series involved 100 patients with cancer. Attributes common to all cancer patients. in the study were: 'basically anticipatory fears and underlying dependency, combined with a trend towards negative reactivity under stress difficulty in making their way in a world of adequate social relationships, they often regard emotional relationships as dangerous'.

4. **Bacon, Renneker, and Cutler**, 1952.[24]
   Tumour: Breast cancer (40 patients). These patients had six major behavioural characteristics: masochistic character structure; inhibited sexuality; inhibited motherhood;

inability to discharge or deal appropriately with anger; an unresolved hostile conflict with the mother, handled through denial and unrealistic sacrifice; and delay in securing treatment. 'The predominant characterological picture which centred around the unresolved conflict with the mother appeared to be the most essential dynamic denominator in this group of patients'.

5 **Stephenson, and Grace**, 1954.[25]
Tumour: Cancer of the cervix (100 patients) compared with 100 patients with other types of cancer. The authors found poorer sexual adjustment in the patients with cancer of the cervix.

6 **Greene**, 1954.[26]
Tumour: Lymphoma and leukaemia in 16 males. The patients had experienced occurrence or threat of personal loss before the diagnosis of leukaemia or lymphoma.

7 **Greene, Young, and Swisher**, 1956.[27]
Tumour: Lymphoma and leukaemia in 32 females. The patients had experienced the occurrence or threat of personal loss before the diagnosis of leukaemia or lymphoma.

8 **Greene**, 1966.[28]
Tumour: Lymphoma and leukaemia in 61 males. The patients had experienced the occurrence or threat of personal loss before the diagnosis of leukaemia or lymphoma.

9 **Greene, and Swisher**, 1969.[29]
Tumour: Leukaemia which was discordant in three sets of monozygotic twins. 'In each twin pair, the symptoms of leukaemia developed in a setting of major psychological stress – one that was stressful for the entire family, but particularly so for the affected twin'.

References

1. Doll, R., *Brit. med. J.*, 1965, 1: 471.
2. Walshe, W. H., *The Nature and Treatment of Cancer*, Taylor and Walton, London, 1846.
3. Kowal, S. J., *Psychoanal. Rev.*, 1955, 42: 217.
4. Triolo, V. A., *Cancer Res.*, 1964, 24: 4.
5. Triolo, V. A., *Cancer Res.*, 1965, 25: 75.
6. Parker, W., 1885 (quoted by Pelletier, K. R., *Mind as Healer, Mind as Slayer*), Dell, NY, 1977.
7. Paget, J., *Surgical Pathology*, 2nd edition, Longmans Green, London, 1870.
8. Leshan, L, L., and Worthington, R. E., *Brit. J. med. Psychol.*, 1956, 29: 49.
9. Anonymous, *Brit. med. J.*, 1925, 1: 1139.
10. Evans, E., *A Psychological Study of Cancer*, Dodd Mead and Co., New York, 1926.
11. Leshan, L. L., *J. Nat. Cancer Inst.*, 1959, 22: 1.
12. Crisp, A.H., *Brit. J. med. Psychol.*, 1970, 43: 313.
13. Surawicz, F. G., Brightwell, O. R., Weitzeld, W. O., et alii, *Amer. J. Psychiat.*, 1976, 133: 1306.
14. Haney, C. A., *Soc. Sci. Med.*, 1977, 11: 223.
15. Fox, B. H., *J. Behav. Med.*, 1978, 1: 45.
16. Anonymous, *Science*, 1978, 200: 1363.
17. Labarba, R. C., *Psychosom. Med.*, 1970, 32: 259.
18. Jensen, M. M., *Proc. Soc. exp. Biol. Med.*, 1968, 127: 610.
19. Labarba, R. C., *Psychosom. Med.,* 1970, 32: 259.
20. Riley, V., *Science*, 1975, 189: 465.
21. Miller, F. R., and Jones, H. W., *Blood*, 1948, 8: 880.
22. Tarlau, M., and Smalheiser, I., *Psychosom. Med.*, 1951, 13: 117.
23. Cobb, B. A., *Social-Psychological Study of the Cancer Patient*, Ph.D. thesis. University of Texas.
24. Bacon, C. l., Rennecker, R., and Cutler, M., *Psychosom. Med*, 1952, 14: 543.
25. Stephenson, J. A., and Grace, W. J., *Psychosom. Med*, 1954, 16: 267.
26. Greene, W. A., *Psychosom. Med.*, 1954, 16: 220.
27. Greene, W. A., Young, L E., and Swisher, S. N., *Psychosom. Med.*, 1956, 18: 284.
28. Greene, W. A., *Ann. NY Acad. Sci.*, 1966, 125: 794.
29. Greene, W. A, and Swisher. S. N.. *Ann. N. Y. Acad. Sci*, 1969, 164: 394.
30. Foque. E., *Gas Hop.* (Paris), 1931. 104: 827.
31. Leshan, L., *Ann. NY Acad. Sci.*, 1966, 125: 780.
32. Butler, B., *Cancer.* 1954, 7: 1.

33 Leshan, L., and Worthington, R., *J. J. Clin. Exper. Psycholpathology*, 1955, 16: 281.
34 Cutler, West, Ellis, and Blumberg, in *The Psychological Variables in Human Cancer*. edited by J. A. Gengerelli and F. J. Kirkner, Berkeley. University of California Press, 1954.
35 Kerr, T. A, Schapira, K., and Roth, M. *Brit. J Psvchiat.*, 1969. 115: 1277.
36 Kissen, D. M., *Psychosom Med.*, 1960, 22: 118.
37 Bahnson, C. B., Ann. NY *Acad. Sci*, 1969.164: 313.
38 Schmale, A. H., and Iker. H. P., *Psychosom Med.*, 1964, 26: 2034.
39 Schmale, A. H., and Iker. H. P., Ann NY *Acad. Sci.*, 1966, 125: 807.
40 Greer, S. and Morris, T. J. *Psychosom Res.*, 1975, 19: 147.
41 Greer, S., *Psychol. Med.*, 1979. 9: 81.
42 Kissen, D. M., Ann. NY *Acad. Sci.* 1966, 125: 820.
43 Schmale. A. H., and Iker. H. P., *Soc. Sci. Med.* 1971, 5: 95.
44 Snell, L., and Graham. S., *Brit. J Cancer.* 1971, 25: 721.
45 Graham, S., Snell, L. M., Graham, J. B. and Foro, L., *J. Clin. Dis.* 1971. 24: 711.
46 Hagnell, O., Ann. NY *Acad. Sci.*, 1966, 125: 846.
47 Keehn, R. J., Goldberg, I. D., and Beebe, G. W., *Psychosom. Med.* 1945, 36: 27.
48 Thomas, C. B., and Greenstreet, R. L., *Johns Hopkins Med. J.* 1973, 132: 16.
49 Thomas, C. S., and Duszynski, K. R., *Johns Hopkins Med. J.* 1974, 134: 251.
50 Thomas, C. B., *Ann. Intern. Med.* 1976. 85: 653.
51 Paffenberger. R., Wing, A. I., and Hyde, R. T., *J. Nat.* Cancer Inst., 1977. 58: 1489.
52 Foulds, L., *Neoplastic Development*, Volume 1. Academic Press, London, 1969.
53 Foulds, L., *Neoplastic Development*, Volume 2, Academic Press, London. 1975.
54 Weiss, D. W., Ann. NY *Acad. Sci*, 1969. 164: 431.
55 Shaw, H. M., Milton, G. W., McCarthy, W. H., et alii, *Med. J. Aust.*, 1979, 1: 208.
56 Meares, A., *Med. J. Aust.*, 1976, 2: 184.
57 Meares, A, *Med. J. Aust.*, 1977, 2: 132. (see also *Med. J. Aust.*, 1979, 2: 539).
58 Weisman, A D., and Worden, J. W., *Int. J. Psychiat.*, 1976, 7: 1.
59 Todd, P. S., and Magarey, C. J., *Brit. J. Med. Psvchol.*, 1978, 51: 177.
60 Cassel, J., *Amer. J Public Hlth.* 1974, 64: 1040.
61 Bartrop, R. W., Luckhurst, E., Lazarus, L., et. alii., *Lancet*, 1977, 1834.
62 Berenblum. I., *Cancer Res.*, 1977, 37: 1.

III

CARE OF AGED PERSONS: PRIVILEGE AND RESPONSIBILITY
1981

Edited version of The Clive Hamilton Memorial Address, Hobart. Australian Rehabilitation Review Vol 6, No2, 1982. The Clive Hamilton Memorial Address – Nurses Graduation Ceremony 1951, St John's Park, Hobart.

> Three passions, simple but overwhelmingly strong, have governed my life: the longing for love, the search for knowledge, and unbearable pity for Mankind.

wrote Bertrand Russell (1872–1970) in his autobiography.[1] The passion of 'unbearable pity for Mankind' is present in the heart of all those who embrace a career involving care of the frail elderly within our community – or the care of any who are for some reason weak among us who are the strong.

Kenneth Galbraith (1908–2006), in *The Age of Uncertainty*,[2] alleged that notable leaders have been characterised by their capacity to confront unequivocally the central anxieties of the people. What are our central anxieties – those of us who are concerned with the care of aged persons?

1
The inadequacy of resources for aged persons in the midst of an affluent society

There is a serious imbalance in our system for caring for people in need. There is, for several reasons, an increasing ratio of chronic to acute illness within our community. Neither the hospitals nor the insurance systems have reflected this shift. The poor elderly and the chronically ill have the greatest need of medical care but available information suggests that they do not have access to a necessary proportion of the health care resources of the whole community. It is disconcerting to realise that, on recent projections of the aged population in Australia by the year 2000, the resources available will need to be doubled by that time.[3]

There are pressures for more resources to be allocated in several areas of the health-care system. What should be the principles which guide decision making in the face or competing needs? Contributions from three sources appear relevant: the Maxwell inquiry;[4] the recent major contribution by social philosopher, John Rawls (1921–2002); and concepts of contemporary philosopher, Karl Popper (1902–1994).

Maxwell, in 1974, undertook a detailed study of the health care systems of over twenty Western nations – with Australian statistics incorporated in a second edition in 1975.[5] in the preamble, Maxwell noted that:

> In *every* nation, the demand for health care is growing and the balance of needs is changing towards less tractable problems associated with handicap, affluence and age.

The Maxwell inquiry considered many other facets of the health care delivery system: patterns of supply of health professionals, their geographical distribution, patterns of use of hospitals and the cost effectiveness of the systems prevailing in the various countries. It was clear that 'each country requires a means of confronting and resolving the question of priorities'.

In every health care system there are organisational problems which the Maxwell inquiry lists as: (1) barriers to patient access (simple non-availability, financial problems, the complexity of the health system); (2) inflexibility of resource use (e.g. by boundaries between hospital services and services outside hospital, professional demarcation); (3) ill-defined responsibilities with inadequate planning; and (4) excessive complexity and cost.

The Maxwell inquiry concludes that 'four kinds of shifts in strategy will be widely called for', and details these as:

1) greater attention to, and expenditure on, prevention and health education;
2) building and maintaining stronger systems of primary care;
3) upgrading the treatment of long-term illness and handicap; and
4) streamlining the acute hospitals as an integral part of the total pattern of provision.

The Maxwell report has been mentioned, not because the points it makes are new nor unexpected but because it represents, from an international perspective, a useful discussion of health care.

John Rawls of Harvard, in his seminal work *A Theory of Justice*,[6] in merely ten years has evoked so much interest, discussion and debate that the contribution has been styled the most significant since the 19th century utilitarians represented by JS Mill. His central idea is a revised version of a contract approach to the distribution of resources, with the principles being worked out by a consensus of persons who do not know their own social status, age, needs etc. under the so-called 'veil of ignorance'. Rawls argues that under such circumstances principles will emerge which ensure the *fair* distribution of resources:

> We are to imagine that those who engage in social cooperation choose together, in one joint act, the principles which are to assign basic rights and duties and to determine the division of social benefits.

> Men are to decide in advance how they are to regulate their claims against one another and what is to be the foundation charter of their society.
>
> Among the essential features of this situation is that no one knows his place in society, his class position or social status, nor does any one know his fortune in the distribution of natural assets and abilities, his intelligence, strength, and the like. I shall even assume that the parties do not know their concept of the good or their special psychological propensities. The principles of justice are chosen behind a veil of ignorance. This ensures that no one is advantaged or disadvantaged in the choice of principles by the outcome of natural chance or the contingency of social circumstances. Since all are similarly situated and no one is able to design principles to favour his particular condition, the principles of justice are the result of a fair agreement or bargain. For, given the circumstances of the original position. the symmetry of everyone's relations to each other, this initial situation is fair between individuals as moral persons, that is, as rational beings with their own ends and capable, I shall assume, of a sense of justice. The original position is, one might say, the appropriate initial status quo, and thus the fundamental agreements reached in it are fair. This 'explains the propriety of the name justice as fairness': it conveys the idea that the principles of justice are agreed to in an initial situation that is fair.

A basic concept in Rawls' work is that 'all social primary goods – liberty and opportunity, income and wealth, and the bases for self-respect – are to be distributed equally unless an unequal distribution of any or all of these goods is to the advantage of the least favoured'.

We can reasonably ask what principles for allocation of health resources would emerge if the parties charged with reaching consensus did not know their age, economic status, health status, ethnicity nor their place in the health system – whether patient, cook, nurse, general practitioner, hospital specialist, health administrator, and so on. Some discussion of applications of Rawls' ideas to the health system is beginning elsewhere (for example, in the USA[7]) and debate is essential in Australia.

If a sign of the significance of a philosopher is the seminal nature of his ideas, in that his concepts stimulate progress in thought across a broad range of other disciplines, then Karl Popper, currently in retirement in England and maybe with some of his finest work still to be published, is a highly significant philosopher in our times. His thought is rich and out of this rich ness may be distilled many lines of inquiry of relevance to medical practice.[8]

Popper pointed out that logically a scientific law is conclusively falsifiable although it is not conclusively verifiable. Popper therefore urges that we do not systematically evade refutation but that we formulate our theories as unambiguously as possible so that they may be exposed to refutation. Where an observation is made which refutes the theory by methodology which is truly rigorous then we must search for a new hypothesis which may then be tested by devising confrontations between its consequences and new observable experience. It is a liberating thing to turn the mind not to defending (even irrationally) what one holds to be correct but to devising means whereby it could be shown to be false or inadequate. He wrote that: 'The man who welcomes and acts on criticism will prize it almost above friendship: the man who fights it out of concern to maintain his position is clinging to non-growth'.

A proposed medical care system is (if planned at all) basically an hypothesis generated in the face of data concerning needs, resources and foreseeable trends. It could be fruitful to seek deliberately for additional data which would demonstrate that the proposed plan (hypothesis) is inadequate, incorrect, 'false' rather than approaching the 'truth' in relation to the content within which it has been generated. A policy, then, according to Popper is an hypothesis which has to be tested against reality and corrected in the light of experience. Once again, the search for multiple pieces of evidence which would confirm the policy may be far less valuable (even though emotionally more comfortable) than the search for one soundly produced piece of evidence which would refute it.

There is a further area of Popper's thought put forward in *The Open Society and its Enemies* as the general guiding principle for public policy, namely, 'minimise avoidable suffering'. Popper bases this on his observation of, as it were, a logical asymmetry: we do not know how to make people happy (as the policy 'maximise happiness' demands) but we do know ways of lessening their unhappiness ('minimise unhappiness'). 'Instead of the greatest happiness for the greatest number, one should demand, more modestly, the least amount of avoidable suffering for all; and further, that unavoidable suffering, such as hunger in times of unavoidable shortage of food, should be distributed as equally as possible.' The relevance of this concept of health planning at the national, regional or local level is singularly obvious, and liberating indeed, capable of giving impetus to the creative spirit of health professionals.

2
Our fear of frailty and our fear of the burden of the frail

A second area of anxiety is related to the first but is centred on more personal and more distressing issues. In our consideration of resources of the elderly, there can arise the sudden realisation that we, ourselves, are (if we survive) the elderly in two or three decades ... and the shock of our possible frailty is considerable.

There will come ringing in our ears the debate concerning whether or not the elderly need more resources – or whether such resources should be centred on those of more obvious future benefit to the community.

Such problems are not new. William Farr (1807–1883), the British statistician, in his 19th century work, *Vital Statistics,* progressed to calculating the value to the state of a life according to future accrued income, that is, setting off investment in early nurture and sanitation against late wages and taxes. He estimated that a Norfolk agricultural labourer was worth £5 at birth; £56 at the age of 5; £117 at the age of 10; £192 at 15; £234 at 20; a peak of £246 at 25; £241 at 30; thereafter declining to £138 at 55: and £1 at 70; and thereafter at a rising cost to the community, until at the age of 80 the old man was costing £41 a year. Smith, after discussing Farr, notes, 'This investment-orientated approach positively discourages expenditure in areas that will not yield a higher return.'[9]

It is clear that care of our frail elderly cannot be based on concepts of economic return to the community. A totally different perspective is necessary.

We are here in the midst of what might be termed the weak–strong dilemma. Much has been written by thinking men concerning the role of the strong in the care of the weak in human society. Charles Darwin (1808–1882), in the *Descent of Man,* wrote:

> The aid which we feel impelled to give to the helpless is mainly an incidental result of the instinct of sympathy, which was originally required as part of the social instincts, but subsequently rendered ... more tender and more widely diffused. Nor could we check our sympathy, if so urged by hard reason, without deterioration in the noblest part of our nature. The surgeon may harden himself whilst performing an operation, for he knows

he is acting for the good of his patient; but if we were
intentionally to neglect the weak and the helpless, it could
only be for a contingent benefit, with a certain and great
present evil ...

Not all agreed with this point of view. Frederich Nietzsche (1844–1900) in Germany in the 19th century propounded the need for men to be strong and the writings of this fiery genius influenced many, including the poet, Rainer Maria Rilke (1875–1926), who, as a young man, after reading some of Nietzsche, wrote in 1896:

> He whom men worship as the Messiah turns the
> whole world into an infirmary. He calls the weak, the
> unfortunate, the disabled His children and His loved
> ones. What about the strong? How are we ourselves
> to climb if we lend strength to the unfortunate and the
> oppressed, to idle rogues with no wits and no energy?
> Let them fall, let them die, alone and wretched. Be
> hard, be terrible, be pitiless! You must thrust yourselves
> forward, forward! A few men, but great ones, will build a
> world with their strong, muscular, masterful arms on the
> corpses of the weak, the sick and the infirm.

It is consoling that this youthful piece of work does not represent Rilke's mature thought but the ideas embodied in it continued to be nurtured in fertile ground. This stream of thinking, glorifying, in some measure, the powerful may have been significantly complemented by ideas emanating from Auguste Comte (1798–1857) and his followers.

In 1847, Comte gave a series of lectures and one of his hearers, Dr Robinet, wrote: 'In those hallowed hours that heralded such great destinies, we felt the breath of Humanity, we caught a glimpse of its reality, its greatness, we bowed before it.' The glorification of humanity as such – not the sheer celebration of man as had been seen in some features of the Renaissance – but a triumphalism concerning humanity continued palpably in the positivist tradition. In the following generation another fervent positivist (addressing Catholics) said: 'We shall convince the men, we shall persuade the women, and the day is not far off when we shall enter your forsaken temples as masters, bearing above our heads the banner of triumphant Humanity'.

A further nuance was expressed by Controt, another positivist, in the 1930s:

> Objectively, the only individual being that surpasses the individual is his species, carrying in it … that extraordinary additive faculty which enables man to outclass the animals. This suggests an inspiring extension of the humanist attitude. We seek to divert religious feelings toward the species, as the Marxians tried to divert it towards class warfare, the dictatorship of the proletariat or the organisation of industrial production.

Once the good of the species moves to the centre of the stage then the context is ripe for the upsurge of ideas that the well-being or individuals especially the weak and apparently unprofitable can be logically sacrificed as a manifestation of concern for the species. We have many precedents is in history for heroic persons to sacrifice themselves so that others may survive but our instinct does not respond with such admiration for persons who made decisions that others should perish to save the strong: the captain of a crowded lifeboat ordering the weak to be thrown overboard so that the others may more readily survive may face charges of homicide rather than receive commendations for heroism. Kant wrote that 'Man is characterised by a moral law within' – and despite the ebb and flow of cultural patterns and the tides of history, there is an instinctive repugnance at the sacrifice of the weak for the sake of the strong, even for the species' sake.

In this context came Adolf Hitler. In *Mein Kampf*, he wrote:

> Defective people (must) be prevented from propagating equally defective offspring ... For, if necessary, the incurably sick will be piteously segregated – a barbaric measure for this unfortunate who is struck by it but a blessing for his fellow men and posterity.

As we know, this logic was mercilessly put into effect without mercy.

Mr Justice Michael Kirby, Chairman of the Law Reform Commission of Australia, in the course of a significant analysis of the rights of the living and the rights of the dying,[10] reminded us that the Nazi euthanasia program began as a means of 'relieving' the severely and chronically sick, with the medical profession advancing the program.

Recent studies show that many of the doctors who presided over the killings saw themselves as idealists – parties in a 'vast revolutionary biological therapy'.

Kirby quoted one of them, recently interviewed:

> It started with the acceptance of the attitude, basic in the euthanasia movement, that there is such a thing as life not worthy to be lived. This attitude in its early stages concerned itself merely with the severely and chronically sick. Gradually, the sphere of those to be included in this category was enlarged to encompass the socially unproductive, the ideologically unwanted, the racially unwanted and finally all non-Germans. But it is important to realise the infinitely small wedged-in lever from which this entire trend of mind received its impetus was the attitude towards the non-rehabilitatable sick.

It will already be apparent that some of these issues are (unfortunately) relevant now forty years later. It is instructive, therefore, to look more closely at the involvement of the medical profession (and others equally informed) in such manifest evil.

Violence, cruelty, for example, attacks on defenceless elderly people – all these are recognised as evil, and we have a criminal code to deal with them. It is the 'evil without horns' which is the danger and it could be that evil may be present wherever and whenever a decision made by the powerful concerning the relatively powerless (the aged, the frail, the chronically ill, the dying or the very young or unborn) benefits the powerful ... and certainly any such decision must be highly suspect.

3
Anxiety concerning the appropriateness of applications of contemporary clinical science in the case of the frail aged

There is much talk today of perpetuation of life of poor quality by the inappropriate application of technology. There is the fear also of being subject to unnecessary and hazardous investigations and of being 'pushed around' in large hospitals with no respect for the priorities and preferences of the individual. Fortunately, the concept of hospitals as impersonal non-caring places is, in most part, a caricature. However, there is indeed a place for re-examination of clinical science.

As a point of departure, let us refer to Ian Kennedy in the 1980 Reith lecture:

> Science has destroyed our faith in religion. Reason has challenged our trust in magic. What more appropriate result could there be than the appearance of new magicians and priests wrapped in the cloak of science and reason? Please understand that it is we; all of us, who have hitched our wagon to the wrong star: scientific medicine as our guiding light.

It can be argued that, in this point, Kennedy has an inadequate view of science. 'Science' is defined by the Oxford dictionary as 'systematic and formulated knowledge' and 'scientific' as 'according to rules laid down in science for testing soundness of conclusions, systematic, accurate.' It is my view that medical practice needs to be *more,* not less scientific, with clearly articulated goals, appropriate processes and recognition of limits – as befits a major science.

What is the principal goal of medical practice? The philosophers and thinkers down the ages have often commented on what they saw as the goals of medicine to be and their comments are uncompromising. Cicero (106BCE–43BCE) was quite clear: 'The art of medicine is valuable to us because it is conducive to Health, not because of its scientific interest'.

The ancient Greeks told us to 'help your patient die young, as late as possible'. Hippocrates wrote:

> I will define what I conceive medicine to be. In general terms, it is to do away with the sufferings of the sick, to lessen the violence of their diseases, and to refuse to treat those who are overmastered by their diseases.

There is, in fact, a whole spectrum of the interplay between symptoms and signs but the fact that this exists should not obscure the key points being made; improving the quality of life now and in the future is the key task of clinical activities and remains a task even though life will be inevitably shortened by a condition which is over-mastering the patient. Dying is part of life and the quality of life in one dying is, as we have seen, still a central issue in care. If, on the whole, we recognise that quality of life is the goal of clinical activity then it is logical to recognise that diagnosis is, where appropriate, a means – not an end. It is very easy for contemporary clinical medicine to see diagnosis as an end in itself. It is unscientific and illogical clinical medicine to threaten the quality of life seriously in any patient by performing any investigation to add just a little information in the endeavour to reach a diagnosis if, in fact, that added information will not materially influence therapeutic decisions.

There is a body of medical knowledge and skills directed unequivocally towards the maintenance or improvement of quality of living and/or of dying which is sometimes, but not necessarily, embodied in separate medical and nursing personnel or even institutions. However, the total practice of clinical medicine wherever practised with regard to elderly persons and/or the dying patient must include awareness that the patient should be as actively involved in decision-making in this phase of life about matters of the moment as in any other phase of life: human medicine is concerned with the personal, and the freedom of a true subject of existence is one of the notes of the personal.

4
Anxiety concerning death

Involvement with aged persons is involvement with those nearer (on the whole) to death than ourselves – our patients will often die – and they themselves are repeatedly bereaved as years go on. We are forced somehow to come to terms with our own mortality in such circumstances.

Acceptance of the fact and even of the proximity of mortality may bring with it profound freedom. However, in accepting death, the philosopher Maurice Merleau-Ponty (1908–1961) in discussing Georg Hegel (1770–1831)) urges that this acceptance 'cannot be separated from the decision to live and to get a new grip on our fortuitous existence', and the poet Rilke (who said it was the poet's mission to bind life and death together) wrote: 'Whoever rightly understands and celebrates death at the same time magnifies life'.

In Freudian terms, Norman Brown (1913–2002) held that the acceptance of death, its reunification in consciousness with life, cannot be accomplished by the discipline of philosophy or the seduction of art but only by the abolition of repression: 'Man who is born of woman and destined to die is a body, with bodily instincts. Only if Eros – the life instinct – can affirm the life of the body, can the death instinct affirm death, and in affirming death, magnify life'.[11]

These concepts are surely in accord with Erik Erikson's (1902–1994) description of integrity by which he means a sense of wholeness of life and acceptance of one's place in space and time (in contradistinction to despair) which is the task of the last phase of life. Erikson's concept of personal growth is sensitive indeed in its consideration of the developmental task of the elderly. He conceives the task as the development of a sense of wholeness, of integrity.

> Only he who in some way has taken care of things and people and has adapted himself to the triumphs and disappointments of being, by necessity, the originator of others and the generator of things and ideas – only he may gradually grow the fruit of the seven stages. I know no better word for it than integrity … It is the acceptance of one's own and only life cycle and of the people who have become significant to it as something that had to be … an acceptance of the fact that one's life is one's own responsibility. It is a sense of comradeship with men and women of distant times and of different pursuits, who have created orders and objects and sayings conveying human dignity and love.

On the other hand, Erikson noted further:

> … the lack or loss of this accrued ego integration is signified by despair and an often unconscious fear of death: the one and only life cycle is not accepted as the ultimate of life. Despair expresses the fear that the time is short, too short for the attempt to start another life and

to try out alternate roads to integrity. Such a despair is often hidden behind a show of disgust, a misanthropy, or a chronic contemptuous displeasure with particular institutions and particular people – a disgust and a displeasure which (where not allied with constructive ideas and a life of co-operation) only signify the individual's contempt of himself.[12]

It has been well said that 'It is when the human heart faces its destiny and, notwithstanding, sings – sings of itself, its life, its death – that poetry is possible'. But no wise sayings can take away the pain of growth in acceptance of our inevitable death nor of the pain of grieving for one loved: such experience both facilitates and is facilitated by care of the frail elderly.

Related indeed to our difficulty in accepting painful aspects of the human condition is a fear that in contact with the frail we have nothing to give – the 'dry well' syndrome. In such a mood one has the option of withdrawing from involvement, but it may be consoling to recognise that even in such states of mind and heart we may be the vehicle of the rebirth of hope in another.

We have glanced at least at some of our anxieties in the face of the pressing human obligation to care for those among us who are old, frail or otherwise weak: there must be a shift of resources; we must recognise the significance of the weak; we must practise precise and appropriate clinical science and we must accept the reminders of our mortality and finitude. Let us face not only our anxieties but also our opportunities.

Kingsley Mortimer has written that it is the task of medicine (by which we understand the whole medical effort involving a whole spectrum of staff) 'to emancipate Man's interior splendour'. In old age, as the exterior splendour may well be fading, the task should bring with it a sharp poignancy and a heightened sense of privilege.

References

1 Russell, B., *Autobiography*, Prologue, 1956.
2 Galbraith, J. K., *The age of uncertainty*, B.B.C., London, 1977, p. 330.
3 Sax, S., The challenge of post clinical medicine. The Richard Gibson Oration, Australian College of Rehabilitation Medicine, Sydney, 1981.
4 Maxwell, R., *Health care: the growing dilemma*, 2nd edn, McKinsey & Company, New York, 1975.
5 Maxwell, R., *Health care: the growing dilemma*, 2nd edn, McKinsey & Company, New York, 1975.
6 Rawls, J., *A theory of justice*, Harvard University Press, Cambridge, 1971.
7 Beauchamp, D. E., 'Public health and individual liberty', *Annual Review Public Health* 1, 1980, pp. 121–36.
8 Popper, K., *The open society and its enemies, Vols 1 and 2*, Routledge, London, 1945.
9 Smith, F. R., *The people's health, 1830–1910*, Groom Helm, London/A.N.U., Canberra, 1979, p. 420.
10 Kirby, M. D., 'The rights of the living and the rights of the dying', *Medical Journal of Australia* 1, 1980, pp. 252–5.
11 Brown, N. O., *Life against death*, Wesleyan University Press, Middletown, 1970.
12 Erikson, E. H., *Identity and the life cycle*, Psychological Issues Monograph, International Universities Press, New York, 1968, p. 58.

IV

ON THE KINDNESS OF STRANGERS;
NOTES ON THE EXPERIENCE OF CARE
2006

*First Barbara Leroy Memorial Address, Orange NSW.
Edited version of the Barbara Leroy Memorial Lecture,
Annual Conference of Palliative Care Association, NSW,
2 November, 2006* [1,2]

Tennessee Williams, in his play, *A Streetcar Named Desire*, explored many dimensions of the human condition. His biographer notes, of the play's central character, 30-year-old Blanche Dubois, that, 'at the end, the complexities of life and death are italicized ... Blanche suffers a complete breakdown and is led away to an asylum, now dependent in a new way – as before in a promiscuous way – on what she calls "the kindness of strangers"'.[3]

Australia has been described as, not a project, but an ongoing conversation.[4] This human conversation, now in progress for over 50,000 years, involves the sharing of life by those who previously may have been strangers, but encounter each other (however diverse) as possessors of, after all, a common humanity. Such human connectedness appears to be acknowledged (especially if the other is in need) as a primordial response unless trauma has blighted perspectives: indeed philosophers have stressed that empathy may be the primary human response to another.[5]

In the course of the long history of Australia, strangers not only lived together but have danced with each other: the historian, Inga Clendinnen, recounts that indigenous men and British soldiers danced together, in 1788 on the beach in Sydney, at the first contacts before hostilities disturbed the harmony.[6] The place of strangers in Australian society today may be more fraught. Yet the inter relationships with strangers are part of the human infrastructure of our society, and this is clearly evident in the health system, a part of the spectrum of care.

Consideration of some of the fundamental concepts, inchoate (but often not articulated) in the intellectual infrastructure and function of a health care system, may be timely. Founding concepts historically relate to many matters: questions about the meaning of the 'good' and the 'good life', the meaning of 'person', the grounds for response to a needy other, the place of responsibility for care (am I my brother's keeper?) and for accountability (to whom?), the relation between individual and community (which is prior?), the basis of the duty of care, the place of the weak in society (is there a right or claim to care?), grounds for limitation of care (are there limits?), the realistic possibilities for enhancement of length of individual life and its quality (and at whose expense?). Furthermore there is always the question (and debate) about where should lines in the sand be drawn regarding both practice and research methodologies, now in our time and place.

These and other cognate questions are not in general answerable by empirical evidence, but on the other hand, communal reflection is called for as a basis for pragmatic unavoidable decisions. Reflection is in short supply, yet the foundations of clinical practice may warrant reflection and examination – in the hope that the winds shaking some of the superstructure may be less harmful. Despite brilliant advances in medical practice, not only administrators, but some patients, notably the elderly, are afraid. Advance care directives, so precious to those who have made them (still fearful that they may be disregarded) are but one indication that patients may have a clearer view of what is their 'good' than the mightiest of clinicians. Yet the health system is specifically organised to advance human good: it is not morally neutral. Such issues matters are relevant, not merely to end-of-life care, but also to mainstream medical care, in acute hospitals, emergency departments and intensive care units, as well as other levels of care, and above all, community practice.

Three areas of enquiry will be considered: first, there will be exploration of the concept of 'person', then, consideration of several dimensions of the interpersonal activity of 'care', and finally an approach to clinical decision-making in situations of complexity on the basis of the foregoing.

1

Exploring the concept of person

Strangers on whose kindness we depend or who depend on us for some dimensions of care are above all persons. The notion of person requires exploration: Jacob Needleman noted in 1969 that, 'what medicine lacks is any fundamental notion of the nature of man and any remotely adequate understanding of that to which we refer as a person.'[7]

Philosophers down the ages have sought to define 'person' with almost all definitions referring to an individual, usually with certain capacities considered specifically human. But Walt Whitman in *Song of Myself*, a defining American poem, wrote (in stanza 7):

> I pass death with the dying and birth with the
>   new wash'd babe,
> and am not contain'd between my hat and my boots.

He wrote further, in stanza 16:

> And these tend inward to me, and I tend outward to them,
> And such it is to be of these more or less I am,
> And of these one and all I weave the song of myself.[8]

Are we in need of recognising more clearly that, whereas the body may indeed be contained between hat and boots, a 'person' cannot be so contained, but is an inherently relational reality?

Philosophers, notably in the personalist tradition, know this well. Continental thinkers (especially) searching for adequate bases for bioethics currently stress the relationality of persons: and stress that an individualistic ethic is incongruent with human existence.[9] Through interaction with others human beings develop subjectivity. Relationality is seen to stem not from the free choice of the subject, but comes as a prior condition and orientation of that free choice. One dimension of ethics, 'care ethics', always starts from a relational view of the human person; care is a basic given in the human existence, a very human way to hold one's own in life and moreover a way that fundamentally 'weaves' people into a network of relationships.[10]

Can the clinical mind approach these issues, and as some philosophers would hope, contribute nuances to some elements of Western philosophical tradition? We have a privileged perspective of and experience within the human condition. Many years ago (1968 –70), in the course of research which involved learning from the indigenous people of Sydney, a paper was noted by Apley describing a child as 'an unique ecological experiment'.[11,12] Subsequently a simple schema was developed, portraying an ecological view of a person: a person is depicted as within and actually constituted by, a web of relationships comprised of present environment, the past as experienced, and inheritance with both biological and cultural dimensions ... all of significance and in constant flux and interaction – like a spider's web. The only addition to that schema was made during a focus on palliative medicine (1985–2005) at a metropolitan teaching hospital: it became imperative to recognise that the way out of an otherwise closed system could be hope. It is impossible to predict what would be, even if given, the response to the question, 'in what (or for what) do you hope?' for the question relates to the core of the self. The schema simply offers assistance for structuring clinical history-taking, practice and research.

A relational view of persons applies not only to patients, family members, friends, but also carers; for care is fundamentally an inter-personal activity (even intersubjective), even if much technical activity is involved in therapeutic interventions. The concept that a person is constituted by relationships adds immeasurably to the richness of clinical practice; as the continental writers put it, 'Care is one way of acknowledging the other as person. Care is not a corollary to rational consideration: rather it starts with respect for the other's dignity and seeing the other as person, as mystery.'[13] Such ideas, rightly not usually articulated in words (though maybe in gestures) in the everyday world of clinical practice, say in a busy ER department, or general practice clinic, do not preclude but mandate urgent focussed attention to a wounded or failing body, styled by some personalists as the 'condensation' of human dignity. In triage situations it may be the significance of each human person within one's gaze which drives the passion to care, with objective aspects of the human person (the vital signs, etc) in close focus.

So 'person' may be best explicitly thought of as a relational reality, and as such each person is unique. Differences may be blurred by statistical techniques, such as randomised controlled trials, which deliberately set out to suppress that which is distinctive about each individual as person: the implications and limitations of such an approach have been recognised by the wise, such as [AR] Feinstein.[14] It is the subjective, the uniqueness of an individual, which is a focus in palliative medicine: the slide into 'over-objectivisation' in the interests of quantification of, sometimes core, personal data, needs to be recognised, and maybe curtailed. It is the inviolable mystery of the human person which is the well of joy, sorrow, hope and wonder, in the exercise or receiving of care: we need to respect that which we cannot adequately measure as of equal if not surpassing value to that which we can measure, even in the context of clinical practice (and research).

Persons are not only intrinsically relational, and unique, but also are continually in process, continuing changing. The processes of personal growth and development have been the subject of much research and writing, but the corpus of Erik Erikson has stood the test of time as a way of thinking about these matters.[15] Erikson portrayed life as a succession of development tasks, with personal change facilitated (for good or ill) by the negotiation of psychological and social crises. Each stage of life offered opportunities for choosing between favourable and unfavourable options. The last stage of life (at any age) offers the opportunity for moving towards 'integrity', that is, for Erikson, a certain acceptance of one's time/place/life, or despair – rejection of these. The risk of a slide into despair is always there for the frail, or irreversibly ill.[16]

Growth of persons occurs from within, just as in the case of a pot plant. Good care may provide a structure within which to grow and nourishment needed, but the form of the growth is not the responsibility, much less expression of the preference of a carer. Some plants go wild, some persons die despairing, and, in the end, however tragic this may be and painful for companions/witnesses and carers, we must bear the sorrow, with our only source of peace the conviction that we have conscientiously done (and been) all that is possible.

A further consideration is the meaning of human dignity, a dimension of the human person which is basic to many major legal documents, including recently the UNESCO Universal Declaration on Bioethics and Human Rights (2005). Serious exploration of human dignity requires interdisciplinary effort,[17] as well as clinical attention given elsewhere.[18] [Harvey Max] Chochinov, on the basis of a body of clinical research, has prepared a valuable guide to the recognition and conservation of human dignity in clinical practice.[19] Suffice to note that an adequate notion of human dignity requires foundations in an adequate anthropology.

2
Considering care
The relationality of the human person is at the core of further considerations of care. Care is a profound and complex concept, even if limiting consideration to the human stratum of our world. One of the exponents of the field of care ethics, defines care as follows: 'On the most general level, we suggest that caring be viewed as a species activity that includes everything that we do to maintain, continue, and repair our 'world' so that we can live in it as well as possible. That world includes our bodies, ourselves, and our environment, all of which we seek to interweave in a complex, life-sustaining web.'[20]

Care of our bodies, especially if seriously failing, often involves strangers in a challenging fashion. The care of those with probably eventually fatal illness, a constant strand in individual lives and in communities because of the nature of the human condition, is but one instance of a larger pattern of human activity, involving so often, at its heart, the kindness of strangers.

Care may be considered as an attitude, or practice. Care as both is pervasive in a human community, and finely focussed in the health care (or medical care) system, as indeed a driver for planning, administration, evaluation as well as clinical activity.

The care of patients with probably eventually fatal illness, involving much of the activity of the health care system and personnel (far more than the relatively small specialist palliative care services) is but one instance; some aspects will be briefly considered. Questions which may be need to be faced, to elucidate some of the complexities of care include: why is care needed? Why care for another?

a) *Why is care needed?*
There are two fundamental reasons why individuals need to be prepared to give and receive care: first, we are radically incomplete, and second, trauma and/or loss are normal components of human life. A third could be added: 'interdependency as an ineliminable feature of human social existence.'[21]

The radical incompleteness stems from the relational quality of persons, not mere biological need. Baby birds need mothers or fathers to care for them or they will die. Primates need far more than food, water and shelter. For growth as persons we need others: 'of these one and all I weave the song of myself. 'We grow as well as exist and experience illness/loss in what Taylor called 'webs of interlocution.'[22,23]

The French revolutionaries had as a goal the elimination of death,[24] and the same appears to be the goals of some zealous junior medical staff (at least as expressed at Grand Rounds) and even of reporters. But death is universal, and part of the human pattern, just as the last movement of a symphony contributes richly to the shape of the whole. Trauma/loss/distress and/or frailty are normal, not exceptional, components of the human condition, however much we seek to prevent and alleviate them.

[E] Cassell, in his landmark paper (1982), prompted reflection on the goal of medicine as the relief of suffering.[25] He gave a memorable definition of suffering as 'a sense of impending personal disintegration', which, in common parlance, may (I think) equate with a feeling of 'being about to go to pieces'. McCosker, Best and Lickiss (unpublished) demonstrated after gentle conversations with over 100 successively referred patients in the course of palliative care consultations, that patients do certainly know if they have ever felt like that in the course of their illness, and if so, what had triggered the feeling. The response was not predictable; the trigger may have been in the area of relationships, or related to medical investigations, uncontrolled symptoms, difficult communication or arduous treatment, or a specific unfortunate episode (such as incontinence), or in areas of life far removed from current health issues. Knowledge of such triggers, and indeed enquiry into them, maybe of much value for carers, including professional carers, lest the patient's suffering be aggravated unwittingly by well-intentioned efforts.

Janice Morse, a professor of nursing whose special expertise lies in qualitative research, has contributed significantly to recent literature on suffering. She and her colleagues on the basis on many hours of meticulous research, especially in trauma situations, developed the notion of two discernible phases of suffering: the phase of 'enduring', to which the appropriate professional response is 'holding techniques' such as eye contact, but not touch or expressions of sympathy, and the phase of 'emotional release' to which the appropriate response is expression of sympathy, maybe supportive touch and so on.[26] The work of Morse needs to be given careful consideration in the context of the care of patients close to death, where persons may be, so to speak, completing a difficult marathon, or being present to a loved one in much difficulty negotiating the last few metres: competence in 'holding techniques' may need to be recognised as the most appropriate response of a professional carer in such circumstances.

Bearing or even perceiving the suffering of another, especially if especially bonded, but even as a fellow human (or even fellow living thing), is a significant source of personal suffering. The cost of professional care may be manifest as suffering (though called other things); attention is increasingly given to the suffering of doctors in relation to the death of patients, and the need for concerted efforts to restore the self in the face of clinical demands.[27]

Responses to the suffering of others, related to professional responsibility, are highly influenced by individual and cultural factors. The cultural diversity within Australia, manifest in both patients and professional carers, calls for both reticence to import ideas from elsewhere without reflection, but also a concerted effort to recognise distress patterns. This may be especially necessary for colleagues of junior medical staff, where suicide may not be merely a sign of overwork or ordinary maturation issues, but deep unarticulated distress at the suffering witnessed, sometimes powerlessly and silently, in emergency departments, intensive care units, general wards, nursing homes, homes and elsewhere. The burden of bereavement borne by physicians (and nurses) often experiencing the death of patients may be inadequately recognised. Medical oncologists in particular often (or usually) develop significant relationships with patients, relationships built on hope for cure or control of life threatening cancer, and yet, sadly, many (even most) patients (except those treated in an adjuvant setting) who receive chemotherapy eventually do succumb to their disease. What then of the grieving of oncologists? Is this bereavement burden a contributor to the burn out documented so frequently in medical oncologists? Does this matter? Does it, could it distort practice as well as private life? Participation in the human condition is sometimes fraught.

b) *Why care for another?*

Care is a characteristic of human life, and is manifest in some manner in all human communities. Why? Is it innate? One has only to observe a colony of non-human primates to see manifestations of caring behaviour, and certainly the bonding of a mother for a new born baby appears an instinctive matter, but still reflection on this is warranted.

Desmond Manderson (then Director of the Julius Stone Institute of Jurisprudence, University of Sydney), gave a lecture at the 9th Annual Symposium of the Sydney Institute of Palliative Medicine in 2000, on the philosophical basis of the duty of care. He carefully examined the case that the duty is based in law, or contract, but concluded with the philosopher Emmanuel Levinas, that the basis of the duty of care is response to 'the call of the other'. This would of course, not preclude the response being instinctive, if untrammelled. It is only 'the call of the other' which may be strong enough to sustain a physician or nurse responding day after day to situations of distress. Only that could sustain persons involved in caring for people in unspeakably distressing situations of civil disaster or war. But the very concept of the power of the call of the other in need, and the power of responsiveness in the carer raises the concomitant issue of the limits to care, of the need to set boundaries (especially for junior clinical staff) and the delineation of the principles from which boundaries may be ethically constructed and maintained.

c) *Are there limitations to the obligation to care?*

Levinas, the philosopher so identified with recent thought about care as response to the other, not as based in universal principles of justice, offers also a basis for setting limits to care. The concept is rooted in the recognition that there are other others, including the self. Care of the self is mandated in order that one may care for the other.[28] This is not narcissism but radical altruism. The implication of such a view is profound, and needs careful teasing out in the context of health care. The stress experienced by carers (of all types) of very ill patients may be extreme, and clarity of thought as well as principles of practice is needed. Clinical decision-making should always include reflection on carer impact ... but often does not.

3
Clinical decision-making in complex situations: some implications of the foregoing considerations with special reference to palliative medicine.

Palliative medicine (whether practiced by palliative medicine specialists or a wide range of other doctors in contact with relevant patients) as an area of clinical science and practice, has several components:

a) symptom relief (the bottom line) throughout the course of an eventually fatal illness, in parallel with anti-disease strategies, resting now on a sound base of clinical science of diseases and therapeutics,

b) personal and family support as needed, and

c) participation in clinical decision-making, preferably from time of the diagnosis of eventually probably fatal illness.

Palliative care (as distinct from palliative medicine) properly involves planning for future care, approaching death, aftercare of bereaved persons and other matters.[29] The landmark Report of the Institute of Medicine based in Washington DC was prepared in response to the travesties in end-of-life-care in some leading USA hospitals, unearthed by valuable and courageous clinical research: it stressed that palliative care should begin with diagnosis of eventually fatal illness, so called 'mixed management'. This implies competence in all aspects of palliative care being available to all diagnosed patients, whether or not specialist palliative care professionals are needed or involved: pain relief is still clearly the bottom line, but other aspects are also of significance, especially to patients.[30] The implications of 'mixed management' are considerable with regard to the practice of palliative medicine, education and training and research.[31] If the mixed management (maybe better termed 'integrated') approach prevails, efforts for evaluation of end-of-life-care (outcome measures at least), should not usually be able to distinguish the contribution of palliative care services or professionals if truly integrated within the whole care enterprise for a particular patient and family – a significant shift. The involvement in clinical decision-making throughout the trajectory of illness of persons with clear perspectives if not specialised competence in palliative care is a wise development.

Textbooks and journals (and websites), notably specialist palliative care resources, are replete with information and directions about the assessment of patients, techniques for relief of pain and other symptoms, particular approaches to the care of patients in special circumstances, and ideas about how to organise care, and so on.

Clinical decision-making may justify more attention. Decision nodes punctuate the experience of illness for both patient and physician, but the impact of right or wrong decisions is hefty for not only the patient: but also for carers and administrators of (finite) resources. Decisions are made by those charged with the care of seriously ill patients (and their families) almost every hour of every day with regard to almost countless matters, including choice of investigation, treatment approaches to be adopted, appropriate consultation procedures, or approaches to communication. Some decisions are easy, almost automatic, according to established protocol, but others require much more scrutiny.

Clinical decision making when a patient is in the last phase of life, and especially if approaching death, may be particularly fraught with difficulties. Matters for decision-making in such circumstances may include not only technical aspects of palliative medicine but also issues with complex ethical content such as how to balance competing strategies and when (and of what process) to allow a patient to die rather than to persist in efforts to prolong life.

Clearly some methodology, which becomes almost instinctive even in situations of complexity, needs to be internalised in the course of medical education and training. How can this be approached? The vast literature in ethics is complex, nurtured by several discernible philosophical streams; the philosophical basis of ethics is getting more attention,[32] and may need a greater presence in Australian medical schools. But it is not ethicists who are the clinical deciders in everyday practice: heightened ethical competence and increased capacity to articulate the processes by which one arrives at a decision (after due consultation) may be required of physicians now. The following is a relatively simple approach which seeks to recognise and embody the main ethical traditions without even using the names. The approach takes cognizance of the relationality of persons: persons as constituted and rooted in relations, to self, to other persons, to the transcendent (however conceived), to personal history, and to cultural and biological inheritance, as well as current environment, and communicable hopes.

Clinical decision-making requires first, the clarification of what are the reasonable options, justifying attention, under the particular prevailing circumstances. Obviously input will be needed at this point concerning not only the objective aspects of the patient's condition (for example, a woman with good performance status with advanced ovarian cancer not responsive to 2nd line chemotherapy), but also more individual and subjective dimensions of the situation as known to clinical staff. Relevant legal requirements and resource restraints must also be known. It cannot be wise or mandatory to place on the table, for further consideration, all possible (even experimental) options: in the real world, respect for the autonomy of patient does not demand that. Judgement, hopefully wise, is exercised in that initial choice of options worth further consideration.

Thereafter, each reasonable option may be considered systematically in terms of the traditional ethical principles (very briefly mentioned here):

autonomy – what do the appropriately informed patient or patient and family prefer?

beneficence – what benefit might be expected from this course of action and what are the chances (on what evidence?),

non-maleficence – what harm could ensue from this course of action, and what is the risk (on what evidence?),

justice (individual and social) – would this proposed course of action be fair to the patient, and also fair to the others concerned, notably carers/family/hospital/community.

Controversy surrounds the role of the four traditional ethical principles in guiding judgement. Each principle needs to be adequately understood in the light of the foregoing discussion concerning to the meaning of persons: this is the case for autonomy especially, in view of the prominence of this element in current deliberations at least in the West. Informed consent is a complex concept indeed, if information is limited to medical data concerning procedures planned, risks entailed, and probability of benefit, considered by an isolated stressed ill patient.

[Jeff] Malpas has recently articulated some aspects of autonomy from a philosophical perspective:

> It is not that autonomy has no relevance to an understanding of human being, but rather that too great an emphasis on autonomy alone threatens to deliver a distorted picture of that in which a human being consists. Who and what we are is not determined solely by our existence as independent beings, but is instead intertwined with the being of those others to whom our lives are shaped, as well as with respect to the wider world in which our lives are played out ... If the principles that determine human being are indeed principles of relationality that place human thinking and acting in an ever-present relation of interdependence with others and with the world, then to think and act autonomously will not be to think and act in separation from others and the world, but to think and act in a way that is attentive to them.[33]

It is clear that the principles alone, narrowly interpreted and in isolation, are not an adequate basis for decision-making: the present approach seeks to avoid these pitfalls. An ecological view of clinical decision-making recognises not only the relational dimensions of the principles, but also the relation between them, but recognises also the human capacity to make wise judgement in situations of complexity – an expression of 'virtue' so emphasised in the virtue ethics tradition. The deontological ethics tradition is recognised as influencing prevailing values, and consequentially, the imperative to examine carefully not only the merits of strategies under consideration but also their foreshadowed outcomes. There is another point maybe worth noting. In a criminal case, judgements are made on the basis of 'beyond reasonable doubt', but in a civil case, on the basis of 'on the balance of probabilities'; it seems that the latter standard pertains to clinical decisions, leaving open the possibility of error, despite all care. And we must be prepared to cope with making errors. There is need for far more articulation of the matters raised in this discussion.

Discussion about strategy is vitiated by unclear goal(s). Goal setting requires care; generic concepts such as relief of suffering or prolongation of life need precision in the circumstances of an individual patient, in a particular time and place and state. Strategies, once the goal is set, also require careful thought.

Care needs to be taken to avoid flat-of-the-curve medicine[34] with diminishing benefit from increasing expenditure of resources (energy, time, even patient distress, as well as finance). Physicians, especially, need to be alert to the possibility of some options being clearly at the flat part of the curve. A schematic diagram with regard to cancer may illustrate this point (see figure below). There are some aspects of cancer care which bring high yield in relation to resources used: pain relief is one example, closely followed by surgery, radiotherapy or chemotherapy in situations where cure is considered, on the basis of available evidence, a likely outcome. On the other hand there are circumstances where benefit may appear less in proportion to resources, and even situations where the more that is done the greater the distress of the patients, with ensuing harm not benefit. Working at the flat-of-the-curve is justifiable in carefully monitored research settings: obviously effort is necessary if advances are to be made in apparently intractable situations, but there is need for continuing ethical transparency. In all circumstances, there must always be consideration of what is meant by benefit and in whose eyes. What is the good is an old philosophical question, and so very relevant. Differing notions of the good may be at the bases of many difficulties in clinical decision-making: there is room for deeper reflection.

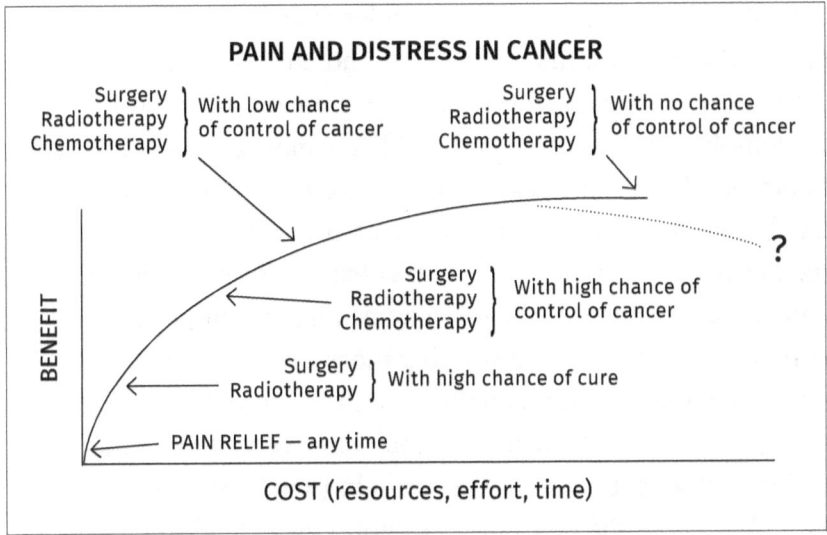

In the course of complex clinical deliberations, implicit and even explicit attention should be given to the values prevailing in the particular circumstances and cultural climate, forming, as it were, a moral horizon. Values may include items such as the following: value of life, human dignity, human possibility, value of last phase of life and of dying, privacy, human fraternity, liberty, equality and other matters held dear. Each has a history and is subject of vast literature, and worthy of close scrutiny with respect to present relevance.

Furthermore, the clinical decision-making occurs on the basis, not only of medical facts (including 'evidence'), but also legal facts, and resource limitations, and social facts. Social facts, often given little attention or not seen as core issues, are also highly relevant: especially facts about likely social consequences of favoured options. As previously mentioned, there is a case for a Carer Impact Statement to be prepared with respect to any option being seriously considered: the impact on carers/family of further treatment of attempts to prolong life, or say, moving the patient to another facility for a perceived benefit, needs to be carefully considered and documented as part of the decision making process, not after a judgement is made: an Environmental Impact Statement prepared if contemplating building an airport is an analogy! An attempt to prolong life for a week or two, or even a month or two, by another course of chemotherapy, with a chance of response of the disease of 5–10%, and an 80% chance of severe side effects increasing the burden of care, may be an acceptable proposal at first sight, for a patient wanting more time if possible, but may appear less wise when the burden to those she loves is considered. And all her life she may have considered others, and would want to now, at this fraught time, if she was informed about the consequences not only to her but to them of an option on the table.

It needs to be kept in mind when striving (laudably) for evidence-based medicine, that not all that is known has been written down in Western European languages, and not all that has been written in these languages has been considered by those formulating statements regarding evidence. Further, the personal and individual aspects of the situation of a person experiencing the illness are deliberately suppressed in clinical trials. The continuing process of reduction needs to be noted, and the limitations as well as the value of 'evidence' kept in mind. Evidence for the potential benefit or harm likely to ensue from a proposed course of action is of course not the decision: evidence for the efficacy and efficiency of clinical manoeuvres is part of the fact base, not the decision. Evidence based guidelines often recognise the need for individualisation, but it needs to be given more emphasis; evidence is not itself judgement or wisdom.

In the face of all of these elements of a complex ecological situation, a decision must be made (unless delay will not be harmful) of what it is most wise to do, a choice between options. This exercise of judgement requires 'virtue' or professional integrity, manifest as clinical wisdom. It is noteworthy that a judgement that a specified course of action (for example, a specific anti-disease treatment) would be futile, is a judgement the patient may need to make in the light of appropriate and comprehensible information about the possibilities of both a favourable outcome and harm, including harm to carers. On the other hand a physician cannot be obliged to implement a decision which he or she considers, on balance, to be unwise, or simply wrong: patient autonomy is not the only autonomy at stake in a complex situation.

Certainly, the way we choose to live the last weeks or days of life is as diverse as the way we choose to live other periods of life. There is surely no correct way to die! The teaching of *ars moriendi* of past times did not wholly specify that! [William Shakespeare's] King Lear was insistent in rejecting attempts to avert his death:

> O let him pass, he hates him,
> That would upon the rack of this tough world
> Stretch him out longer

But the poet noted (considering the impending death of his father), 'Rage, rage against the dying of the light', but we do not know whether the father agreed!

The dignity of difference in this and all things is to be celebrated, whilst celebrating also human connectedness. It is not the role or responsibility of professional carers to attempt to change personal preferences, but it may however be a responsibility to ensure that there is adequate consideration given to the impact of individual preferences on others and indeed that the patient has appropriate understanding of this as well as other implications of treatment options (information hard to impart gently but information which should not be withheld).

Obviously, seriously complex matters are over-simplified in this account, and by this process. Nevertheless, a conscientious, even if brief, systematic consideration of the overtly sensible options may offer a way through a difficult morass, and assist patients and professionals under stress. At the very least, the reasons for a very difficult decision will have been articulated, even written down, for consideration later if the outcome appears to have been unsatisfactory, or unexpected. As Karl Popper stressed, careful examination of error is a tool for the advancement of knowledge, and this idea has been found helpful in the context of palliative care.[35]

An overall ethic needs to be imprinted in the mind of a physician charged with the care of those with eventually incurable illness. With respect to individual patients, I have been guided, over the years, by the traditional Jewish ethic: 'Affirm life! But do not obstruct death!' Furthermore, a fundamental ethic needs to be embodied in a just society – that the weak are to be valued and cared for.[36] It may be timely to note again, 60 years later, the analysis of [Leo] Alexander at the Nuremburg trials, that the travesties of the medical profession (with nurses also involved) arose from an initial devaluing of those who were incurably ill, the weakest in society.

> The beginnings at first were merely a subtle shift in emphasis in the basic attitude of the physicians. It started with the acceptance of the attitude, that there is such a thing as life not worthy to be lived. This attitude in its early stages concerned itself merely with severely

and chronically sick. Gradually the sphere of those to
be included in this category was enlarged to encompass
the socially unproductive, the ideologically unwanted,
the racially unwanted and finally all non-Germans. But
it is important to realise the infinitely small wedged-in
lever from which this entire trend of mind received its
impetus was the attitude toward the non-rehabilitable
sick ...[37]

It has been said, by a professor of anatomy, that, 'the task
of medicine is to emancipate man's interior splendour':[38] it may
be the human task to grow to understand what is that splendour.
Maybe the core is, after all, a web of relationships, a fragile
unique pattern, a complex gossamer, yet the substance and
form of human dignity, embodied in each one uniquely. 'The
longest journey is the journey inward',[39] and we may come to
see that the rock to which we journey is within ourselves, our
human core, and one day we will know it, and enter into it, and
stay there. If this is the fundamental personal reality our care
systems have much to safeguard and to cherish.

In conclusion

At the heart of Australia is a rock – Uluru, and the seeking
of the centre is a constant in Australian culture.[40] The most
difficult journey for the discipline of medicine in Australia
may be the exploration of its own core. It may be that there are
Australian nuances to the concept of person which may yet to
be appreciated: the chequered long history of humankind in this
place, the kaleidoscope of cultural patterns, the hidden personal
and collective often hidden grieving, and the relationship to the
painful beauty of the land may contribute to the configuring
of the human persons here, and to the ongoing conversation.
Maybe, the kindness of strangers, the giving and receiving of it,
is part of our inheritance and a principle of our hope.

REFERENCES

1. An Occasional Paper, Sydney Institute of Palliative Medicine, Royal Prince Alfred Hospital, Sydney. Edited version of the Barbara Leroy Memorial Lecture, Annual Conference of Palliative Care Association, NSW, 2 November 2006.
2. Barbara Leroy (1932–2003) was initially an educator, who later became a remarkable nurse who oversaw palliative care of patients (and their families) in the sparsely populated Far West region and eventually, the Middle Western region NSW. She was an extraordinary leader, innovator, administrator, persuader, and friend, and an inspiration to those who knew her, especially professional colleagues. She died suddenly, soon after her third attempt at retirement. Three years later the decision was made to inaugurate the Barbara Leroy Memorial Lecture.
3. Spoto D. *The Kindness of Strangers: The Life of Tennessee Williams*. London: Bodley Head; 1985.
4. Thornhill J. *Making Australia: Exploring ouDoctor as Leaderr National Conversation*. Newtown: Millennium Books: 1992.
5. *Clinical Ethics*. Omaha: Creighton University Press; 1998. p 87–94.
6. Clendinnen I. 'Dancing with Strangers'. Melbourne: Text Publishing; 2003.
7. Needleman J. The perception of mortality. Ann NY *Acad Sci*. 1969; 164(3):733–8.
8. Whitman W. Song of Myself, no 7, in *Leaves of Grass*, 1891–92 Edition. Philadelphia: David McKay; 1891.
9. Gastmans C, K Dierickx, H Nys and P Schotmans (eds.), *New Pathways in European Bioethics*, Antwerp and Oxford: Intersentia; 2007.
10. Vanlaere L, Gastmans C. A normative approach to care ethics: the contribution of the Louvain tradition of personalism. In Gastmans C, et al (eds) *New Pathways to European Bioethics*. Antwerp and Oxford: Intersentia; 2007. p 99–116.
11. Apley, J. An ecology of childhood. *The Lancet* 1964; 2:1.
12. Lickiss JN. The Aboriginal People of Sydney with Special Reference to the Health of their Children: A Study in Human Ecology. MD Thesis, University of Sydney. 1972.
13. Verkerk M. Care ethics as a feminist perspective on bioethics. In Gastmans C et al (eds) *New Pathways to European Bioethics*. Antwerp and Oxford: Intersentia; 2007, p 65–79.
14. Feinstein AR. Clinical Judgement Revisited: The Distraction of Quantitative Models. Ann Intern Med 1994;120:799–805.
15. Erikson EH *The Life Cycle Completed: A Review*. New York: Norton. 1982.
16. Lickiss JN. Role of the doctor in the care of patients with far advanced cancer. In: *Palliative care for the 90s*. Edited R. Woodruff. Asperula, Melbourne, 1989.

17 Malpas J and Lickiss N (eds) *Perspectives on Human Dignity: A Conversation.* 2007, Springer, Dordrecht.
18 Lickiss N. On human dignity: fragments of an exploration. In Malpas and Lickiss, *Perspectives on Human Dignity: A Conversation.* op cit, p 27–41.
19 Chochinov HM. Dignity and the essence of medicine: the A, B, C, and D of dignity conserving care. BMJ.2007; 335(7612):184–7, 2007.
20 Tronto, J. *Moral Boundaries: A Political Argument for an Ethic of Care.* London and New York, Routledge, 1994, p1030.
21 Verkerk M. Care ethics as a feminist perspective on bioethics, in Gastmans, et al (eds) *New Pathways to European Bioethics,* Intersentia, Antwerp and Oxford, 2007, p 65–79.
22 Taylor C. *Sources of the Self: the Making of Modern Identity.* Cambridge: Harvard Uni Press; 1989.
23 Lickiss JN. The Human Experience of illness. In *Palliative Medicine*: Walsh et al. (ed) Elsevier.
24 Porter R. *The Greatest Benefit to Mankind: A Medical history of humanity from Antiquity to the Present.* London: Harper Collins; 1997. p245.
25 Cassell E. The goal of medicine the relief of suffering. *New Eng J. Med.* 1982; 306:639–645.
26 Morse JM. Toward a praxis theory of suffering. *Advances in Nursing Science* 2001;24:47–59.
27 Meier DE, Back AL, Morrison RS. The inner life of physicians and the care of the seriously ill. *JAMA* 2001; vol 286(23): 3007–3014.
28 Diedrich,WW, Burggraeve,R, and Gastmans C. Towards a Levinasian Care Ethic: A Dialogue between the thoughts of Joan Tronto and Emmanuel Levinas. *Ethical Perspectives* 2003; 13(1):33–61.
29 Field MJ, Cassel CK eds. Approaching Death: improving care at the end of life. Committee on the end of life. Institute of Medicine. Washington: National Academy Press; 1997.
30 Steinhauser KE. Christakis NA. Clipp EC. McNeilly M. McIntyre L. Tulsky JA. Factors considered important at the end of life by patients, family, physicians, and other care providers. *JAMA.* 284(19):2476–82, 2000 Nov 15.
31 Glare PA, Virik K. Can we do better in end of life care? The mixed management model and palliative care. *Med J Aust* 2001; 175:530–533.
32 Ten Have HA, Gordijn B. (Editors), *Bioethics in a European Perspective.* Dordrecht: Kluwer Academic Publishers, 2001.
33 Malpas J. Human dignity and human being. In Malpas J and Lickiss N (eds), *Perspectives on Human Dignity: A Conversation,* 2007, Springer, Dorderchi, p 19–25.
34 Enthoven AC. Cutting cost without cutting the quality of care (Shattuck lecture). *N Eng J Med* 1978; 298:1229–38.
35 Glare PA, Lickiss JN. Quality Assurance in Palliative Care (letter). *Med J Aust* 1992; 157:572.

36 Lickiss JN. On the care of our aged: privilege and responsibility. *Australian Rehabilitation Review* 1982; 2(6):51–57
37 Alexander L. Medicine under dictatorship. *New Eng J Med* 1949; 241:40–47.
38 Mortimer K. The impossible profession: the doctor – priest relationship. *Proc Aust Assoc Geront* 1974; 2:81–82.
39 Forster EM. *A Passage to India*. London: Edward Arnold; 1924.
40 Haynes R. *Seeking the Centre: The Australian Desert in Literature, Art and Film*. Cambridge: Cambridge University Press; 1998.

7

THE PATIENT AS PERSON

I

ON HUMAN DIGNITY: FRAGMENTS OF AN EXPLORATION
2007

in Perspectives on Human Dignity, ed J Malpas and N Lickiss, Springer, Dordrecht, 2007, pp 27–41.

> What counts in the things said by men is not so much what they may have thought or the extent to which these things represent their thoughts, as that which systematizes them from the outset, thus making them thereafter endlessly accessible to new discourses and open to the task of transforming them.
> —*Michel Foucault*[1]

How should we begin to think about human dignity? Rodney Hall, the Australian writer wrote a fascinating novel called *The Island in the Mind*: he wrote, at one level, about the postulated southern land in the mind of seventeenth century Europeans (an 'island in the mind').² Maybe the idea of human dignity is an 'island in the mind': it is there, we are aware of it, it is present to us in the substratum of our discourse, it gets into our writings, it is in the background of all sorts of debates, and, as in Rodney Hall's book, it is a *terra incognita*. There is an island there, a mysterious island indeed, and I propose to try to explore this notion or terrain as if one is exploring an island which beckons for exploration: images of childhood here!

How does one get to an island? We have several possible routes, and many options.

If we had a lifetime, we could consider many streams of human archaeology: what do the traces of the human tell us – especially about the symbolic life? The resources are too rich: even a fragment is fascinating to a non-professional inquisitive explorer, for example, the ancient Upper Palaeolithic images in the Lascaux caves in France are considered to reflect sophisticated Shamanic activities,³ and Aboriginal rock paintings in Australia may well reflect similar thought worlds.⁴ We certainly learn from even a glimpse of archaeological richness that, as Walt Whitman wrote, 'I am not contained between my hat and my boots',⁵ and neither can the concept of human dignity be so contained. The awareness of the social world and symbolic universe immediately appear to be generated within, not outside human consciousness, albeit in response to other realities.

There is an interesting connection here with debates concerning the origin of religious practices and ideas, usually based in major traditions on some revelatory event. [N] Gillman discusses this usefully for the modern inquirer;⁶ he notes that for [B] Kaplan, 'the experience of revelation is very much akin to other forms of human creativity. When we experience within our social order, or in humanity at large, a striving for ever-growing levels of perfection, when we devise means to reach those levels, and when we are personally impelled to put these means into effect, we have experienced revelation'. Gillman notes further that 'salvation' for Kaplan 'denotes the actualisation of all our values and the elimination of all evils that come in the way of personal and social fulfilment', and the word 'God' denotes not a 'personal' being but a 'certain kind of activity … salvational activity'. Could these ideas take forward an exploration of current, possibly difficult, notions of 'human dignity' as: a) conferred from outside (for example, by a creative or revelatory event – man as the image of God, or others (politicians, law-makers, physicians), or b) restricted to the notion of autonomy (after [Immanuel] Kant) or, c) even, as in a recent literature review concerning the illness experience of older adults as 'an individually defined construct involving self – esteem, respect, well-being, and pride'.[7] Extensive medical practice induces restlessness with conventional ideas of human dignity such as mentioned: the notion of 'God' may be obscure in a secular culture (especially contemporary clinical subculture), the limits of autonomy as basis of or defining human dignity become more and more obvious, and even the 'individually defined construct' appears inadequate in the face of the complexity of the human condition. Relationality (or, as we may also refer to it, mutuality) must somehow be recognised as primary in any exploration of human dignity.

Alternatively, we could engage with philology – and semiotics: to try to grasp the notion of the human and human dignity which can be appreciated by an adequate understanding of human language and symbols – over time, and space, in diverse cultures. We quickly recognise that dignity was closely related to status (*dignitas*) in the Greco-Roman period, but in more recent times, for example, since the French Revolution, other notions are included: this touches the realm of the historian.⁸ Extensive studies of contemporary language in diverse cultures could yield a rich harvest of how men, women and children understand human dignity, and meaning, and circumstances, which threaten dignity, and modes of restoration. Any such exploration would at least touch on human rituals for recognition of and restoration of respect for dignity, with the actions themselves pointing beyond language.

As another option, we could ponder the physical universe, to try to comprehend more of the meaning, place and possibility of man: we would be within a long tradition if we did so, especially if we can accept that the sacred concepts and writings of most people appear to have been a response to such reflection, for example, in the Hebrew scriptures.⁹ But even some of these writers considered that a search for wisdom is 'chasing of the wind'!¹⁰ One of the matters, which can frustrate, especially the young seeker after the 'meaning of man' and by inference 'our dignity' is the enigma of our place in the universe. The physicists no longer cut us down to size, but in their best moments (like the poets) they seem to help us cope with the size we are, a speck, but a precious speck, even immortal diamond.¹¹ We do participate in the matter of the universe; and, even as matter, we share in whatever immortality (or not) the physical universe has, being maybe, each of us, a unique but passing pattern, rendered coherent for a time (or forever) by or whatever spirit is, came from, or means.

Cultural anthropology (obviously cognate with linguistics and semiotics) offers another route to this island of the mind. What is understood by human dignity in one culture may be considered indignity in another. Or we could examine formally the historical dimensions of the idea of human dignity, even in one culture, or place, over time, and in relation to other events/trends/pressures. Or sociologists could be consulted: what do we know of the social dimensions, origins, implications or the idea of human dignity, in our time and in past times …? And how do political scientists and legislators view human dignity?

There are so many prisms through which the gaze may pass! It is obvious that the sciences concerning the human necessarily interpenetrate, with permeable boundaries. The situation is like the story of many men feeling part of an elephant and each trying to describe first (easy), then interpret (harder) what they have felt or experienced. [Wilhelm] Dilthey, in his introduction to the human sciences (as distinct from natural science), stressed the historical dimension in any approach to understanding the human, since man is an historical being, in evolution.[12] It can be contended that medicine is fundamentally a human science, however a significant place the natural sciences hold in the study and practice of medicine: there is much to learn from the consideration of the writings of Dilthey who was, as a philosopher, 'totally consumed with that most universal of beings in the universe, man himself, all his manifestations … and Dilthey's pursuit of man took him in all the directions that man himself has taken.'[13] It may be said that the entire philosophical tradition has been obsessed by the human seeking understanding,[14] with the ill-defined idea of the dignity of the human, as a driving force, continuing to press the search for knowledge if not comprehensive understanding of man.[15]

In addition to sociology, philosophy, and anthropology, where the idea of human dignity is if not often articulated, but always implicit, conventional theological and religious studies often specifically focus on 'human dignity' as explicitly linked with concepts or reality of a supreme being, however, named. I have already alluded to Kaplan's notions, which might not find much acceptance in more conventional religious cultures, but on the other hand, may prove to be a useful bridge. The Second Vatican Council (notably in the document the Church in the Modern World, in the writing of which the late Pope John Paul II, the Bishop Carol Wojtyla, was much involved) devoted a chapter to 'The Dignity of the Human Person', detailing the concept that man is made in the image of God, with dignity lying in observing the law 'in his heart', in response to conscience, and that dignity 'rests above all in communion with God'.[16] [Wolfhart] Pannenberg, a Protestant Professor of Theology, nearly 20 years after the Vatican Council, sought to examine the disciplines concerning the human (the 'anthropological disciplines') with reference to such themes. The result is a weighty tome the writer of which might consider that human dignity is part of its 'raison d'être', but he does not analyse 'human dignity', nor include it in the index.[17] By contrast with Pannenberg, contemporary literature in ethics, especially but not only, emanating from continental Europe in relation to medicine, frequently explicitly attends to the concept of human dignity.[18,19,20] [DN] Weisstub and [DC] Thomasma, ask the question: 'Why then has dignity become so central to our moral-liberal thinking at the beginning of this (twenty-first) century?', and respond, 'It is incontestable this the western preoccupation with dignity was accelerated after the degrading experiences of the Holocaust, that shocked democratic observers who previously had come to the naïve conclusion that enlightened values were our best protection against evil. In the years after World War 2 and in view of widespread cynicism with regard to transcendental metaphysical assertions about absolute values, many democrats, in order to avoid the punishing consequences of radical relativism, turned to human dignity as the one arching protector value'.

These writers went on to note: 'It is no accident that the German constitutional system fashioned human dignity as the basic and absolute value of the entire constitutional structure' – in the Basic Law of Federal Republic of Germany, 1949 ('The dignity of man is inviolable. To respect and protect it shall be the duty of all public authority'). Reference to human dignity is frequent in other European writings, and is explicit in documents of the Council of Europe: the history of indignity on European soil has surely compelled the highlighting of dignity. The German Basic Law, after specifically stating that 'the dignity of man is inviolable', continues by linking it clearly with human rights, and articulates that universality of the concept as a systematising idea: 'The German people therefore uphold human rights as inviolable and inalienable and as the basis of every community, of peace and justice in the world.[21]

What can be added to this treasure of scholarship by the experience and musings of a practicing clinician? I take as my standpoint the here and now, the everyday experience of men and women often in limit situations, articulating in their actions if not in speech or writing (though empirical research can yield rich results what is implied by 'human dignity'). What, do we as clinicians, experience about the human condition? – and what, of that which we experience and know, could be a resource for philosophy?[22]

What can be a starting point?

Those at the coalface of the care of fellow citizens experiencing grave illness and/or frailty do speak, and sometimes write about human dignity?[23] and undertake research which explicitly mentions human dignity.[24,25] In addition, the voluminous research which though not explicitly referring to dignity, is highly relevant, for example the vast corpus of research on pain, suffering, abuse and so on.[26] Human dignity as a concept is there in the depths of the mind, and its violation causes distress to staff, especially nursing staff. But, those same staff do have difficulty in defining any measure of dignity, as was found in a small study which focussed on retained (not lost) capacities in the last 3 days of life. It was also found however, that staff can identify matters they regard as of high rank with regard to human dignity. It was noted that two 'retained capacities' (continence and cognitive) rate at the top in the minds of experienced professionals – and at least offer a challenge to contemporary medicine. Patients' lists may be statistically analysed, but for the individual patient the elements in a concept of dignity may be unexpected, unpredictable and indeed change from time to time as experience, loss and wisdom concurrently accumulate: serious illness or the last phase of life may be a period of rapid personal growth.

But items on lists are not portraits – just impressions giving teasing glimpses of the underlying reality, worth pondering and exploring to try to find some coherence in the emerging portrait(s) of human dignity.

What *is* human dignity? What is that which yields the notions in patients and staff as observable phenomena, facilitating expression of or giving testimony to an underlying complex reality?

There may still be value in considering, through the prism of clinical practice, some further notions relevant to the idea of human dignity, to try to find structures on which a coherent frame can be built. There are so many facets: how can they be held together? What is the shape of the image, the schema, the symbolic frame, the construct, the idea, the place in the mind, underlying all? It seems that, even to approach this place, we need to explore many matters including what we mean by 'person', what is 'suffering' in relation to dignity, and a way of considering human dignity, however understood, in the processes of clinical decision-making.

1
Towards an adequate view of a person for purposes of clinical practice

Jacob Needleman famously remarked: 'What medicine lacks is an adequate view of the person ...'[27] Continental philosophers, notably [Henk] ten Have,[28] are taking up that challenge. Experience in seeking to understand some health aspects of indigenous people in Sydney in the late 1960s led this author to develop a schema, a frame to support the thinking of a clinician.[29] This frame, slightly modified, served as an instrument for both thinking and teaching in the ensuing decades. It could be styled as an ecological view of a person, and is, hopefully, in accord with some fundamental contemporary philosophical insights.

Fundamental to the schema or frame is the conviction that a person is a relational reality. Initially, the relation is recognised to exist with the current environment, personal and non-personal, in a continuous dialectic. [Charles] Taylor[30] among others has stressed that personal identity is: 'defined by the commitments and identifications which provide the frame or horizon' ... 'I am a self only in relation to certain interlocutors: in relation to those conversation partners who were essential to my achieving self-definition ... A self exists only within 'webs of interlocution'. Taylor writes further: 'To ask what a person is, in abstraction, from his or her self-interpretations, is to ask a fundamentally misguided question, one to which there couldn't in principle be an answer ... We are only selves insofar as we move in a certain space of questions, as we seek and find an orientation to the good.' The place of language in all this is critical, and of core importance – and its presence for cognition, even if not articulation in speech needs to be recognised. We may have difficulty in expressing the critical importance of retaining language (comprehension or expression) for human dignity – but it is clear that a capacity for language (not necessarily speech) must be close to the core of the dignity of being human (an immense subject for consideration).[31]

A person is a relational reality with respect to present *Sitz im Leben*, but also in relation to a personal past: the essential historicity of a person stressed so profoundly by twentieth century philosophers such as Heidegger, is a practical consideration for medical staff. Not only the facts of the past (medical, social, psychological) but also the manner in which the patient understands, incorporates and interprets the past, is of immediate importance to the clinician seeking to understand in order to restore, rehabilitate or to continue to care for a patient even in situations of predictable deterioration even approaching death. (The role of language and narrative in psychiatry is obvious and recognised). 'Narrative medicine', currently being recognised again[32,33] as a strand of clinical endeavour, is that perspective on clinical medicine which emphasises that the patient understands him or herself as narrative – and the substance of this needs to be grasped by listening especially (rather than providing boxes to tick!), in addition to judicious questioning and prompting, and the telling of the narrative, especially if received attentively is itself a healing process. Neglect of the historicity of the patient, with so many dimensions inevitably will reduce the possibility of, for example, relieving suffering, a goal which is core business for medicine.[34]

The inheritance of a person, the platform so to speak on which and within which one's personal history is constructed, may be considered to have two dimensions: a) biological (obviously relevant for genetic influences on disease development, but also for much of personal significance, even stature or musical ability or social significance (so often tied to ethnicity)) and b) cultural. Volumes have been written on the former, and there will be no further comment here save to note that in medical circles, an emphasis on eugenics proved a tragic disaster in the early twentieth century, and the present emphasis on genetics in medical education, research and converse needs to be balanced by a regard for persons adequately understood (influenced but not determined by genetics); the humanities are a crucially necessary companion for medical lore, and their relative absence is of grave moment.

Culture is a complex reality and has been variously defined. The cultural matrix in which a child is born, and continues to be embedded, includes not only, what has been termed the 'womb of language' but so much else which will not only influence what happens to this developing person, but how this person will interpret what happens – and all this includes disease and illness and treatment, and health care, and this has been widely researched.

Thus far, the frame might be seen as a closed system, with an internal dynamic as the parts, current environment, history, inheritance and the medical state (health or illness) continually interact in describable ways. It has seemed (in my clinical experience) that the person can move out of such a closed system by means of hope. One can call hope a strategy of transcendence, but we need to be aware of the complexity of that term (and facile aberrations) and some sensitive philosophical literature.[35] One of the most painful questions one can ask (gently) of a person in a limit situation is, 'Can you tell me what you most hope for now?' and the answer is unpredictable. Hope has been given attention by countless writers, poets, novelists, playwrights, theologians and philosophers, but also (formally) by nurse researchers[36,37] and physicians (to a less extent);[38] for present purposes in our consideration of what we mean by 'person', it may simply be noted that hope,[39] the arrow as it were, which leads out of the possibly closed relational system appears to be closely related to human dignity, at least to the awareness of self-worth (as the last vestige of hope), even in extremis. Articulated hope for an ill person may be for recognisable things (and even measurable things): to be cured, to be out of pain, to get home again, to walk, to sleep, to see a particular person again, to be reconciled, to observe some ritual, or, as one man said to me, to see Halley's comet. But the hope may be anchored in other domains: the hope may be for immortality, or that I mean something to you, to others, to an Absolute, to God (however understood), or have significance in the universe: the fostering of such hope is very deep in a clinical care relationship, where there is responsibility to assist the patient (and those in the 'web of interlocution' in which she/he is constituted and lives) to fix hope on things or personal fidelity which will not fail, lest the fostering of false hope engender death in despair. It is worth recalling that in Erikson's schema of personal development[40,41] the choice of the last phase of life is between 'integrity' (a sense of the wholeness of life) and despair; clinicians or others bent on giving hope need to be aware of the tragic consequences of falsely orientated hope.

The 'going out' to the other, however conceived, even simply by the awareness or articulation of hope, appears to be part of human dignity-as-process, as a dynamic construct, as a living, evolving idea in the mind. Human dignity, the living idea, may be manifest in action, but that action is not, in the last analysis, directed inward, but outward, in relationship, even in surrender. Absolute autonomy may the antithesis of dignity, the self-locked in (truly no exit). Human dignity is not, then, a static entity, nor property, but process, always a becoming and moving to what is not yet ... as is life.

In sum, after recognition of the complexity of person as a relational reality, it can be conceded that to consider a patient in a bed or a clinic chair as contained within his/her hat and his/her boots, is gross error – and impoverishment. Some glimmer of the role of the personal (and place) relationships, which not only contain, restrain, but also constitute what this person is needs to be appreciated by a physician and nurse – however busy.

2
Understanding 'suffering' and its relation to dignity

Human suffering is a core activity, and deserves mention: consideration of current concepts of suffering may throw light on human dignity.

Clinical experience forces the conclusion that dignity is not to be equated with comfort or absence of fear, pain, or suffering, however much these human experiences may threaten or even impinge on dignity. Emotions are core experiences in human life – and in the lives of other animals. Contemporary philosophers such as Nussbaum[42] have stressed the value of emotional intelligence, and the place of emotions in the totality of personal life: we are not just rational animals. We can simply attest to the role of human emotional responses in response to powerful stimuli – and to the complex cognitive, processes concerned with self-interpretation and critical decision-making in times of personal crises, with profound effects on personal development, as emphasised in Erik Erikson's corpus. As previously mentioned, Erikson portrays the last developmental phase of life as characterised by either a movement/choice towards a sense of 'integrity' (by which he means wholeness of life) – or despair: Erikson does not imply that what he deems the negative choices at critical points of personal development equate with loss of dignity. Health professionals indeed can observe individuals with seriously flawed personal development, even with seriously identifiable psychopathology, who retain in the midst of it, human dignity, not merely intrinsic because they remain fully human, but even a stance expressing that dignity … this, even in despair, even in face of approaching death as well as in the midst of life. Serious psychopathology may threaten but not negate even the observable expression of human dignity.

Similarly, doctors and nurses and others closely involved in the care of very ill and distressed persons can and do distinguish human dignity from 'suffering': human dignity, even as observable, is not necessarily negated or depleted by suffering. Many seek to define suffering in a clinical context[43,44] but world literature is replete with images. Job suffered from the withdrawal of persons and goods, from what appeared to be constitutive of who he was: in the drama (it is surely a drama) the pursuit of meaning follows several well-worn paths, ending with the bursting in of absolute transcendence and the forceful statement that merely human effort cannot construct meaning or the reason why in the midst of such suffering. But there is no hint of Job losing 'dignity', even as he lost his bearings – 'footing', so to speak: food for thought.

Cassell, in his landmark paper,[45] offered an operational definition of suffering: a sense of impending personal disintegration. It is to be noted that the suffering is in the sensing of a possibility of, in common parlance, 'going to pieces'. Patients can attest to ever having felt like this in the course of a serious illness and, if so, can define the 'trigger' (McCosker, Best, Lickiss, unpublished study). May the 'sense' of impending personal disintegration imply also a fear of loss of dignity, as if dignity is dependent on radical cohesiveness, or even a statement of it? It appears that one of the 'triggers' named may be very close to this: for example, one woman could cope with everything (a poor prognosis, pain, stress of complex investigations, side effects of arduous treatment) but she said that a bout of faecal incontinence made her feel like going to pieces … Sometimes the comment is 'broke my spirit'. We are close to the human core here. Patients may be conscious of an interior cohesiveness, which may, in limit situations, be threatened. For others the 'cohesiveness' stopping disintegration is related to the presence of others (the webs of interlocution of Taylor) maintaining their structural integrity. This idea appears close to the 'general resistance resource' critical to well-being when health is under threat described (on the basis of major fundamental research) by [Aaron] Antonovsky:[46] he wrote about the role of the general resistance resource in maintaining 'a sense of coherence'. He, from a sociological perspective, may have been throwing light on factors such as supportive relationships which assist the person to cohere: the impending sense of personal disintegration (Cassell's 'suffering') may be relieved, if not prevented, by relationships, as well as or in concert with individual cognitive processes. It appears that personal integrity/integration/non-disintegration is not equated with 'human dignity', but the concepts appear to inhabit the same space, so to speak, and a threat to personal coherence can certainly be interpreted, if not experienced by a patient – as a threat to dignity. Human dignity is, like a person, intrinsically relational, and may be intimately concerned with the cohesiveness of relationships, which constitute the person. Antonovsky later wrote also of *salutogenesis* (restoration of health) and the significance of others:[47] very recent work indicates that outcomes for women with breast cancer are more influenced by friendship networks than many other apparently more obviously relevant factors.[48]

Two other related comments arise from clinical experience. A patient who has lost a sense of self-worth (a far more telling state than a psychiatric diagnosis of depression) and articulated by such words as, 'I am not worth bothering about', is a challenge for the clinician – who, merely by staying in the same space for a time may assist the return of self-affirmation.

Similarly, the patient who has no sense of continuing control over medical interventions, however benevolent, offers a challenge to create an opportunity not merely for respite and but also decision-making.[49] These two scenarios from real life, rare in good circumstances, but unforgettable, appear to be in the same conceptual space as 'suffering and 'dignity'. There appears to be a layer of human reality far beneath (or deep within) that which is the readily visible, and articulated, stuff of everyday: it is this that a physician is privileged to know, touch and feel – and ponder on.

Philosophers will be able to articulate, place in an intellectual frame, and trace even the traditions of thought, to which such instances and articulations relate: clinicians must experience them, be sensitive to them, and respond basically through the instrumentation of one's own humanity to the other, face to face, not merely physically but in the sense of Levinas,[50] as interpersonal encounter with the other. The Levinasian corpus points to the philosophical basis for the duty of care as not being law, social or individual contract, but the call of the other.[51] Dr Rieux in *The Plague*, the allegorical novel by [Albert] Camus, comments at the close of the book, after a harrowing experience of plague in the city, that there is more good in men to admire than evil to despise. What the experienced physician, even battered and bruised by decades of privileged concourse with fellow citizens in difficult circumstances, often notes is that human dignity may be threatened but is not negated by fear, pain, suffering, passivity, powerlessness or dying – and that, in all circumstances, there is the imperative for the physician to be the unfailing advocate of the weak.[52] This unfailing commitment to radical human worth, which we might term 'dignity', should be considered part of that which 'systematises' (in Foucault's terms) the thought worlds of clinical practice and discourse.

The debate about whether or not dignity in dying is facilitated by deliberately accelerating death by physician assisted suicide, or by euthanasia will not be entered into here, but the comments of [Daniel] Callaghan[53] should be remembered as a background to this difficult discussion: our dignity should not rest on the actions of others asked to put us to death. If one accepts the traditional Jewish ethic that a physician should strive to affirm life, but not obstruct death,[54] then there is much room for scrutinising carefully the circumstances even in great hospitals, where dying is sometimes apparently occasionally 'obstructed'.

3
Human dignity as a value in the context of clinical decision-making

Human dignity as an idea, with its appreciation as a value, is part (or should always be part) of the matrix of clinical decision-making.

The decision will usually involve a choice of options, made in the light of: a) the fact base, b) recognition of the relevant values in the cultural environment where the health care is occurring, and c) respect for the traditional ethical principles, autonomy, beneficence, non-maleficence, justice (individual and social). Awareness of values is part of the adequate consideration of beneficence, and the perspective should include matters considered by the patient as pertaining to his/her dignity; this may of course include issues related to the body, for example, care, comfort, respect, having life prolonged at reasonable cost, or being allowed to die, with death not being obstructed, but also freedom for the spirit to express relationships, to move toward another, or even Absolute other in prayer. Decision making in this perspective justifies extended consideration elsewhere.

What are the implications for medical education in the twenty-first century? Memories of the ghastly failures of the medical profession in twentieth century haunt the mind: actions especially specifically with respect to all aspects of human dignity, in the form of unspeakable aberrations and grossly unethical experimentation on the relatively powerless, (citizens in camps, prisoners, the elderly, handicapped children, not only in Europe) considered as means not ends, even in the land walked by Kant who declared how unethical is would be to do so. The most massive moral collapse of medical authorities (including senior academics) began apparently with apparently slight misjudgements, a salutary point for today, outlined in the conclusion of Alexander, medical observer at the Nuremburg trials:

> The beginnings at first were merely a subtle shift in emphasis in the basic attitude of the physicians. It started with the acceptance of the attitude, that there is such a thing as a life not worthy to be lived. This attitude in its early stages concerned itself merely with the severely and chronically sick. Gradually the sphere of those to be included in this category was enlarged to encompass the socially unproductive, the ideologically unwanted, the racially unwanted and finally all non-Germans. But it is important to realise the infinitely small wedged – in lever from which this entire trend of mind received its impetus was the attitude toward the non-rehabilitatable sick …[55]

Palliative medicine, the branch of clinical science and practice concerned especially with the subjectivity of the patient and especially with the care of the non-rehabilitatable sick, needs to be seen not as marginal but central to medical practice, indeed as core business: the touchstone of the quality of a health service or hospital, as well as the practice of an individual clinician. Disregard by doctors of the dignity of the powerless

is a grave omen: involvement in torture of prisoners falls under the same condemnation.[56] In mainstream health care practice there is need to recognise the danger of the conjunction of
a) absorbing intellectual interest in what is genetically possible (even designer babies), b) almost fixation or adulation on what is physically perfect (models, sports heroes), c) an almost obsession to remove from society, render invisible, or prevent the occurrence of marred human beings, and d) excessive respect for efficiency in administration/business/health care:[57] all four being understandable, but complex and ethically risky approaches to thought and action. Any idea of creating others to serve solely for the survival of others (for example, as source of organs for transplantation) jars a sense of fittingness in relation to human dignity, the social as well as personal implications require deep reflection, not only by novelists.[58] If such currents of thought (and even medical enthusiasms) are not combined with well-founded moral principles and unfailing respect for the dignity of persons more adequately understood, and sound medical academic leadership, a repeat of the moral collapse of the medical profession in the West could occur. 'Never again' applies to the medical profession, with its oldest contemporary members still reeling from the shocks of what happened in Europe in 1930–1945, and many of its youngest members totally oblivious to the events – and therefore vulnerable to be deflected gradually into ways of practice which should be unthinkable.

Medical education involves leading out (from *educere*) and nourishing (from *educare*) – a stretching and feeding not only with concepts of the natural sciences, but also in humanness: and this must not fail in the West (or anywhere) again. Can we educate the medical profession to recognise human dignity as inhering in the life of every man, woman and child, to be respected while life lives and after death; that this dignity and awareness of it may be increased or jeopardised (though not destroyed) the actions of others, and that respect is due not only to the body, but also relationships with other persons, personal history, place and cultural context, and finally, with whatever is perceived as the absolute other (and personal rituals expressing this relationship)? It needs further to be imparted that deliberate non-recognition or disrespect of the dignity of another (by humiliation, torture or violence) is never fitting for a physician; and that physicians in society should be trustworthy (even if all else has failed, with structures of society in ruins) as the ultimate guardians of human dignity – no greater privilege, nor more onerous responsibility: how can we teach this? Is this the radical charge to medical education for twenty-first century, so that what happened in twentieth century at the hands of physicians will never happen again?

[Michel] Foucault (in a book concerned with medical practice) issued a challenge: What counts in the things said by men? What systematises their thoughts, 'making them endlessly accessible to new discourses and open to the task of transforming them?'[59] Maybe the idea of human dignity, 'the island in the mind', if allowed to expand to its fullness, and be firmly rooted in the depths of the mind, may restore and refresh the heart (even of a burned out physician)[60] and sustain the humanity of the physicians of the future, helping them to justify the trust their fellows need to place in them. And an island, even in the mind, has its beauty, as noted in the words of an anonymous Australian poet responding to Rodney Hall's novel, *The Island in the Mind*:

> O there are
> islands in the mind !
> clouds of unremembered dreams,
> cliffs, crevasses, waterways

of spent tears sea seeking,
and a forest clearing, charred wood
of past fire, and caves
still lantern lit, flaming
the lost fire still,
and the sound of a day breaking on a quiet shore.
And you are there !

If it be said that the idea of human dignity is, after all, merely poetry, how much do we need poets to 'redress' the balance of our times.[61] [Ruth] Macklin has noted the vagueness of the notion of human dignity and questions its usefulness,[62] but vague ideas, even rumours, can begin fires! What if health services, or individual hospitals were dedicated to 'Human Dignity'? Dedication to 'The Glory of God' is commonplace in some cultures, but it is to be noted that Irenaeus, Bishop of Lyons in the second century wrote that 'the glory of God is man fully alive', not too far from a paen to human dignity! We may have run full circle. We may arrive at a radical humanism, after all. It has been said, by a professor of anatomy, that 'the task of medicine is to emancipate man's interior splendour'.[63] It may be a lifetime's task to understand what this means, but it is surely something to do with the dignity, however obscured, of every man, woman and child, everywhere.

REFERENCES

1. M. Foucault, *The Birth of the Clinic: The Archaeology of Medical Practice*, (New York: Vintage, 1993).
2. R. Hall, *The Island in the Mind*, (Sydney: Pan Macmillan, 1996).
3. D. Lewis-Williams, *The Mind in the Cave*, (London: Thames and Hudson, 2002).
4. G. Chaloupka, *Journey in Time*, (Sydney: New Holland Publishers, 1999).
5. W. Whitman, 'Song of Myself', no 7, *Leaves of Grass*, (Philadelphia: 1891–92 edition), David McKay.

6. N. Gillman, *Sacred Fragments: Recovering Theology for the Modern Jew*, (Philadelphia: The Jewish Publication Society, 1990), pp. 18–24.
7. D. A. Gruenwald and E. J. White, 'The illness experience of older adults near the end of life: a systematic review', *Anaesthesiology Clinics of North America*, 24 (2006), pp. 163–180.
8. See Milton Lewis's essay in *Perspectives on Human Dignity*, ed J. Malpas and N Lickiss, Springer, Dordrecht, 2007.
9. Hebrew Scriptures, for example, Gen 1, Psalm 104, Job.
10. Hebrew Scriptures, Ecclesiastes 2: 17.
11. G. M. Hopkins, That Nature is a Heraclitean Fire, (1918).
12. W. Dilthey, *Introduction to the Human Sciences*, (1923) trans R. J. Betzanos, (Detroit: Wayne University Press, 1988).
13. B. J. Betzanos, Wilhelm Dilthey: an introduction, in Dilthey W, op cit. p 16.
14. R. Tarnas, *The Passion of the Western Mind: Understanding the Ideas that have shaped our World View*, (New York: Ballantyne Books, 1991).
15. P. H. Rhinelander, *Is Man Comprehensible to Man?* (Stanford, California: Stanford University Press, 1973).
16. A Flannery (ed.), The Church in the Modern World (1965),Vatican Council 11: The Conciliar and Post Conciliar Documents, (Dublin: Dominican Publications, 1975), p. 903.
17. W. Pannenberg, *Anthropology in Theological Perspective*, trans M. J. (Edinburgh: O'Connell, Clark, 1985).
18. L. Nordenfeldt, 'Dignity and the care of the elderly', *Medicine, Health Care and Philosophy*, 6 (2003), pp. 103–106.
19. D. Beyleveld and R. Brownword, *Human Dignity in Bioethics and Biolaw*, (Oxford: Oxford University Press, 2001). (See also review by M. E. Sokalska, *European Journal of Health Law*, 9 (2002), pp. 413–421).
20. L. Gormally, *Euthanasia, Clinical Practice and the Law*, (London: Linacre Centre, 1994).
21. D. C. Thomasma, D. N. Weisstub and C. Herve (eds.), *Personhood and Health Care*, (Dordrecht: Kluwer, 2001).
22. K. W. M. Fulford, 'The potential of medicine as a resource for philosophy', *Theoretical Medicine*, 12 (1991), pp. 81–85.
23. A. Street and D. Kissane, 'Constructions of dignity in end-of-life care', *Journal of Palliative Care* 17 (2001) pp. 93–101.
24. K. Turner, R. Chye and G. Aggawal et al, 'Dignity in dying: a preliminary study of patients in the last three days of life', *Journal of Palliative Care*, 12 (1996), pp. 7–13.
25. T. F. Hack, H. M. Chochinov, T. Hassard, L. Kristjanson, S. McClement and M. Harlos, 'Defining dignity in terminally ill cancer patients: a factor analytic approach', *Psycho-Oncology*, 13 (2004), 700–7–8.

26 D. Doyle, G. W. Hanks, N. Cherney, and K. Calman (eds.), *Oxford Textbook of Palliative Medicine*, (Oxford: Oxford University Press, 3rd Edition, 2004).
27 J. Needleman, 'The perception of mortality', *Annals of the New York Academy of Sciences*, 164 (3), pp. 733–738.
28 Ten Have H. 'Images of man in philosophy of medicine' *Advances in Bioethics*, 4 (1998), pp. 173–193.
29 J. N. Lickiss, The Aboriginal people of Sydney: a study of human ecology, MD Thesis, (Sydney: University of Sydney, 1972).
30 C. Taylor, *The Sources of the Self: The Making of Modern Identity*, (Cambridge, Massachusetts: Harvard University Press, 1989).
31 J. N. Lickiss, 'Speech and community', *Proceedings of Annual Convention of Australian Association for Speech and Hearing* (1978), pp. 4–12.
32 T. Greenhalgh and B. Hurwitz (eds.), *Narrative Medicine*, (London: British Medical Journal Books, 1998).
33 B. Hurwitz, 'Narrative and the practice of medicine', *Lancet*, 356 (2000), pp. 2086–89.
34 E. Cassell, 'The goal of medicine and the relief of suffering', *New England Journal of Medicine*, 306 (1982), pp. 639–6.
35 F. Kerr, *Immortal Longings*, (London: SPCK, 1997).
36 J. M. Morse and B. Doberneck, 'Delineating the concept of hope', *Sigma Theta Tau International*, 27 (1995), pp. 277–285.
37 J. R. Cutcliffe and K. Herth, 'The concept of hope in nursing1: its origins, background and nature', *British Journal of Nursing*, 11 (2002), pp. 832–840.
38 C. L. Nekolaichuk and E. Bruera, 'On the nature of hope in palliative care', *Journal of Palliative Care*, 14 (1998), pp. 36–42.
39 J. Hockley, 'The concept of hope and the will to live', *Palliative Medicine*, 7 (1993), pp. 181–186.
40 E. H. Erikson, *Identity and the Life Cycle. Psychological Issues Monograph*, (New York: International Universities Press, 1969).
41 E. H. Erikson, *The Life Cycle Completed: A Review*, (New York: Norton, 1982).
42 M. Nussbaum, *Upheavals of Thought: The Intelligence of the Emotions*, (Cambridge: Cambridge University Press, 2001).
43 J. M. Morse, 'Toward a praxis theory of suffering', *Advances in Nursing Science*, 24 (2001) pp. 47–59.
44 N. I. Cherny, 'The problem of Suffering', D. Doyle G. Hanks, N. Cherny and K. Calman (eds.), *Oxford Textbook of Palliative Medicine*, (Oxford: Oxford University Press, 3rd edition, 2004), pp. 7–14.
45 E. Cassell, 'The goal of medicine and the relief of suffering', *New England Journal of Medicine*, 306 (1982), pp. 639–6.

46 A. Antonovsky, *Health Stress and Coping*, (San Francisco: Jossey Bass, 1979).
47 A. Antonovsky, *Unravelling the Mystery of Health: How People Manage to Stay Well*, (San Francisco: Jossey Bass, 1987).
48 C. H. Kroeke, L. D. Kubansky, E. S. Schernhammer, M. D. Holmes, and I. Kawachi, 'Social networks, social support, and survival after breast cancer diagnosis', *Journal of Clinical Oncology*, 24 (2006), p. 1105.
49 J. N. Lickiss, 'Care of the patient close to death', J. Klastersky, S. Schimpff and H. J. Senn (eds.) *Supportive Care for Oncologists: a Handbook for Oncologists*, (New York: Dekker, 2nd edition 1999), pp. 677–692.
50 E. Levinas, *Basic Philosophical Writings*, A. Peperzak, S. Critchley and R. Bernasconi (eds.) Bloomington: Indiana University Press, 1996), p. 8.
51 D. Manderson, 'Philosophical basis of the duty of care', unpublished lecture, Annual Symposium, Sydney Institute of Palliative Medicine (2001).
52 J. N. Lickiss, 'On the care of our aged: privilege and responsibility', *Australian Rehabilitation Review*, 2 (6) (1982), pp. 51–57.
53 D. Callaghan, *The Troubled Dream of Life: In Search of a Peaceful Death*, (New York: Touchstone, 1993).
54 A. L. Mackler, *Jewish and Catholic Bioethics: a Comparative Analysis.* (Georgetown University Press, 2003).
55 L. Alexander, 'Medical Science under dictatorship', *New England Journal of Medicine*, 241 (1949) pp. 39–47.
56 R. Farberman, 'A stain on medical ethics', *The Lancet*, 366 (2005), p. 712.
57 J. N. Lickiss, 'Late lessons from Auschwitz: is there anything more to learn for the 21st century?', letter, *Journal of Medical Ethics*, 27 (2001), pp. 137–8.
58 K. Ishiguro K, *Never Let Me Go*, (London: Faber, 2003).
59 M. Foucault, *The Birth of the Clinic: The Archaeology of Medical Practice*, (Vintage?, 1993).
60 D. E. Meier, A. L. Back, S. Morrison, 'The inner life of physicians and the care of the seriously ill' *Journal of the American Medical Association*, 286 (2001); pp. 3007–3014.
61 S. Heaney, *The Redress of Poetry*, (London: Faber, 1995).
62 R. Macklin, 'Reflections on the human dignity symposium: is dignity a useless concept?' *Journal of Palliative Care*, 20 (2004), pp. 212–216.
63 K. Mortimer, 'The impossible profession: the doctor – priest relationship', *Proceedings of the Australian Association of Gerontology*, 2 (1974) pp. 81–82.

II
HUMAN EXPERIENCE OF ILLNESS
2009

First published as an edited version in Palliative Medicine, ed. D Walsh et al. Saunders, Philadelphia. 2009, pp 42–46.

Human Experience of Illness

> Illness is the night side of life, a more onerous citizenship. Everyone who is born holds dual citizenship, in the kingdom of the well and in the kingdom of the sick. Although we all prefer to use only the good passport, sooner or later each of us is obliged, at least for a spell, to identify ourselves as citizens of that other place.
> —*Susan Sontag*[1]

1
What is illness?

Illness is a personal not medical reality, defined usually as a deviation from 'health'. Adequate definitions of health go far beyond medical facts, for example Johannes Bircher[2] stresses the facet of 'potential', by defining that 'health is a state of well-being characterised by a physical, mental and social potential, which satisfies the demands of a life commensurate with age, culture and personal responsibility'.

Although 'disease' has some subjective connotations (lack of 'ease'), the word refers in the main to an objectively verifiable disturbance of bodily structure or function, whereas 'illness' connotes subjective awareness of a state deviating from the normal state of well-being for that individual. Illness is intrinsically experiential, related etymologically to 'peril': the experience may be easy or difficult to communicate, describe or explain. Disease may be manifest in imaging, biochemical studies, histopathology and so on, in life or in death, but illness is not so demonstrable: the behavioural concomitants of illness may, of course, be observable, but not the illness itself.

It may be worth noting that illness may occur without demonstrable disease, and also that disease may be present without illness. There are many examples of the latter, even just in oncology; for example, rising levels of tumour markers heralding recurrence of symptomless ovarian cancer; but illness may appear, in the form of severe anxiety or depression if not awareness of other symptoms, simply as a result of the conveying of such information – a cancer survivor may go to a follow up appointment feeling very well, but identify as a citizen of the kingdom of the ill (and even approaching death) when leaving the consulting room.

Illness, as an aspect of the human condition in all places and times, may be looked at through any one of several prisms: history, art, literature, philosophy, sociology, psychology, theology, economics, political science – through all the prisms which can be used to refract the light impinging on the human intellect. The study of disease relates medical science to the natural sciences, but the consideration of illness marks medicine as a 'human science', requiring adequate understanding of the foundations of the human sciences, a key exponent of which was the German philosopher, Wilhelm Dilthey (1833–1911).[3] For the experience of illness is not marginal to the human condition, nor an aberrant marginal optional extra at the edge of human affairs, but central: illness is core business for a human person, almost always embedded in the pattern of a life, save maybe in the lives of those having sudden traumatic deaths at a young age (like young soldiers, but even on the battlefield illness used to be almost the norm –

more soldiers died of disease than trauma in wars until very recently, and the same situation prevails even in natural disasters).

2
Towards an adequate view of person
Illness is an intensely personal, subjective reality, and a consequence of this fact is that medical practice requires an adequate concept of a person, despite age-old difficulty in defining what is meant or defined by the term 'person'.[4] There is need for adequate philosophical anthropology as part of the 'furniture of the mind' (as John Dewey would say) of a clinician and clinical teacher. The philosopher, Jacob Needleman, pointed out in a contribution to the New York Academy of Sciences that 'what medicine lacks is any fundamental notion of the nature of man and any remotely adequate understanding of that to which we refer as a person'.[5]

In addition to the sacred writings in various traditions addressing the meaning of the human condition in the shape usually of powerful myths embodying deep truths and issuing in wise counsels, vast tomes have been written over the centuries, in the East as well as the West concerning 'the nature of man', the 'meaning of man', 'images of man', or formal studies in philosophical anthropology in a religious framework[6] and so on. But, even in a secular world, there needs to be a frame, a way of considering the human person in a manner accessible to medical (and other health) practitioners (and students) who may lack formal philosophical training but who are immersed in the human condition, not merely as individual human persons, living lives but also in the midst of others in need of their skills and often in situations of extreme distress. A simple frame has proved useful in clinical teaching: a frame to hold in the mind and to which may be attached new knowledge as well as new questions or reflections; it could be termed an ecological view of a person, which emphasises that 'person' is intrinsically a relational concept. The schema applies, of course, not just to patients, but also to carers (lay or professional).

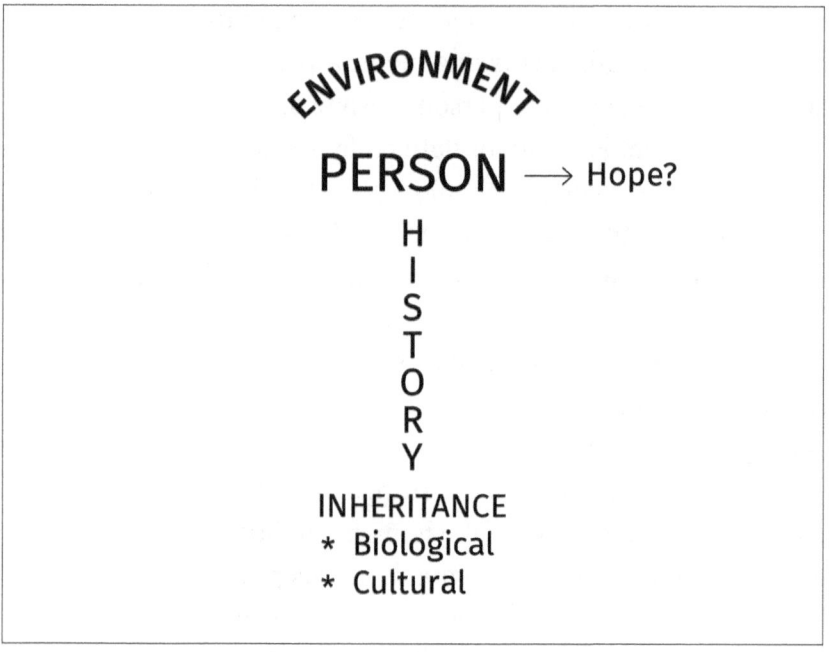

Fundamental to the schema is the conviction that a person is a relational reality. Initially the relation is recognised with the current environment, personal and non-personal, in a continuous dialectic. Charles Taylor, among others, stressed (of relevance to the current environment) that personal identity is: 'defined by the commitments and identifications which provide the frame or the horizon' ... 'I am a self only in relation to certain interlocutors: in relation to those conversation partners who were essential to my achieving self-definition ... A self exists only within 'webs of interlocution'. Taylor wrote further, 'To ask what a person is, in abstraction, from his or her self-interpretations, is to ask a fundamentally misguided question, one to which there couldn't, in principle, be an answer ... We are only selves insofar as we move in a certain space of questions, as we seek and find an orientation to the good'.[7]

A person is a relational reality with respect to the present life-situation, but also in relation to a personal past: the essential historicity of a person stressed so profoundly by twentieth century philosophers such as Martin Heidegger, is a practical consideration for medical staff.

Not only the facts of the past (medical, social, psychological) but the manner in which the patient understands, incorporates and interprets the past, is of immediate importance to the clinician seeking to understand in order to restore, rehabilitate or to continue to care for a patient even in situations of predictable deterioration, even approaching death. Neglect of the history of the patient may reduce the possibility of relieving suffering.

The inheritance of a person, the platform or scaffolding, so to speak, on which and within which one's personal history is constructed, may be considered to have two dimensions: a) biological (obviously relevant for genetic influences on disease incidence, but also for much of personal significance or social significance), and b) cultural. Culture has been variously defined. Culture related to ethnicity, occupation, social circumstance or religious tradition, the atmosphere which a person breathes from cradle to grave, but which a person also embodies will influence not only what happens, but how what happens is interpreted, and will give shape to the self and to emotional response, whether it be anxiety, fear, hope or despair.

It is to be noted that hope may be considered a way out of a closed system, a means of transcendence which is part of the core reality of the person. It will be noted (below) that the task of the last phase of life is to move toward a sense of the wholeness of life (rooted in hope in what will not fail, like the fidelity of others or one's own worth), or to despair: clinicians or others bent on giving hope need to be aware of the tragic consequences of falsely orientated hope. Some glimmer of the complexity of the relationships which not only contain, restrain, support function, but also constitute what this person is needs to be appreciated by a physician or nurse, however busy.

Walt Whitman, of course said all this, very succinctly, in mid-nineteenth century, 'I am not contained between my hat and my boots',[8] and Henry James (1892) – 'a man's "me" is the sum total of all that he can call his, not only his body and his mind, but his clothes and his house, his wife and his children, his ancestors and his friends, his reputation and his works, his lands and horses, his yacht and his bank account'.[9] Ernest Becker, who influenced a generation, wrote colourfully:

'You get a good feeling for what the self 'looks like' if you imagine the person to be a cylinder with a hollow inside, in which is lodged his/her self. Out of this cylinder the self overflows and extends into the surroundings, as a kind of huge amoeba, pushing its pseudopodia to a wife, a car, a flag, a crushed flower in a secret book. The picture you get is of a huge invisible amoeba spread out over the landscape, with boundaries very far from its own centre or home base. Tear and burn the flag, find and destroy the flower in the book, and the amoeba screams with soul-searing pain.'[10]

Western concepts arising in affluent societies are not necessarily applicable in other cultural contexts. There is room for research (compassionate and ethical) regarding, for example, the personal response to AIDS in different cultural contexts (even within one nation). But humanity is one, and some matters are universal. There is debate concerning any image of the person or of the self, and the concept of an 'inner' and 'outer' to a human person (or of 'soul') is contested, but Ernest Becker's rather dramatic portrayal of the extended self rings true everywhere in the kingdom of the ill (even if there is no wife, car or flag –just the crushed flower of a precious memory) ... illness may cause soul-searing pain by touching unexpected aspects of the self.

A note on personal development
A person is not only an intrinsically relational reality, but also a dynamic reality, ever changing, perceptibly or not, not merely structurally (by cell turnover etc) but as a functioning whole. The self is constantly being fashioned: tomes have been written concerning how persons develop and change:[11] the large discipline of developmental psychology has contributed richly. Once again, some accessible schema is needed by the practicing clinician (and teacher) to help make sense of the tapestry of phenomena expressing personal change and development to be appreciated in the everyday stuff of clinical practice. It is necessary for a clinician without formal training in psychology or psychiatry to have some grasp of the way persons (including oneself) develop, especially in response to life crises, in order that one's mode of practice might be facilitatory and not deleterious with respect to personal growth.

The ideas of Erik Erikson have stood the test of time.[12] Erikson saw human growth as taking place by negotiation of development tasks through the resolution of crisis. The growing human being is continually faced by options, each life stage being characterised by its own options which, while they confront one throughout life, do come to a point of ascendancy in a given stage. For example, the favourable outcome of infancy is an attitude of basic trust, rather than that of basic distrust, and on this basis the child goes on to face confidently the choice of autonomy rather than be afraid of decision. Where the life process is characterised by the embracing of favourable options, the personality becomes characterised by trust, reasonable autonomy, initiative, capacity for effort, a sense of identity (to be oneself and to share being oneself) rather than confusion, capacity for intimate personal relationships (to lose and find oneself in another) instead of isolation, fruitfulness rather than stagnation, and finally a sense of integrity or wholeness of life rather than despair.

The negotiations of these developmental tasks involve inevitably personal relationships and the whole spectrum of human communication, both within the present (verbal and non-verbal) and between the past and present.

In the course of such communication, life cycles, as Erikson called them, are interlocked, cog wheeled as it were, welding together the human community into a matrix in continuous process or movement.

Erikson's analysis of personal growth is sensitive indeed in its consideration of the developmental task of the elderly and, by analogy, to those of any age approaching death. He conceived that task as the development of a sense of wholeness, of integrity:

> Only he who in some way has taken care of things and people and has adapted himself to the triumphs and disappointments of being, by necessity, the originator of others and the generator of things and ideas – only he may gradually grow the fruit of the seven stages. I know no better word for it than integrity ... It is the acceptance of one's own and only life cycle and of the people who have become significant to it as something that had to be ... an acceptance of the fact that one's life is one's own responsibility. It is a sense of comradeship with men and women of distant times and of different pursuits, who

have created orders and objects and sayings conveying human dignity and love.

On the other hand Erikson noted further:

[...] the lack or loss of this accrued ego integration is signified by despair and an often unconscious fear of death: the one and only life cycle is not accepted as the ultimate of live. Despair expresses the fear that the time is short, too short for the attempt to start another life and to try out alternative roads to integrity. Such a despair is often hidden behind a show of disgust, a misanthropy, or a chronic contemptuous displeasure, which (where not allied with constructive ideas and life of co-operation) only signify the individual's contempt of himself.[13]

Erikson has been quoted at length, not only because the source is relatively inaccessible, but also because the shape of the task needs to be understood by those in contact with patients who are approaching death. Patients may well vacillate between wholeness and despair and need to be supported gently. They may long and need to try to express their internal states, explore the threat of despair and through dialogue with significant others, reach out again towards the wholeness which is possible. If it is the task of each man to explore the limits of his own possibilities, it is surely the task of the doctor to free a very ill patient from obstacles (such as pain) to such an exploration. Palliative medicine is concerned with the facilitation of free being, with liberation.

Erikson's sensitive portrayal of the developmental task of the final phase of life as being the movement towards integrity and away from despair calls for a consideration of the clinician's role in the sustaining and reconstruction of hope. No one can live without hope – but in what my hope be anchored, if it is not to be doomed to fail?

No person should die in despair – and it is clear that the doctor should surely assist the patient to centre hope not on what will in the end probably fail (e.g. 10th line chemotherapy, radiotherapy, surgery) but in what will not fail. The clinician's commitment to care, the control of pain, the intrinsic value of the patient as a unique irreplaceable subject of existence: these matters call for such pondering if we are not to add to the despair of those dying in 'high-tech' contexts – or anywhere.

It is significant to stress that in Erikson's schema, the last choice is between a sense of wholeness of life (termed by Erikson 'integrity', acceptance of one's place and time and oneself) and despair. The last phase of life (on this schema) is an opportunity for growth in wholeness, with growth occurring (as in a pot plant) from within, but influenced (as for a pot plant) by context.

3
The 'seasons of illness'

Fitzhugh Mullan, a physician survivor of cancer, coined the term, in a landmark paper, 'seasons of survival'.[14] The concept of seasons could well also be applied to the different phases of illness, which might be experienced by one person in the course of one disease (for example, lung cancer), which may or may not prove fatal. The trajectory of chronic disease has long been recognised to have definable phases,[15] but until recently the cancer trajectory has not been so readily considered.

Each phase or season of illness, as the experiential dimension of a disease, has definable though variable features, challenges and opportunities for influence by carers (lay or professional). The following 'seasons' may be delineated: the experience of diagnosis, treatment, surveillance, favourable response, non-response, relapse, surveillance, progression, approaching death, with challenges to be met as well as opportunities to be grasped.[16] Each phase may include many 'perils' – symptoms, uncertainty, ambiguity, delay, difficulties in decision making, loss of many kinds, relationship stress, and the experience of needing, as one approaches death, to trust 'the kindness of strangers', to use the felicitous phrase of Herbert Anderson (after Tennessee Williams).[17]

The 'seasons of survival' have been differentiated by Mullan into: 'acute survival',' extended survival' or 'permanent survival' (surely cure rather than immortality). Mullan considered, after describing the features of each season, that an appreciation of the seasons of survival will help both patients and health professionals to develop better strategies. He stressed also the need for further consideration and research about survivors, and attention has indeed been given by nursing personnel[18] and Australian ethicists[19] who have highlighted particularly the characteristics of liminality, a feature recognised in other contexts, for example, in the context of chronic pain.[20] Liminality is redolent of the classic studies of Everett Stonequist (1937) describing the characteristics of the 'marginal man', 'uneasily poised in psychological uncertainty between two (or more) social worlds, reflecting in his soul the discords and harmonies, repulsions and attractions of these worlds, one of which is 'dominant' over the other':[21] Stonequist was concerned with marginality due to ethnicity, but marginality in the sense of Sontag[1] (above) appears relevant.

The seasons of survival may be best and most fruitfully seen as part of this larger diverse spectrum. The needs of survivors and their experience of liminality may be mirrored in other seasons of illness: there appears need for far more research into such matters. Much has been written concerning the definable side effects of, for example, anti cancer treatments such as surgery, chemotherapy and radiotherapy,[22,23] and efforts continue to reduce the price of benefit by improvement in techniques as well as better attention to symptom management during therapy. However, it is apparent that more emphasis is needed, and that the core competence of palliative medicine practitioners (symptom relief, personal and family support, and clarification of goals – which cannot include immortality) should be available in parallel with all treatment programs, even if curative in intent, in potentially lethal conditions such as lung cancer. The more radical the treatment (justifiable if cure is a reasonable possibility) the more the skills of palliative care personnel, and necessary access to specialist palliative care services should be ensured. This may mean a seismic cultural shift, not just semantic, within oncology (and other medical services) and in specialist palliative care services as well as health administration (and insurance) circles. Only reliable parallel care may bring the benefits of contemporary treatments to patients in such a way that after the treatment phase and in survivorship they do not feel that they resemble a battlefield.

One practical issue (as oncology practice goes 'global') is the irresponsibility of introducing potentially toxic or hazardous anti-cancer treatments into contexts where there is not equal competence in symptom relief (and surveillance) and provision for personal and family support. It can be further argued that, in any culture or circumstances, when decisions are being made concerning treatment options concerning a very ill patient, for example, whether or not to try further chemotherapy with the goal of trying to prolong life, a 'carer impact statement' is needed, as well as careful consideration of the patient's wishes (preferably known for some time through a process of advance care planning instituted as soon as it looks possible that the illness will be eventually fatal, not merely when attempts to control it are failing).

These matters require urgent discussion, and research; the experience of illness is not individual, for the personal is relational with impact on the whole personal field and notably on carers.

The facing of death is one of the seasons of illness – the final season indeed. Great literature describes it; Tolstoy, in *The Death of Ivan Illich*, has provided a disturbing (for doctors) literary icon. Medical texts need to be supplemented by the humanities. No empirical medical research can capture the entirety of the experience, any more than can philosophers, or poets, or theologians, or sacred writings of all peoples: some uncertainties are at the core of human experience, and that aspect of the human experience of illness which involves facing death, though in part accessible remains part of the 'riddling essence' of human existence.

4
Psychological responses of patients to illness

The field of psycho-oncology has developed as a clinical as well as theoretical discipline, of benefit to those seeking to understand the human experience of illness in general.[24,25]

Emotions are respectable, and essential! Martha Nussbaum in her consideration of emotional intelligence, stresses from the outset that emotions shape the landscape of our mental and social lives, intimately related to thought, here echoing (and quoting) Proust who called the emotions 'geological upheavals of thought'.[26] The 'upheavals' (which may be related to new knowledge or awareness) are features of the illness of many persons and need to be recognised by others as manifestations of underlying tensions, not negative features of personalities. The changing patterns of emotional responses in the same patient over time, through the different seasons of illness, are less amenable to study than portraits in time in cross – sectional studies; there is however much value in longitudinal studies. However, narrative approaches, more common in qualitative studies, may yield precious information, even if applicability to other patients in other cultures may be limited.

The response of patients to serious life threatening disease, in all the 'seasons of illness', may be influenced not only by the particularities of the disease but also by many personal factors: personality, support structure, previous history, inheritance, culture, all the elements previously considered in the ecological view of a person. Part of the response may take the form of observable and communicable emotions, severe global distress, or states/complexes defined as post-traumatic stress disorders. Although each person is unique, some patterns are discernible.

Loss and the responses associated with grieving, are to be expected. The self may keenly feel many losses in the course of a serious illness, with the profile of loss changing with the changing season of illness: initially loss of time, finance, capacity for gainful employment, but later loss of mobility and eventually of exercise of autonomy, except to express it (as the highest exercise of autonomy) in the handing over of oneself to 'the kindness of strangers'. There is need, in such serious situations of potential or actual loss, for the professional carer to ensure not only good symptom relief – pain relief is always prominent in research studies as high priority need [27] – but also to facilitate as far as possible retention of highly significant personal capacities (speech, cognition, recognition, continence) even in the last days of life – a measurable facet of care,[28] maybe (though simple), of more value than complex quality of life indices.

Loss and grieving may not necessarily take centre stage in the array of emotions of a seriously ill person: fear may do so. Fear is not easy to investigate. An informal study concerning the pattern of elderly patients' wished-for activities in the face of obstacles caused by their (various) medical conditions or treatment demonstrated that patients (in an ambulatory care clinic) had no difficulty (except if depressed – an interesting point) in formulating things they would like to be able to do. However when the investigators attempted to look at the obverse side of the coin and asked the patients to indicate what they most feared, it was clear very quickly that this question caused much distress, and the study was aborted within one day of commencement: the naming of fears is distressing, whereas the articulation of hopes appeared to be a pleasant task.

Fear of recurrence is understandable and has been amenable to study: Lee-Jones and colleagues have reviewed this field [29] and proposed a formulation to facilitate further understanding. Their model proposes that 'stimuli, both external and internal play a role in activating cognitive responses associated with fears of recurrence', which thus comprises cognitions, beliefs and emotions; they note that possible consequences of high fears of recurrence include: anxious preoccupation, limited planning for the future, and/or misinterpretation of bodily symptoms. Fear of death has been more extensively considered [30,31,32] indeed from time immemorial, but there is less formal study of fear of other things which are spoken of in consulting rooms and even around dinner tables, such as fear of prolonged life (against one's wishes or even disregarding advance directives), fear of loss of core capacities, fear of pain, fear of abandonment; data on these things are harder to capture, because the context (and trustworthiness) of the context in which such painful questions could be asked, as well as the variability even for the same person, as well as the enormous diversity, may so affect the responses that the 'truth' may not be findable.

Hope has had more prominence in health research. Hockley stressed the relationship between hope and the will to live.[33] Kaye Herth and colleagues, also in UK, have published extensively concerning the concept of hope in nursing in various contexts, from intensive care units to the circumstances of palliative care.[34] Cheryl Nekolaichuk and Eduardo Bruera define hope as 'a multidimensional life force characterised by a confident yet uncertain expectation of achieving a future good which, to the hoping person, is realistically possible and personally significant'.[35] Morse and colleagues have analysed the 'seven abstract and universal components of hope: a realistic initial assessment of the predicament or threat, the envisioning of alternatives and the setting of goals, a bracing for negative outcomes, a realistic assessment of personal resources and of external conditions and resources, the solicitation of mutually supportive relationships, the continuous evaluation for signs that reinforce the selected goals, and a determination to endure', and some implications for nursing practice.[36]

It might be expected that the content of hope as well as its articulation by very ill patients in non-Western and resource poor countries would differ markedly from that in affluent Western contexts. Humanity is one, and hope may have some constant components, but expectations of the fulfilment of hopes may vary unless hope is centred, in the end, and at base, on matters which are not context determined such as enduring love of significant others, non-abandonment and one's own intrinsic worth: matters for reflection indeed. What is fairly evident everywhere is that the fostering of unrealistic hope ('of course you are cured', or 'there is no chance of recurrence', or 'this new treatment is sure to control your cancer'), that is, hope vested in things which may fail, may lead to despair: clinical effort needs to be expended in helping the patient to place hope in those things which will not fail, and in the end (if there is nothing else) his/her own intrinsic dignity.

Attention to suffering in the context of health care was given impetus by the landmark paper of Eric Cassell.[37] Cassell offered not only a perspective on the significance of the relief of suffering (a subjective concept), as well as the induction of improvement in a disease, as a crucial goal for clinical practice. Cassell further gave a useful operational definition of suffering, namely a sense of impending personal disintegration. Such a concept could well correspond with the colloquial 'feeling about to go to pieces': an informal study (McCosker, Best and Lickiss, unpublished) indicated that patients could readily identify a time when they felt like that, and also an event which triggered it. The identified trigger could be (as might be expected) in the field of relationships, particular loss, an unpleasant investigation, uncontrolled symptoms especially pain, dyspnoea or nausea, experience of incontinence, psychological trauma or poorly communicated 'bad' news. Clarification of such triggers in an individual patient are clearly of practical significance, offering opportunities for either reparation, support or prevention, and certainly need to be taken into account in clinical decision-making.

There are other formulations of suffering in recent medical literature; Nathan Cherny stresses the complexity of the concept of suffering,[38] Richard Chapman and Jonathan Gavrin point to the relationship of suffering to persisting pain,[39] David Kissane and colleagues describe the closely associated 'demoralisation syndrome'.[40] Janice Morse and colleagues, on the basis of a large body of research, differentiate the phase of 'enduring' from the phase of suffering characterised by emotional release, and point to the need for professional carers to recognise the distinction, lest efforts to relieve suffering be seriously misplaced.[41] In the course of an exploration of the philosophical basis of clinical ethics, Welie examines the philosophical tradition concerning sympathy in the face of suffering.[42] All such authors enhance the growing recognition of the subjective dimensions of disease, encapsulated in the illness experience.

'Cumulative adversity' has been recognised as a factor significant in the etiology of psychiatric illness.[43] The accumulation of adverse events in the course of eventually fatal illness may add up to be an unbearable burden, especially if concurrently there is reduced personal and social support. Some investigators have concluded that some patients with cancer manifest the features of Post Traumatic Stress Disorder, and it may occur at a higher rate than in the general community:[44] this might usefully be studied in relation to measures of 'cumulative adversity'.

Cancer is increasingly a chronic disease, and the considerable corpus of research concerning the experiences of patients with chronic disease[45,46,47] is relevant to the understanding of patients with chronic illness related to cancer. Maybe the universe of discourse and research concerning chronic disease needs to be juxtaposed to the conceptual frame within which cancer-as-illness (rather than disease) is considered. Knowledge (concentrated in rehabilitation literature) concerning the relationship between disease, disability and handicap is relevant, with modes of treatment influencing the resultant disability, but with social and psychological factors largely determining whether a definable disability will lead to handicap. Such ideas could be readily applied to persons with cancer, from time of diagnosis, not when disability, or (worse) handicap is established for want of intelligent preventive measures.

There is no doubt that the subjective dimensions of the cancer trajectory need far more attention, and in any cancer centre, just as much intellectual effort and resources as expended on anti cancer treatment should be brought to bear on the experiential dimensions of cancer: relief of symptoms throughout the experience, personal and family support and care planning for care, including but not only in situations of disease progression with death on the horizon. Such notions echo the recommendations of World Health Organisation two decades ago, with respect to distribution of resources in developed/affluent countries (equal expenditure on the elements of palliative care as on anticancer treatment) and in developing countries (90% of all cancer expenditure to be devoted to the elements of palliative care, especially but not only pain relief):[48] advice seriously disregarded the world over.

Conclusion

The human experience of serious illness, at any age, and in any place is one of the ordinary elements of the human condition: part of the pattern of life as we know it. The philosophical basis of the duty of care is, in the end, not law, or contract, but the call of the other, face to face: the required response of physicians involve an unfailing commitment to beneficence (which may well imply measures to cure or control disease), to the relief of suffering in so much as it arises from factors amenable to clinical measures, and to respect and guard human dignity in every circumstance, especially in those who are the most vulnerable.

REFERENCES

1 Sontag S., *Illness as Metaphor*. Vintage Books, New York, 1979.
2 Bircher J., Towards a dynamic definition of health and disease. *Health Care and Philosophy* 2005; 8:335–341.
3 Dilthey W., *Selected works: Vol. 1. Introduction to the human sciences.* (RA Makkreel & F. Rodi, Eds. and Trans.). Princeton, NJ: Princeton University Press, 1985. (Original work published 1893).
4 Thomasma DC, D.N. Weisstub and C. Hervé (eds), *Personhood and Health care*. Kluwer, Dordrecht, 2001.
5 Needleman J., The perception of mortality. Ann NY *Acad Sci.* 1969; 164(3):733–8.
6 Pannenberg W., *Anthropology in Theological Perspective*. Westminster Press, Philadelphia, 1985.
7 Taylor C., *Sources of the Self: the Making of Modern Identity*. Harvard Uni Press, Cambridge,1989.
8 Whitman W., Song of Myself, no 7, in *Leaves of Grass*, 1891–92 Edition. Philadelphia, David McKay, 1891.
9 James H., 1892, quoted in Becker E *The Birth and Death of Meaning: An Interdisciplinary Perspective on the Problem of Man*, 2nd edit, Penguin Books, Harmondsworth, 1971, p 43.
10 Becker., op. cit, p 44.
11 Siegel J., *The Idea of the Self: Thought and Experience in Western Europe since the Seventeenth Century*. Cambridge University Press, Cambridge, 2005.
12 Erikson EH., *The Life Cycle Completed: A Review*. 1982, Norton, New York.
13 Erikson EH., *Identity and Life Cycle*. Psychological Issues Monograph. International Universities Press, New York. 1969.
14 Mullan F., Seasons of survival: reflections of a physician with cancer *New Eng J Med* 1985; 313:270–273.
15 Corbin JM., Strauss A: A nursing model for chronic illness management based on the Trajectory Framework. *Scholarly Inquiry for Nursing Practice* 1991; 5:155–174.
16 Vachon MLS., The meaning of illness to a long-term survivor. *Seminars in Oncology Nursing* 2001; 17:27–283.
17 Anderson H., Living until we die: reflections on the dying person's spiritual agenda. *Anaesthesiology Clinics of North America* 2006; 42:213–225.
18 Dow KH., The enduring seasons of survival. *Oncology Nursing Forum* 1990; 17:511–6.
19 Little M., Chronic illness and the experience of surviving cancer. *Internal Medicine Journal* 2004; 34:201–202.

20 Honkasalo ML., Vicissitudes of pain and suffering: chronic pain and liminality. *Medical Anthropology* 2001; 19:319–353.
21 Stonequist EV *The Marginal Man: A Study in Personality and Culture Conflict.* Charles Scribner's Sons, New York, 1937.
22 Loescher LJ., Welch-McCaffrey D, Leigh S, Hoffman B, Meyskens FL. Surviving adult cancers. Part 1: Physiologic effects. *Annals of Internal Medicine* 1989; 111:411–432.
23 Welch-McCaffrey D, Hoffman B, Leigh SA, Loescher LJ, Meyskens FL., Surviving adult cancers. Part 2: Psychosocial Implications. *Ann Internal Medicine* 1989; 111:517–524.
24 Holland JC., An international perspective on the development of psycho-oncology: overcoming cultural and attitudinal barriers to improve psychosocial care (IPOS Sutherland Memorial Lecture). *Psycho-Oncology* 2004; 13:445–459.
25 Gibson CA, Lichtenthal W, Berg A, Brietbart W., *Psychological issues in palliative care.* Anaethesiology Clinics of North America 2006; 24:61–80.
26 Nussbaum M., *Upheavals of Thought: The Intelligence of Emotions.* Cambridge University press, Cambridge, 2002, p1.
27 Steinhauser KE., Christakis NA, Clipp EC, et al: Factors considered important at the end of life by patients, family, physicians, and other care providers. *JAMA* 2000; 284:2476–2482.
28 Turner K, Chye R, Aggarwal G, et al., Dignity in dying: a preliminary study of patients in the last three days of life. *J Palliat Care* 1996; 12:7–13.
29 Lee-Jones C, Humphris G, Dixon R, et al., Fear of cancer recurrence – a literature review and proposed cognitive formulation to explain exacerbation of recurrence fears. *Psycho-oncology* 1997;6:95–105.
30 Cicirelli VG., Personal meanings of death. *Death Studies* 1998; 22:713–733.
31 Penson RT, Partridge RA, Shah MA, et al., Fear of death. *Oncologist.* 2005; 10:160–9.
32 Spiro HM, McCrea-Curnen MG, Palmer Wandel L (eds), *Facing Death: Where Culture, Religion, and Medicine Meet.* Yale Uni Press, New Haven, 1996.
33 Hockley J., The concept of hope and the will to live. *Palliative Medicine* 1993; 7:181–186.
34 Cutcliffe JR, Herth K., The concept of hope in nursing 1: Its origins, background and nature. *British Journal of Nursing* 2002; 11:832–840.
35 Nekolaichuk CL, Bruera E., On the nature of hope in palliative care. *J of Palliative Care* 1998 14: 36–42.
36 Morse JM, Doberneck B., Delineating the concept of hope. *Sigma Theta Tau International* 1995; 27:277–285.
37 Cassell E., The goal of medicine the relief of suffering. *New Eng J. Med.* 1982; 306:639–645.

38 Cherny NI., The problem of suffering. in Doyle D, Hanks G, Cherny N and Calman K (eds) *Oxford Textbook of Palliative Medicine*, 3rd Edition Oxford Uni Press, Oxford, 2004,pp 7–14.
39 Chapman CR, Gavrin J., Suffering: the contributions of persistent pain. *Lancet* 1999; 353:2233–2237.
40 Kissane D, Clarke DM., Street AF: Demoralisation syndrome – a relevant psychiatric diagnosis for palliative care. *J Palliative Care* 2001; 17:12–21.
41 Morse JM., Toward a praxis theory of suffering. *Advances in Nursing Science* 2001;24:47–59.
42 Welie JVM., *In the Face of Suffering*. Crighton Uni Press, Omaha, 1998, p 125.
43 Turner RJ, Lloyd DA., Lifetime traumas and mental health: the significance of cumulative adversity. *Journal of Health and Social Behaviour* 1995; 36:360–376.
44 Alter CL, Pelcovitz D, Axelrod A, et al., Identification of PTSD in Cancer Survivors. *Psychosomatics* 1996; 37:137–143.
45 Ironside PM, Schekel M, Wessels C, et al., Experiencing chronic illness: creating new understandings. *Qualitative Health Research* 2003; 13:171–183.
46 Delmar C, Bōje T, Dylmer D, et al., Achieving harmony with oneself: life with a chronic illness. *Scand J Caring Sci* 2005; 19:204–212.
47 Thorne SE, Paterson BL., Two decades of insider research: what we know and don't know about chronic illness experience. *Annu Rev Nurs Res* 2000; 18:3–25.
48 World Health Organisation Expert Committee Report. Cancer pain relief and palliative care. WHO, Geneva, 1990.

III
MEDICAL PRACTICE AND SPIRITUAL CARE
2016

Professional 'spiritual care' has burgeoned in Western affluent societies in the last decades, with formal associations (with conferences with impressive programs), research programs, vast literature (in professional journals, bookshops and on line), guidelines with considerable status. Yet in this turbulent 21C there is some disquiet concerning spiritual care – not only among health professionals and not only the frail. Why? The contributory factors may include societal and individual mistrust of institutions, notably religious institutions (whilst respecting individual practitioners), confusion regarding the links between 'spiritual care' (or 'spirituality') and 'religion', and a withdrawal from certain dimensions of the self. And yet bookshops, media and cyberspace are replete with words and images about 'spirituality'.

Furthermore, experienced professionals in health services, notably palliative care services but also doctors and nurses involved in care of patients with chronic illness, may well consider the total care of patients as within their area of responsibility and find the intrusion of other professionals (with expansion of the 'team') rather difficult; a team involved in the care of one very ill patient may include now not only doctors and nurses, but nurses' assistants, physiotherapists, occupational therapists, advance care planners, and professionals for 'spiritual care'. Boundary problems may arise. But above all, very ill patients may be overwhelmed by such complexity – and seriously deprived of the two resources most in short supply, namely time and energy (for all the personal tasks in the last phase of life) and of the privacy fitting for a unique person involved in the most personal of all activities – the task of life completion.

Amidst this cacophony is there anything worth saying? Are new perspectives possible?

A perspective is simply a way of looking – at issue is an aspect of the care of persons. The implication is that there are several dimensions, levels or layers, or segments of care – vaguely in response to various dimensions of human need. So in trying to interpret more adequately the current explosion, in health services especially, of 'spiritual care' (by designated persons possibly with formal religious affiliations) as part of services charged with improving the care of patients, there is need to have a large view embracing ideas of 'person', 'spirit', 'ritual', and 'religion' – as well as ideas about human possibility and human flourishing.

The practice of medicine has a long history! The care of persons with particular needs has always involved other persons with socially recognised competence – called by many names, and with varying social status. Archaic medicine engaged the early 20C historian, Henry Sigerist. He found no reliable information about unquestionable non-shamanic medical practice in the Paleolithic period, but in the Neolithic (from around 8000 years ago) relevant traces of activities are to be found, not only trephining (opening the skull) but other surgical procedures, and other therapeutic measures.[1]

A process of evolution of medical practice is discernible over the ages, not only with respect to increasing capacity to treat afflictions but also in modes of delivery of care. From a concern about the well being of a whole person and a response by another with recognised relevant competence – a one-to-one professional relationship between a 'patient' (a 'sufferer', usually supported by kin) and a 'professional' supported by colleagues, and all with the approval of society, there has been a process of continuing differentiation with the delineation of special activities as branches of the mainstream of practice; examples include the selection of some, maybe dying, patients to leave the Hippocratic clinics to go for healing to the temple of Aesculapius, later the splitting of medical practitioners into physicians and surgeons, and later again, the recognition of public health as a designated field. Each new branch often split into further subspecialities, and the process continues with considerable momentum, within the central thrust and also the branches. The trend to continuing differentiation into separate branches is understandable, even if somewhat regretted (and protested) but why this continuous surge within the soul, as it were, of medicine, of a beneficent stream of energy leading (on the whole) to improving human flourishing? Is there a pull factor as if the universe and human history were teleological, with a defined purpose and goal? There are various ways of conceiving it all – Baruch Spinoza's 17C concept of *conatus* (striving of a living thing – person or institution to continue in being) in a non-teleological universe may be worth pondering. This portrayal of the human thrust has been reinforced in our time by recent philosophers such as Ernst Bloch[2] and has the potential to be a central notion in the present inquiry.

The resolution of tensions concerning spiritual care within the complexus of clinical, notably medical, practice (and there are tensions) may rest on a sounder conception of comprehensive care in relation to human flourishing. Whatever else, medical practice is concerned with the flourishing of persons. It is necessary for medical practitioners of today, especially in those specialties in immediate contact with very ill and/or distressed persons to have some frame in which to consider what is 'spiritual care' in relation to the whole enterprise of the care of persons. So there are several questions in play. What do we mean by 'person'? What is 'human flourishing' – a term beloved of philosophers? What *is* spiritual care?

At stake may be, especially, an adequate understanding of humanness – what differentiates the human from non-human animals? Arguments continue concerning the mark of the human: there may be a case for going back to the first glimmers of modern humanness! What do we mean by the human spirit? The complexity of the term 'spirit' is profound, even if qualified by 'human' and focussed on a dimension of person and prescinding from some usages recognised in standard dictionaries.

The following comments are recognisably limited. Can reflection on our beginnings, on our earliest modern human ancestors illumine the path to understanding? It appears reasonable, as a start, to try to discern, in the traces of the first emergence of humanness, those activities of modern humans which seem to go beyond the demands of the body, and suggest a dimension of human life which is not contained in the physical or instinctive emotional lives of our nearest non-human ancestors or contemporary associates.

The human march is long, barely understood (certainly not by this writer). It is generally agreed that Homo erectus (early modern humans) emerged maybe around 1.5 million years ago, and modern humans, Homo sapiens sapiens, at least 100,000, maybe up to 200,000 years ago. Thereafter there appear to have been critical phases: the emergence of language at a time still disputed – maybe as late as 40,000 years ago, the cultural explosion in the (so called) Middle/Upper Palaeolithic transition, the emergence of agriculture and cities – and writing. Later came the so-called 'Axial Age' from around 1000 BCE with new currents of thought burgeoning in divers regions. Later, in the West, followed the emergence of Christendom, the ambiguities of the Middle Ages, the restructuring of sense of self and world in the Renaissance, the exploration of the globe, the Enlightenment, the crash and 'terrible beauty'[3] of the 20C, and the chaos of the present 21C. The choice of what is worth noting is utterly subjective (and clearly Western-centric here): professional world historians, including those focussed on 'big history' like David Christian[4] have the task of illumination of the long path for the rest of us.

The first features of modern 'humanity' (a matter distinct from human evolution) are accepted to be noted around 60,000–30,000 years ago. Archaeologists agree that whilst early modern humans had been around for over 100,000 years (maybe 200,000) leaving evidence of tool making and other manifestations of practical intelligence and some language, there was a cultural explosion (likened to a big bang) 60,000–30,000 years ago, during which period art and, religion emerged, and other practices appeared, for example, critical changes in burial practices (the oldest modern human burial found thus far in Australia, at Lake Mungo NSW, dates from around 30,000 years ago).[5] Also this is the period of origin of the now famous European cave art: the cultural explosion (notably in the period 30,000–12,000 years ago) gave rise to cave art of sheer magnificence.

Why this 'explosion'? It was probably not due to dramatic changes in brain size or macro-structure: from the first appearance of modern humans brain size changed very little. Archaeologist David Mithen, in his exposition of the evolution of the human mind, regards a change in brain *function*, in cognitive capacity, which he terms 'cognitive fluidity', as the critical seminal factor in the genesis of the explosion.[6] He considers that archaeological evidence suggests that human thought ceased to be compartmentalised – and synthetic capacity enabled the modern human to relate one area of observation and information to another.

Synthetic activity is indeed fruitful – and serious interdisciplinary encounter is one form of this. It may be useful to pay attention to the conclusions of recognised relevant specialised seminal scholars in archaeology: such as David Lewis-Williams,[7] Jean Clottes,[8,9] Aujoulat,[10] Steven Mithen (already mentioned), David Whitely[11] and anthropology: notably Clifford Geertz,[12] and David Rappaport;[13] and sociology, particularly Emile Durkheim.[14] The ideas of these significant thinkers, and if brought together, may facilitate the emergence of a view which can enrich the 21C mind searching to enhance the flourishing of humankind.

There is abundant documentation now available in the scholarly works by original investigators noted above and those carefully compiling the findings – and undoubtedly far more material to be found by ongoing research, including work in Australia.

But *why* such human feats? What do these artworks, sometimes deep in almost inaccessible hypoxic caves, painted by candle light *mean*? Many theories abound; the simple idea that the animals depicted related to those being hunted has not stood the test of time or prolonged scrutiny. Mithin sees the cave art in a simple light – simply the documentations of certain animals for utility and educational purposes – as well as evidence of cognitive fluidity – for example in fusions of animal form with human. Whitely surmised that the artists were subject to mental illness which was expressed in outbursts of energy. Some notable archaeologists (for example, Lewis-Williams, Clottes, Whitely) see shamanism as at the root of the ancient Paleolithic cave art – the artists may have been in a trance-like state. Shamans – persons with particular capacities to heal (maybe associated with trance) are traceable in most cultures, including Australian Aboriginal cultures, as noted by Elkin[15] – and must have been perceived to be of human benefit.

The search for explanation continues. It is noteworthy that ancient Australian rock art (some almost as old as, or maybe older, than Chauvet) has stylistic differences – for example, far more frequent portrayal of human forms and activities and less magnificent portrayals of beasts; there is an extensive and growing literature now concerning not only Australian indigenous history in general, but also ancient Australian rock art, documented in, for example, the volumes of AE Worms,[16] George Chaloupka,[17] John Mulvaney and Johan Kamminga,[18] Elaine Godden,[19] Mike Donaldson,[20] and countless articles in academic journals and elsewhere. The history of the Australian people is long (at least 50,000 years – there is very recent clear proof of that – Flinders ranges in South Australia, 2016), and probably over 60,000 years, and recorded in fact deep in the land.[21]

Art of the Paleolithic transition is striking evidence of established symbolic thinking accepted as a mark of the human. Language, so obviously dependent also on symbolic thought, may have emerged not long before the first rock art – dating is still unclear (and unlikely to be clarified), and language is continually 'unfolding'.[22]

Rappaport, an eminent anthropologist, notes that our forebears became what may loosely be termed 'fully human' with the emergence of language composed largely of symbols:

> When discourse can escape from the concrete as well as the present, and when it is empowered by grammar, it finally becomes free to search for such worlds parallel to the actual ... It can ... explore the realms of the desirable, the moral, the proper, the possible, the fortuitous, the imaginary.[23]

The emergence of language and, later, writing offered new possibilities of portrayal of the personal – and a glimpse of a dimension other than the physical or instinctive. A handful of narratives drawn from ancient texts, will be mentioned: from The Epic of Gilgamesh, from the Hebrew 'Torah', and from Homer's *Iliad*.

The first writing was on cuneiform tablets written in Mesopotamia by 2600 BCE, first in Sumerian; texts in Akkadian (a Semitic language) appeared about 2300 BCE. The Epic of Gilgamesh which had some elements of both languages is recognised as one of the masterpieces of world literature, and may be the earliest story committed to writing. The finding of cuneiform tablets in the royal libraries of Nineveh in mid 19C, and further major finds a few decades later led to an explosion of interest in Gilgamesh and the epic is of extraordinary power – and contemporary relevance. The epic of Gilgamesh may have taken final form (in multiple copies by assiduous scribes) by around 1000 BCE – at the dawn of the Axial Age (see below).

Gilgamesh, the central character, is a young powerful, flawed and ruthless King who has arduous adventures and rich experiences on his way to wisdom; he undertook, in response to an interior impulse (shades of Spinoza's conatus?), an arduous journey replete with challenges, really of personal discovery. In the course of the narrative he experiences the death of his beloved companion ('best mate') and there is documented unforgettably the human experience of grief.

Andrew George, a noted English scholar, in his informative introduction to his new translation of Gilgamesh in 1999 notes that Assyriologist William L Moran describes the epic as 'a document of ancient humanism'. George comments further as follows on the content:

> [I]n examining the human longing for life eternal, it tells of one man's heroic struggle against death – first for immortal renown through glorious deeds, then for eternal

life itself; of his despair when confronted with inevitable failure, and his eventual realization that the only immortality he may expect is the enduring name afforded by leaving behind some lasting achievement.

The fear of death may be one of the epic's principal themes but the poem deals with so much more. As the story of one man's 'path to wisdom', of how he is formed by his successes and failures, it offers many profound insights into the human condition, into life and death and the truths that touch us all ...

As a poem which explores the truth of the human condition the epic bears a message for future generations ... Maturity is gained as much through failure as success. Life, of necessity, is hard, but one is the wiser for it.[24]

George asserts that the epic is not strictly 'myth' (which is centred on stories of the gods or has purpose to explain the origin of some feature of the natural or social world). George comments further (and relevantly to the present considerations) that the epic is not a religious poem like Newman's Gerontius: 'Gerontius in his anguish puts himself in the hands of his God ... Gilgamesh, however, in his terror and misery spurns the help of his gods ... and, even at the last, turns for solace to his own achievements rather than to his creator.'

The Hebrew scriptures also evolved over many centuries (with some activity contemporaneous with the Gilgamesh project) and were undoubtedly written and redacted over and over again, before reaching a final form around 200 BCE. There is a vast literature about all of this. The thought of Lord Jonathan Sacks (philosopher and former Chief Rabbi of UK) is fruitful for clinicians: he stresses that Torah (notably the first five books of the Hebrew Bible) is not about history or science but 'never deviates from its intense focus on the questions: What should one do? How should one live? What sort of person should one strive to become?' and 'The Torah is a sustained exploration of human freedom.' Sacks asserts that 'the great truth of Genesis 1 remains as the most powerful statement of religious humanism'.[25]

The Hebrew scriptures are indeed a library of stories concerning the human condition: in fact a work of philosophy and specifically philosophical anthropology.[26] As pointed out by contemporary scholars such as Yoram Hazony, there are complex historical and cultural factors in play influencing the nuances of the narratives, but the bare stories are still worth pondering as glimpses of humanness. A few examples will be noted from the first books.

The first pages, the creation stories, have elements in common with ancient near eastern writings (including Gilgamesh) but transcend these in grandeur and simplicity, and in freedom from a view of the cosmos as dualistic. The creation narratives in the first chapters of Genesis (especially the second story, chronologically the oldest) portray the emergence of the human as ontologically and intrinsically complex – rooted in the earth (Adam) but with an element from elsewhere (*ruah* – 'spirit/breath') and awareness of a life of dialogue or dialectic, prompted by conscience. Note also that the idea of man being the image of God, in a tradition where it is forbidden to construct images might imply that the only place ultimate reality is to be found is in the human; the human being embodying and reflecting the meaning of all that is. There are surely the building blocks of a radical humanism here.

But there are other seminal stories in the Torah which not only give further portraits of human complexity but offer glimpses of another dimension of person which may be called spiritual; one may think of Adam and Eve in the garden – of the earth but infused by *ruah* (spirit/breath) not of the earth, of Cain angry in rejection, of flawed Noah building a boat for no other reason than an inward compulsion – a sense of duty to respond to a command, and of the tower of Babel with implied uniformity of aspiration to encounter the whole (a 'spiritual' aspiration, surely) having to make way for radical diversity, Abraham conflicted concerning the idea of an imperative to kill his son – his only hope; of Jacob wrestling in the night (with himself? with an Other? with self as other?) before meeting a justly aggrieved brother; of Moses in a difficult career place shaken by an unusual happening – a bush burning in the desert – and a changed view of his life responsibility. These stories (worth reading in full over and over again in our rare reflective moments and reinterpreting) have entered into our stream of consciousness in the West.

It may be that one spends a lifetime coming to answer the two radical human questions: who am I? and who or what is the Other, Ultimate Reality, for me – who/what is 'God'? We know that, deep down, we live a life, not only impelled from within – Spinoza's conatus again, but also, mysteriously, of responsiveness to the other: this is at the heart even of clinical responsiveness and we do not need philosophers to tell us. The clinician who cannot feel the call to 'respond' is truly burnt out. This is not the place to consider concepts of 'God' save to recognise a huge range, from a personal creative being transcending the cosmos, ready to intervene in human affairs and alter the course of a river or history (or football match), and an object of belief, to (on the other hand) the unity of all that is and immanent as pattern in all that is, including the human person, a presence worthy not of petition but of praise – albeit silent. The range of meanings of the word 'God' need to be kept in mind as one considers the ancient stories in the Hebrew scriptures and the centuries of reflections on them.

The Prophetic and Wisdom Literature within the Hebrew tradition also enriched thought and influenced conduct. The prophets like Jeremiah told it 'as it was', not as the powerful might have preferred: there is a rich literature on the prophetic tradition – it may be acutely relevant as the globe shakes with challenges to power. The Wisdom literature is also too vast to do more than to note the significance in the human literary heritage. The drama of Job (and it is surely a drama not 'history') emphasised the limitations of glib philosophy or theodicy concerning human suffering – the comments of the 'friends' (spokesmen of ideas of the time) were of no solace to the anguishing man. Each person will interpret Job (as all great literature) in his or her own way, influenced by personal experience, cultural milieu or state of mind. For clinicians pondering the depths of human suffering (and finding most 'answers' woefully inadequate) the drama of Job may be precious indeed.

Contemporaneously with the Jewish literary activities, vigorous activity was occurring in Greece. In the last millennium BCE oral traditions in Greece took written form – and the works of Homer (or the Homeric tradition) became known – notably the Iliad and the Odyssey. The Iliad depicts events of the battles between the Greeks and Trojans concerning the city of Troy, and is bloodthirsty indeed, but with glimpses of further dimensions of humanness.

The portrayal in the Iliad of the aged King Priam asking for the body of Hector who had been killed by Achilles gives a glimpse of a human negotiation far beyond the ordinary. Wikipedia (the impeccable source accessible to those other than specialists in the humanities!) offers the following concise comment concerning one poignant episode:

> Priam begs Achilles to pity him saying 'I have endured what no one on earth has ever done before – I put my lips to the hands of the man who killed my son'. Deeply moved, Achilles relents and returns Hector's corpse to

the Trojans. Both sides agree to a temporary truce and Achilles gives Priam leave to hold a proper funeral for Hector.[27]

Was Priam right – that such a demonstration of pleading was *new* for humanity? It bears pondering, as does the relevance of such exchanges for the unspeakable conflicts currently raging in the Middle East. The ancient Greek Tragedies which flourished a few centuries later, portrayed very richly the moral dimensions of human life and the complexities of persons. By 6C BCE what we know as the Greek tragedies became a feature of ancient Greek culture – and contain in their turn poignant glimpses of humanness, especially regarding morality: notably individual responsibility for decision and the consequences of decision, the repercussions of flawed heroes, ethical conflict, the place and price of disobedience (for example, Antigone placing her duty to bury her brother above prohibition by the King of Thebes), the possibility for effecting harm under the influence of passion such as revenge, the possibilities of nobility. The influence of the ancient Greece is not spent yet.[28]

Harold Bloom attributed to Shakespeare the 'invention of the human', particularly by his portrayal of inwardness, say in Hamlet's soliloquies.[29] But it may be that reflective pondering on the ancient Hebrew and Greek stories may yield a richness of concept of humanness hitherto not adequately recognised.

The art of the later Palaeolithic points to the emergence of some change in human awareness of the human context. Millennia later there is evidence of further seismic change, in what historian Karen Armstrong calls the Great Transformation.[30] Jaspers had called it the Axial Age, because it was pivotal in the spiritual development of humanity:[31]

> [F]rom about 900–200BCE, in four distinct regions, the great world traditions that have continued to nourish

humanity came into being: Confucianism and Daoism in India; Hinduism and Buddhism in India; monotheism in Israel; and philosophical rationalism in Greece. This was the period of the Buddha, Socrates, Confucius and Jeremiah, the mystics of the Upanishads, Mencius and Euripides. During this period of intense creativity, spiritual and philosophical geniuses pioneered an entirely new human experience.

Armstrong further asserts that:

The Axial Age was one of the most seminal periods of intellectual, psychological, philosophical, and religious change in recorded history; there would be nothing comparable until the Great Western Transformation, which created our own scientific and technological modernity.

Why did the Axial Age happen? Was it a further development of cognitive capacity? Of responses to technological changes influencing modes of living? or a response to overwhelming suffering (as Jaspers suggests)? A quantum leap in awareness so that human inwardness came into view more clearly? Homer's heroes (at the beginning of the Axial Age) are persons of action, and display little 'inwardness', but Jeremiah certainly testifies to it ('a fire burning within me') and calls for the searching of the heart. Armstrong begins her magnum opus by noting that, 'The first people to attempt an Axial Age spirituality were pastoralists living on the steppes of southern Russia, who called themselves Aryan; they were influenced by Zoroaster around 1200BCE to become less violent. Armstrong clearly regards these efforts as presaging what was to come: 'When – centuries later – the Axial Age began, philosophers, prophets and mystics all tried to counter the cruelty of their time by promoting a spirituality based on nonviolence'. Radical ethical consciousness is being manifested in the traditions being founded – though diluted in subsequent iterations of the traditions, according to Armstrong.

It is not surprising that Armstrong stresses the relevance of the Axial Age for our own times and urges a rediscovery of the 'Axial vision'. At the very least the explosion of that millennium needs to be recalled alongside the extraordinary Palaeolithic Cave art as articulations of the human spirit. Contemporary wise thinkers, urge, in the face of unspeakable violence and distress even in affluent contexts (for example, domestic violence, youth suicide – both impinging on clinicians), a reconsideration of the (neglected) spiritual, even sacred (in the radical sense), dimension of the human person.[32]

In Australia it needs to be noted that, although our first inhabitants (the oldest continuous culture on earth, dating from maybe 60,000 years ago) do not find mention in discussions of the Axial Age or the Great Transformation there is clear evidence of not only a richly symbolic world view but profound spirituality, and an ethical system, increasingly appreciated: the classic account of Aboriginal Religions by AE Worms, translated into English only in 1973, deals (among other things) with perceptions of the world as evidenced by the extraordinary rock art, and still extant oral traditions concerning sacred objects:

> The cult objects of the Australian continent are extremely diverse in kind. Behind this lies a common belief ... in the permanent proximity of supernatural beings, a proximity mediated precisely by these objects ... To the Aborigines [sacred objects] are a means of localising and making present both a spirit and his creative energy.[33]

Stanner, another revered authority on Aboriginal affairs noted:

> The truth of it seems to be that man, society and nature, and past, present and future, are at one together with a

unitary system of such a kind that its ontology cannot illumine minds under the influence of humanism, rationalism and science. One cannot easily, in the mobility of modern life and thought, grasp the vast intuitions of stability and permanence, and of life and man, at the heart of Aboriginal ontology.[34]

Maybe contemporary thinkers and writers like Nicholas Rothwell[35] demonstrate that Stanner was too pessimistic; we moderns can and need to enter into these intuitions of our forbears in this ancient land, and be enriched thereby. Many generations and millions of men and women have walked with unshod feet where we tread in our time – maybe our foot, being shod, has yet to feel the pulse of the past.

Thus far comments and considerations have been made concerning the marks of the modern human. Underlying all the forgoing consideration is the supposition that there is clarity regarding what we mean by 'person' What *do* we mean by 'person'? Is there any problem? Maybe.

Philosopher Jacob Needleman, some decades ago, in a communication to NY Academy of Sciences asserted that, 'what medicine lacks is any fundamental notion of the nature of man and any remotely adequate understanding of that to which we refer as a person'.[36] These are fighting words!

Art and literature are replete with various images of persons – and there are compendia of such notions. There is a distinct philosophical tradition concerning the human (philosophical anthropology). 'Person' may be considered from several points of view, defined conventionally by various intellectual disciplines: biology, psychology, geography, history, anthropology, sociology, philosophy, theology – and the arts – a formidable array. The primary discipline of such thinkers influences the lens through which 'person' is viewed but, not surprisingly, concurrence of ideas is discernible. The landscape is large, the terrain sometimes difficult (with vocabulary and constructs utterly unfamiliar to a relatively illiterate clinician) but sometimes there are glimpses of meaning worth the effort of exploration.

There have been many concepts of 'person' in the history of human thought, even just in the West, about the human and the human condition.[37] The word 'person' derives from the Latin *persona,* or Greek *prosopon,* the mask which actors wore to portray a given character in a play – and thus to the roles. The Oxford English Dictionary indicates various nuances: person as role or character (from persona – a mask or guise), person as an individual human being, person as the actual self (present 'in person'), the living body of a person ('my person'), an individual or group with rights. In fact, there are many nuances of the word 'person' in contemporary usage, which bear traces of the history of the word.

Recently Simone Plourde has usefully outlined, (tellingly) in an ethics text, the evolution of the concept of person.[38] She noted that, for the ancient Greeks, the term *prosopon,* was close to the notion of *anthropos* and *soma* (the animated individual), and initially designated the human face before it came to signify the mask worn by actors on the stage. In Latin, the terms *homo, caput* and i*ndividuum* are to be found next to persona to designate man-in-general, the human subject and the mask, respectively. With Cicero the full meaning of the Latin word *persona* is established and could imply a judicial role, a social role, a collective reality, an outstanding personality, the philosophical notion of the person as strictly individual or as gifted with reason. The complexity of the notion is manifest even then!

Plourde further notes that in Christian antiquity the notion of *persona* was deepened, notably in relation to debates about the Trinity. By the Middle Ages there was prominence of the principle of unity and identity, and the philosopher Boethius introduced the ontological notion by his definition of person as 'an individual substance of a rational nature'. Thomas Aquinas (13C) regarded 'person' as 'the being insofar as he subsists, who finds in himself, and not in another, the bases of his existence': this notion, maybe, presages the modern concept of personhood considered from the perspective of self consciousness. The discipline of 'philosophical anthropology' (the term was introduced by Immanuel Kant) is flourishing: a rapid literature search will yield tomes, thus named, on the subject. But philosophical themes relevant to humanness are of course not confined to writings categorised as 'philosophical anthropology', and a clinician is soon lost at sea or at best treading water.

Formal theological ideas abound in the Christian tradition. In the Encyclopedia of Theology edited by the German Jesuit theologian, Karl Rahner and H Vorgrimler, one finds many complex statements, for example, classical metaphysical definitions of person: 'the person is the permanent de facto unity of the absolutely individual (a freedom which can be exercised by none but itself) and the most comprehensively universal (the spiritual)' and so on, and 'Man as a spiritual being is ... located in space and time in his bodily reality'. It is to be noted, by the way, that the attempt to differentiate 'philosophical' from 'theological' perspectives may be fruitless in the Christian tradition at least; and the term' 'theological' has indeed a very narrow application in the history of thought, even within a religious frame of reference. Recent Australian initiatives are noteworthy, such as those of the Anthropos in the Antipodes Project at Australian Catholic University.[39]

The Jewish tradition of thought concerning 'person' is rich indeed, inchoate in the Hebrew scriptures, notably in the portrayals in Genesis and Exodus. The Jewish tradition comprises far more that the Hebrew scriptures: the rabbinical tradition is also a rich vein, as well as generations of philosophers. In the 20C alone, thinkers such Rosensweig, Buber, Heschel, Soloveichik, and notably more recently Jonathan Sacks, have contributed contemporary thought of high relevance to present considerations of the personal. The complex strands of modern Jewish thought may be further illuminated by Yovel's fine writing[40,41] and that of Hazony. Some aspects of this tradition have been recently outlined by Alan Mittleman:[42] Mitttleman articulates the concept of human personhood as an emergent phenomenon: 'Personhood *emerged* from a natural, biological substratum, from the elements of our human nature.' He highlights the thought of Joseph Soloveitchik, one of the critical (Orthodox) Jewish thinkers of 20C, noting that 'Soloveitchik argued that a philosophical anthropology stressing our distance from nature, unnaturalness, and possession of divine, immortal souls is profoundly misguided. The medieval view that treats the natural world as carnal, material, a snare, and a temptation for the divine element within us is, for him, completely wrong': strong words.

Just as corals rooted in the same rock (even if the roots may not be easily seen) may be influenced by not only intrinsic qualities but also nutrition patterns and the currents buffetting them, and may manifest a diverse array of corals; so persons rooted in the Jewish tradition, influenced by powerful currents, may embody that tradition in a plethora of ways. Yirmiyahu Yovel, in his sensitive historical and philosophical analysis of Marranism – that intellectual, emotional and spiritual layering (or is it amalgam?) of many 'worlds', to be found in so many gifted persons (including many physicians) even of only partial Jewish descent, offers a rich understanding of this diversity and of the personal experience of what he calls 'The Other Within'.

Spinoza, one of the truly seminal philosophers now being increasingly recognised as such, was merely one of many such persons: the study by Australian philosopher Genevieve Lloyd offers valuable insight.[43] The rich lode of the ancient Jewish tradition, born initially in the deserts of Mesopotamia, then in places of dispersal such as Babylon, and with accretions from the ages sometimes even obscuring the origins, still bears gold – and like invisible yeast giving vigour to dough, can be (albeit unrecognised) light to the nations. There is need of light, now. It may be, for example, that the concepts of Marranism – and 'The Other Within' as expounded by Yovel may be profoundly applicable to many persons, notably but not only those with indigenous ancestry, in Australian society; such Marranism may be a well-spring of personal rediscovery and creativity.

Anthropological perspectives offer possibilities for deepening understanding. Marcel Mauss in 1938 opened debate on the nature of person in different societies. In anthropology, the individual is agent of institutions in society – the term 'person' is used to refer to the individual as a social actor. In the West, 'person' has been contrasted with 'self' which refers to the individual as the locus of experience (stress on agency). In other societies there is no distinction between the self and social agent. Cultural anthropologist Clifford Geertz offered rich perspectives and not only cautioned about generalisations concerning human nature but also about a static view of the individual.[44]

So thinkers down the ages have sought to define 'person', with almost all definitions referring to an individual, usually with certain capacities considered specifically human. However, some erudite philosophical writing seems not to resonate with the mundane experience of modern persons, especially those not immersed in the language of the humanities (including health professionals).

Is there another way to envisage what we mean by 'person'? A concept of use to clinicians?

There may be value in putting forward a relational view of 'person' simply expressed but in accord with concepts embedded in several philosophical strands and in accord also with clinical (and indeed everyday) experience. It is to be stressed that the comments concerning 'person' which follow are not a formal philosophical consideration but an attempt to introduce some concepts which may offer an anchor for the mind not of one versed in the humanities but a clinician expert in his or her own field of knowledge and action, and in a culture with its own vocabulary and web of meanings.

Poetry has a role in enlarging, as well as expressing, perceptions of humanness, and the poets have something to say. Walt Whitman in *Song of Myself*, a defining American poem, wrote (in stanza 7): 'I pass death with the dying and birth with the new wash'd babe, and am not contain'd between my hat and my boots'.[45] Australia's Noonuccal (Kath Walker) also points to another way of thinking: 'This accidental presence is not all of me' ...[46]

There is so much more to this person in front of me – in hospital, at home, in a residential care facility – anywhere. Can this be conceptualised in a way which assists the clinician's thinking – and deciding? Maybe. A relational view of person, expanded elsewhere,[47] may offer a way into a rich and useful concept of human personhood: with relations recognised as, not merely supplementary and noteworthy, but *constitutive* of 'person' – just as the array of filaments of a spider's web are what a spider's web *is*.

In this view, 'person' may be considered to be *constituted* (not *complemented*) by relationships – with persons, place, things, culture, personal aspirations, with the totality of all that is, recognising the unity of the fabric of reality (even fundamentally mathematical?), even the pattern (or even energiser) of the whole, whether or not conceived as radically benign and beneficent, and whether or not named 'God'. Is the *awareness* of such a relationship, and acting transparently in accord with such consciousness, the face of 'redemption'? The radical relationship with (beneficent) transcendence is portrayed in the creation of man in Genesis – dust of the earth is energised by what is beyond the dust. 'Person' may be considered as a relational reality with respect to the present life situation, but also the personal past (what is done and also experienced); not only the facts regarding the past but how the past is interpreted and incorporated in the present. These relationships are 'embodied', 'incorporated' (note the imagery!) in this person at this time. A person is as it were, a complex system.

So, each of us may be conceived as *constituted* by relationships, at any moment – a cross sectional view, if you like. But, furthermore, there is a temporal dimension also: each constitutive relationship has its own history and each of us, as persons, is a moving strip, as it were, constantly in flux in the ocean of time. The pattern (not our material constitution) is somehow the constant, even as the whole evolves. I, the person, am still responsible for what I did 30 years ago, for good or ill. The law has words for such! Philosophers argue about the form or means of continuity – the word 'pattern' will do for now.

Furthermore, should a constitutive relationship, even one, be strained or broken, 'personal' damage is inevitable (as we experience 'distress') – and if the whole is significantly disturbed we call it 'suffering', defined by Eric Cassell as a 'sense of impending personal disintegration'.[48] If one's car is stolen, or one breaks one's leg, or loses a precious object, or is separated from a significant person or place or receives a difficult diagnosis or other news – some 'distress' is fairly inevitable – and may proceed to suffering; but if one's whole family and house is lost in bombing or bush fire it is an exceptional person – whose 'spirit is not broken' (we say those things) and who may not 'suffer', in Cassell's sense. Suffering is wholly subjective and immeasurable. No-one else can predict what will trigger or has triggered the sense of impending personal disintegration ('suffering') of another or whether another is simply distressed or actually 'going to pieces' (that is, suffering): some suffering is 'unspeakable' – the suffering person may be wordless. These matters are critically significant for clinicians, not idle 'talk'.

What then can we understand by 'human spirit'?

On the relational view of person, the vector which is hope/aspiration which impels exploration may be at the root of art, even the impetus in Chauvet; for some individuals to explore even in the dark, deep in the earth to almost inaccessible places, is surely an urge to test the boundaries of human possibility. This may be a way of looking at the phenomenon whether or not the circumstances of making the art included shamanism (supported by many scholars) or even (Whiteley's proposal) involving mental illness. One may also discern a working out of this interior impulse in Gilgamesh – impelling him to explore beyond limits. All this is (to me) redolent of the *conatus* (striving) of Spinoza – the striving to continue in being. For a human to 'continue in being' implies not simply staying on the spot but exploring new possibilities – and this may be conceptualised as an exercise of the human spirit. Resilience is clearly a quality of the human spirit – the person is not irrevocably broken because the spirit has endured. Spirit, then, in this schema of a relational view of person, is being formulated as the principle of integration – that which holds the living complexus together, that is, 'animates' during life. and impels towards the future.

It is suggested by some thinkers that what holds the complexus together is intention, but it is hard to see that this could be the case in a sleeping or unconscious or otherwise cognitively impaired individual, even though there is clear evidence in such person of complex brain activity: the animating principle (termed here 'spirit') continues to act.

A short excursus. The term 'person' is used in the context of health care – we strive for 'personal' or 'person-centred' care (without very much analysis of what is meant), not the care of 'selves', but the word 'self' is worth at least a glance. The term 'self' has other connotations – including a move to particularity. Jerrold Seigel in a recent masterly study of the history of the idea of the self usefully clarifies his understanding of 'self':

> By self we commonly mean *the particular being any person is*, whatever it is about each of us that distinguishes you or me from others, draws the parts of our existence together, persist through changes, or opens the way to becoming what we might or could be.[49] (Emphasis added)

Jerrold Seigel notes, in fact, that 'all these terms – self, subject, identity, person ... form a vocabulary of selfhood ... and are permeable and sometimes merge into each other'.

Seigel's massive and complex work is relevant and noteworthy, particularly because he conceives of the self as multidimensional – and distinguishes the bodily (or material), the relational, and the reflective dimensions of the self and embarks on extensive analysis of each of these dimensions and their interrelationship as documented in the thoughts of major philosophers: his work is a quantum leap from the present brief and simplified consideration of 'person' as ontologically relational but resonates with it, and complements it, whilst going far beyond it.

It has been noted that there is some disquiet concerning spirituality and spiritual care, some of it because of tensions and ambiguities about traditional religion and religious institutions in the West – and apprehension concerning expressions of spiritual authority. However, some focus on 'religion' despite the taints of history (even recent history) is necessary, because religion is a quintessentially human reality. An adequate humanism for 21C simply must take the religious dimension of the human into account – and this demands a new perspective in face of the polemic and travesties of the past and of our time. The following remarks are trite but may be pointers to a negotiation of this difficult terrain.

Rappaport, at the close of a distinguished career in anthropology, wrote of the seminal role of ritual and religion, not in the evolution of humankind, but in the development of humanness. He wrote (knowingly) his last book, "about the nature of humanity, a species that lives, and can only live, in terms of meanings it must construct in a world devoid of intrinsic meaning but subject to physical law'.[50] In this lauded magnum opus, he asserted that 'in the absence of what we, in a common sense way, call religion, humanity could not have emerged from its pre or proto-human condition'.

Hart, in his foreword to Rappaport, also made comments on religion:

> Religion belongs to a set of terms which also includes art and science ... If science may crudely be said to be the drive to know the world objectively and art is pre-eminently an arena of subjective self-expression, religion typically expresses both sides of the subject-object relationship by connecting what is inside each of us to something outside. Religion, etymologically speaking, binds us to an external force; it stabilizes our meaningful interaction with the world, provides an anchor for our

volatility ... Through ritual, Durkheim argues, we worship our unrealized powers of shared existence, society, and call it God.[51]

Geertz in his consideration of religion as a cultural system wrote that 'religion tunes human actions to an envisaged cosmic order and projects images of cosmic order onto the plane of human experience'. He defined religion as 'a set of symbols which acts to establish powerful, pervasive, and long lasting mood and motivations in men by formulating conceptions of a general order of existence and clothing these conceptions with such an aura of factuality that the moods and motivations seem uniquely realistic'.[52] It is to be noted that the lens (disciplinary and personal) through which 'religion' is regarded profoundly influences the concept which emerges; this is unavoidable.

For William James whose classic study (*Varieties of Religious Experience*, Gifford Lectures 1901–2, printed 2000), is quoted by Rappaport:

> Religion ... shall mean for us the feelings, acts, and experiences of individual men in their solitude, so far as they apprehend themselves to stand in relation to whatever they may consider to be divine.[53]

However, it is worth recalling that according to Rappaport, for Durkheim, 'the fundamental context of the numinous experience is social rather than individual, and ... the social, characteristics of rituals themselves constitute the characteristics of the divine spirit ... The revelation of the hidden oneness of all things and of one's participation in such a great oneness may be the core meaning of *communitas*.'[54]

It will be noted that our seminal thinkers – Geertz, Rappaport (considering James and Durkheim), and Hart – articulate a wide range of meanings of the term 'religion'. And many more thinkers and writers could be introduced – showing striking diversity in concept.

There are other strands in contemporary thought concerning 'the religious' which may enrich our exploration, such as a collection of essays, mainly by European scholars, edited by Caputo.[55] Caputo, in his introduction, notes the ideas of Marion concerning the religious as involving the 'emptying out' of the subject (surely redolent of the Christian concept of 'kenosis'). The ultimate stance of the human person, especially when facing death, may be not fiercely guarded autonomy (at the root of the quest for total control of the circumstances of one's death through changes in law), but simply 'here I am', in Hebrew, *hineni,* without being able to name the source of the call to which this is a response. There is surely redolence here of Moses before the burning bush responding to a presence articulated as only 'being': Moses could not name the call to which he responded.

Furthermore, Sharon Welch, a professor of religious studies, wrote remarkably:

> I am an atheist, not just in the sense of the binary opposition of belief/unbelief, but in the sense of the symbolics of desire. I write as one of those who do not desire God. We do not desire to become divine, but rather, we *work to be human*, "spirit and dust", and our prayers are venues opening us to our embeddedness in nature, in history, with all their peril and promise. The horizon of our being is not "becoming divine", but being human, "vibrantly imperfect" …[56] (emphasis added)

'Working to be human' is hard work. It may be noted that much of the literature concerning 'burnout' in a clinical context includes a sense of not being able to 'strive' anymore; it may well be that burnout is specifically an ailment of the spirit, a notion hard to accept if spiritual need is identified with 'religious' in a professional culture in which formal religion has little currency. Furthermore, Lisa Rosenbaum, national correspondent for the New England Journal of Medicine, wrote recently of empathic care for dying patients, and concluded (highly relevant to present discussion):

> The nature of prognostication means we will sometimes be wrong. And the nature of disease means we will often have no cure to offer. But the nature of hope requires a sort of empathy that is not about feeling what our patients feel, but instead about seeing in them *what they can be*.[57] (emphasis added)

Maybe, in the search for an approach to thinking about all these closely inter-related ideas it may be worth simply stressing the following fundamental notions:

a) The human person is complex, and increasing consciousness (*awareness*) of the web of relations which constitute me as a person, including my relation to the whole, is a measure of my personal growth – at any age. It is a question of awareness of my whole being, my whole truth. (It is fair to consider whether, in the face of the intrusion of virtual reality, there is deflection of awareness – or is it expansion?)

b) Ritual is an essential part of my life and every human life, and is relevant to each of the relations which constitute me as a person in society. (The relational view of person, considered above, includes, as one of the constitutive relations of person, the relation with totality – all-that-is, however named or conceived. Ritual, such as Sabbath observance, may refresh the awareness of this, as well as of persons and community – and the past.) Meditation practices are clearly concerning with the relation with the self as well as the Whole – and it is to be expected that attentiveness to the deep self and the Whole in practices such as yoga induces bonding with other persons – the making of community.

c) My ritual expression of my awareness of the Whole, may, especially if expressed with others, be called (by some) 'religious' … maybe identifiable with long established traditions, but also may be in new forms. Freedom is essential – and there is no place for persuasion. Religion is essentially about awareness and action, about way of being human, not a matter of belief: this is acknowledged in the Jewish tradition but may be problematic in belief-based traditions.

d) The spiritual dimension of my human life comprises all that is essentially and distinctively human – all that is beyond the capacity of the most gifted non-human animal – and so includes my thoughts, words, inner impulses, creativity, imaginings, hopes, dreams, resilience, endurance, aspirations, ideas, rituals – including my awareness of my place in the universe: and it is my spirit – the 'breath' which may come from beyond (I cannot know), which holds me together while-ever I live, stops me from going to pieces in the face of my complexity, and energises my striving.

What, then, keeping in mind the foregoing discussion, can we mean by 'care of the spirit' – or 'spiritual care? What can be the processes? And whose responsibility? And how measure failure or success?

Care, as such, for one in need is not a mark of the human! Care of the needy, the powerless, notably in a context of bonding, is a feature of the animal kingdom. Care is instinctive, innate – with an impulse to care for one in need unless vitiated. There is a large literature about care in clinical practice, not further discussed here. It is worthy of note though that according to Manderson, following Levinas, and concerning humans, the philosophical basis of the duty of care is not law, or contract, but the call of the other:[58] the implication is radical altruism.

But what of *spiritual* care?

In fact, an evolutionary model with continuing differentiation may be the best frame to understand the recent burgeoning of health service based spiritual care, with 'spiritual care' as a defined area of professional activity.

At the outset it is to be recognised that 'spiritual care' is in no way new – the recent Western efflorescence is rooted in the long experience of humankind, expressed in myriad traces. The orally transmitted stories, myths in all cultures, earliest written narratives, sayings of the wise or those with ability to understand the human condition, both in its glory, possibility and threats, the sages of all cultures, the prophets of Israel, the ancient Greek philosophers – all of these contributed to the wisdom tradition embodied in human societies, and as such are the frame or context of anything which may be called 'spiritual care'.

Shamanism may be the prototype of inchoate professional 'spiritual care'. Traditional Australian Aboriginal society, the oldest surviving culture on earth, had what Elkin termed of medicine men 'of high degree' whose role in the community clearly went far beyond the care of the physical or emotional needs of members – and was exercised in the realm of symbol and meaning which is the world of the human spirit. Fine writings of Worms and other early authorities on Aboriginal culture that that there was a rich spirituality manifest in, for example, the recognition of sacred objects and places as well as actions; 'spiritual care' for a person embedded in the Aboriginal cultural tradition could have nuances worthy of respect. To deprive such a person of proximity to sacred objects (including places) may grossly increase suffering.

Indeed, in multicultural Australia spiritual concepts may increasingly diverge markedly from European notions, and detailed investigation may be fruitful in developing appropriate approaches to 'spiritual care' far removed from conventional, notably Caucasian, understandings: discussion of the myriad of contemporary iterations of spiritual care within most Western societies, and mainly outside the formal health services, is beyond the scope of this essay.

...

What has all this to do with the lives of busy clinicians? Are there practical clinical applications of the foregoing? Has a glance at our distant ancestors and some thoughts of the wise aided understanding about the care of the human spirit – for short, 'spiritual care' – in 21C, wherever human persons live, but especially when in our health services, in hospitals, offices, homes? And not only of patients but of each other and oneself? The following are some notions or footholds.

1   Recognise the human spirit as manifest in striving – in wanting to explore the self and beyond the self, beyond 'sensible' boundaries, in thought, in relationships, in action (including creative action – art, crafts, thinking, learning, writing) – and facilitate such striving.

    Further, if one holds a non-teleological view of human life, that is, that there is no predetermined goal to which the human person journeys, but rather that living is a continuing response to an impulse (intuition) from within, then diversity (if not divergence) of expressions of striving is to be expected, rather than (spiritual) conformity to any norm. If so it appears even more unreasonable to try to formulate a measure of spiritual health or well-being: Jacob struggling in the night, on the way to his deeper truth (Genesis 32:24), may have scored abominably, as would the poet Dylan Thomas raging 'against the dying of the light', and, maybe, the crucified man calling *eli, eli, lama sabachthani.* Spiritual diversity is a manifestation of the richness of humanness.

Kingsley Mortimer, a professor of anatomy, urged that 'It is the task of medicine to emancipate man's interior splendour';[59] the human spirit is many splendored indeed.

2. Strengthen the spirit as 'principle of integration'.

    Give attention to constitutive relations – with the self (for example, through remembering, musing, meditating), with the body, persons, place, memory, culture, or desired ritual) under strain; careful questioning in a private situation may be justified to establish where strains or fractures ('breaking me') are occurring, but such very personal information is not for sharing though, or documentation without specific consent. If a relationship under strain is identified, there may be possibilities of creating situations for repair – for example, being with a particular person, or attending an event, undertaking a ritual, whether religious or not, for example, getting to a church or synagogue or mosque or having contact with persons from those sacred places – or getting out into a personally special place (for example, a building or tree or bushland), or attending to a desire for proximity to a particular object held dear.

3. Emancipate the 'interior splendour' of persons (to express Kingsley Mortimer's suggestions in rather more contemporary language).

    Respect the uniqueness, complexity, depths, immeasurability and incomprehensibility of every person. Cease to want to understand, and rest in respecting each other as other.

Accept that the spirit of each unique person, that which animates and integrates, is unique, subject to no measurement or rules. And so it is right (however difficult for others) that some persons may die raging at the dying of the light, whilst others may welcome the coming darkness or even see it as dawn. It is for each to follow his/her own flame – that is all. It is no accident that fire is so close to the early history of humankind. Spiritual care of another is care of the other's flame, even when and especially when flickering. The care of the spirit is ordinarily one's own responsibility – the guarding of one's own fire is a lifelong task. But others, traditionally a trusted doctor par excellence, maybe a cherished nurse, or maybe a designated religious person, may at times be admitted to the personal place where the spirit is languishing, finding hope hard.

As has already been noted, the philosophical basis of the duty of care is not law, or contract but the response to the call of the other. Discerning of the call of the other when the centre is not holding, when the spirit is in distress, is of all human tasks, the most delicate and costly: there is a real possibility of being burned in the other's flame. If one's own centre is not holding (in a situation of personal suffering for whatever reason) response to the call may be difficult but the resilience of a clinician may suffice, with the cost paid later.

But what of the person in whom any splendour seems hard to discern? That is, if the gaze is fixed on the capacity of the person to function in ways characteristic of humanness: to walk, to be continent, to speak 'normally' or at all, to interact 'normally' with the world of persons and things, to make judgements, to indicate consent ... Such persons are familiar, present in the everyday world (even if often hidden) and prominent in health services, and intensive effort to achieve the identified objectives is mandatory. But what is 'spiritual care' then?

There is a sense in which the principles are no different:

a) Discern and encourage 'striving', recognising that this person may be able to communicate desires only by bodily gestures, but these gestures may be the stuff of consent or refusal – making the case for measures such as tube feeding often inappropriate in persons with advanced Alzheimers disease making gestures suggestive of refusal, as pointed out sensitively by Dekkers.[60]

b) Again, respect the uniqueness, complexity, depths, immeasurability and incomprehensibility of every person; the *person* is fully present though not fully functioning. The evidence is pressing that intensive brain activity is continuing even in patients wholly non responsive, even in the so-called vegetative state, and there is no place for talk *about* such patients to occur in their presence, *as if they were not present.*

c) Attend to each of the constitutive relations, including the presence of a bonded other person even if not recognised or acknowledged by the patient, respectful care of the body (including attention to pain which cannot be explained in words but may be expressed in behaviour – a major issue about which there is much concern), careful thought about particular actions or words or other associations which trigger painful memories – and so on. In fact the expertise in care of such afflicted persons is largely directed, when basic needs are met, to the care of the spirit holding together the fragile and eventually flickering flame. One can only express gratitude and respect to those who do so care. One of the core tasks of medicine is the advocacy for the most powerless,[61] and if doctors fail in this, society is impoverished – and in great danger of repeat of the aberrations of the mid 20C. An observer at the Nuremburg trials of the Nazi doctors caught up in the moral collapse surmised that the very first step was 'a shift in attitude towards the non rehabilitatable sick'.[62] A salutary note.

4   Demonstrate concern for privacy: privacy for all those in need of care should extend to spiritual privacy.

There was/is a vogue for developing a scale regarding spiritual health – of measuring even that most private of aspects of the self – that which is the well spring of personal life, that which may express the person's sense of meaning and relations, not only with persons, places, things, the past as remembered, inheritance – roots in culture, hopes/dreams and with oneself, but also relation with all-that-is, with transcendence extrinsic to the world, or whether immanent in this world, and whether or not called 'God' or anyway recognised in treasured ritual. There is a case for refraining attempts to measure spiritual health: let researchers or carers measure 'distress' (for example in distress scales or 'thermometers') – but not what is of the spirit, for that is sacred ground.

It is a poet who powerfully articulates such notions: Christopher Brennan (1870–1932), a Professor of German and Comparative Literature (University of Sydney), whose life crashed around him – and he walked the Bondi area hills in Sydney, sometimes in despair. He includes, in the Epilogues of his 1913 edition of his poems, a moving image from 1897 of his personal core – and articulates its supports and relationships, including that with a beloved woman and with God:

> Deep in my hidden country stands a peak,
> and none hath known its name
> and none, save I, hath even skill to seek:

> thence my wild spirit came.
> Thither I turn, when the day's garish world
> Too long hath vexed my sight,
> And bare my limbs where the great winds are whirl'd
> And life's undreaded might.
> ...
>
> The gift of self is self's most sacred right;
> only where none hath trod,
> only upon my most secret starry height
> I abdicate to God.[63]
>
> Sacred ground indeed. And no carer should seek to explore it – or tread on it unless unshod and explicitly invited.

The truly seminal thinkers in the western tradition, some of whom have been brought together briefly in this somewhat rambling exploration, indicate the significance of the ground of our exploration, the human core, while maintaining diversity in the language and concepts they use to express it.

Appendix

An excursus: The phenomenological tradition in philosophy may be relevant to clinicians. Eugene Kelly in the Introduction to a translation of *The Human Place in the Cosmos* by Max Scheler (1874–1928) – Scheler's last formulation of his rich ideas – notes what is meant by phenomenology:

> Phenomenology is not the attempt to give the necessary and sufficient meaning or application of a term as was sought in the Socratic *elenchus*. Nor is it the observation of the form, behavior, origins, or causal properties of things ... [nor] concerned with as such with semantics or metaphysics. As contrasted with science, phenomenology is nonreductive; it attempts to exhibit the fullness of the essential phenomena we perceive as "carried by" the

things of the world rather than to trace their attributes or behavior to general laws, substances, or categories. Phenomenology is rather the grasping *in mente*, the cognition, of the meaning-elements we encounter in the world; it requires intuitive reflection upon the meaning-contents of term in an attempt to exhibit their essential relations with each other and their order of foundation ... Accordingly Scheler describes the meaning-structures found in association with such terms as *life, psyche, self,* and *spirit*, drawing on what we know through science about these phenomena, bringing them before the eye of the mind ...[64]

REFERENCES

1 Sigerist HE, *A History of Medicine Vol 1. Primitive and Archaic Medicine*, Oxford University Press, Oxford, 1951.
2 Bloch E, *The Principle of Hope* (1938–1947), trans N Plaice, S Plaice and P Knight, Blackwell, Oxford, 1986.
3 Watson PA, *Terrible Beauty: The People and Ideas that Shaped the Modern Mind. A History.* Weidenfeld and Nicolson, London, 2000.
4 Christian D, *Maps of Time: An Introduction to Big History*, University of California Press, London, 2011.
5 Mulvaney J, and Kamminga J, *Prehistory of Australia*, Allen and Unwin, St Leonards, 1999.
6 Mithen S, *The Prehistory of the Mind: A Search for the Origins of Art, Religion and Science*, Thames and Hudson, 1996.
7 Lewis-Williams D, *The Mind in the Cave: Consciousness and the Origins of Art*, Thames and Hudson, London, 2004.
8 Clottes J, *Return to Chauvet Cave: Excavating the Birthplace of Art, The first full report*, Thames and Hudson, London, 2003.
9 Clottes J, *What is Paleolithic Art?*, Bradshaw Foundation, 2016.
10 Aujoulat N, *The Splendour of Lascaux: Rediscovery of the Greatest Treasure of Prehistoric Art*, Thames and Hudson, London, 2005.
11 Whitely DS, *Cave Paintings and the Human Spirit: The Origin of Creativity and Belief*, Prometheus Books, NY, 2009.
12 Geertz C, *The Interpretation of Cultures*, Basic Books, NY, 1973.
13 Rappaport D, *Ritual and Religion in the Making of Humanity*, Cambridge University Press, Cambridge, 1999.
14 Durkheim E, *The Elementary Forms of Religious Life* (1912), trans. C Cosman, Oxford University Press, Oxford, 2001.
15 Elkin AP, *Aboriginal Men of High Degree: Initiation and Sorcery in the World's Oldest Tradition*, Queensland University Press, St Lucia, 1977.
16 Worms AE, *Australian Aboriginal Religions*, trans MJ Wilson, D O'Donovan, M Charlesworth, Nelen Yubu Missiological Unit, Kensington, 1986.
17 Chaloupka G, *Journey in Time: The 50000 Year Story of Australian Rock art of Arnhem Land*, Reed New Holland, Sydney, 1993.
18 Mulvaney J and Kamminga J, op cit, *Prehistory of Australia*, Allen and Unwin, St Leonards, 1999.
19 Godden E, J Mainic, *Rock Art of Aboriginal Australia*, Frenchs Forest, NSW, New Holland Publishers, 2001.
20 Donaldson M, *Kimberley Rock Art*, 3 Vols, Wildrocks Publications Mount Lawley, 2012–2013.
21 Blainey G, *The History of Australia's People: The Rise and Fall of Ancient Australia*, Random House, Australia, 2015.

22 Deutscher G, *The Unfolding of Language; the Evolution of Mankind's Greatest Invention*, Random House, London, 2005.
23 Rappaport, op cit, p5.
24 *The Epic of Gilgamesh*, Translated with introduction by A George, Penguin Books, London, 1999.
25 Sacks J, *Conversations and Covenant. Genesis: The Book of Beginnings*, Koren, Jerusalem, 2009.
26 Hazony Y, *The Philosophy of the Hebrew Scripture*, Cambridge University Press, Cambridge, 2012.
27 Wikipedia. *The Iliad*, Consulted 20 November 2016.
28 Hall E, *The Ancient Greeks: Ten Ways They Shaped the Modern World*, Vintage, London, 2016.
29 Bloom H, *Shakespeare and the Invention of the Human*, Rivershead Books, NY, 1998.
30 Armstrong K, *The Great Transformation: The World in the Time of Budda, Socrates, Confucius and Jeremiah*, Atlantic Books, London, 2006. (See also *The Axial Age and its Consequences*, ed by R Bellah and H Joas, Harvard University Press, London, 2012.).
31 Jaspers K, *The Origin and Goal of History*, trans M Bullock (London, 1953), pp1–70, cited by Armstrong, p xii.
32 Joas H, *The Sacredness of the Human Person: A New Genealogy of Human Rights*, trans, A Skinner, Georgetown University Press, Washington, 2013.
33 Worms AE, op cit.
34 Stanner WE, quoted by Wilson in Epilogue, *Worms*, op. cit.
35 Rothwell N, *Quicksilver*, Text Publishing, Melbourne, 2016.
36 Needleman J, 'The perception of mortality', *Annals of the New York Academy of Sciences*, 164 (1969), pp 733–738.
37 *Bloomsbury guide to human thought*, McGleish K (ed), 1993 Bloomsbury, London. (See also *The Shorter Routledge Encyclopedia of Philosophy*, ed Craig E. Routledge, London, 2005.)
38 Plourde S, 'A key term in ethics: the person and his dignity', in Thomasma DC, Weisstub DW and Hervé C, (eds), *Personhood and Health Care*, Kluwer Dordrecht, 2001, pp137–148.
39 Kirchoffer D, Horner R and McCardle P (eds) *Being Human: Groundwork for a Theological Anthropology for the 21st Century*, Mosaic Press, Preston, 2013.
40 Yovel Y, *Spinoza and Other Heretics, Vol 1: The Marrano of Reason*, Princeton University Press, Princeton, 1989.
41 Yovel Y, *The Other Within – The Marannos: Split Identity and Emerging Modernity*, Princeton University Press, Princeton, 2009.
42 Mittleman A, *Human Nature and Jewish Thought: Judaism's Case for Why Persons Matter*, Princeton University Press, Oxford, 2015.

43 Lloyd G, *Routledge Philosophy Guide to Spinoza and the Ethics*, Routledge, London, 1996.
44 Geertz C, *The Interpretation of Cultures: Selected Essays by Clifford Geertz*, Basic Books, New York, 1973.
45 Whitman W, *Leaves of Grass*, the first (1855) edition. Penguin Books, New York, 1986.
46 Oodgeroo Noonuccal (Kath Walker), location uncertain.
47 Lickiss N, 'Facing Human Suffering', in Malpas J and Lickiss N (eds). *Perspectives on Human Suffering*, Springer, Dordrecht, 2012, p 245–260.
48 Cassell E, 'The goal of medicine the relief of suffering', *New England Journal of Medicine* 1982; 306: 639–645.
49 Seigel J, *The Idea of the Self: Thought and Experience in Western Europe since the Seventeenth Century*, Cambridge University Press, Cambridge, 2005.
50 Rappaport RA, *Ritual and Religion in the Making of Humanity*, Cambridge University Press, Cambridge, 1999, p1.
51 Hart K, in Rappaport D, *Ritual and Religion in the Making of Humanity*, Cambridge University Press, Cambridge, 1999, p xv.
52 Geertz C, op cit, pp 87–124.
53 James, quoted by Rappaport, op cit, p 374.
54 Rappaport RA, op cit, p 378.
55 Caputo JD (ed), *The Religious*, Blackwell, Oxford, 2001.
56 Welch S, Return to Laughter. in Caputo, op cit, pp301–317.
57 Rosenbaum L, 'Falling together – empathic care for the dying', *NEJM* 2016; 374:6, p 587 –590.
58 Manderson D, Proximity, *Levinas and the Soul of Law*, McGill, Queens University Press, Montreal, 2006.
59 Mortimer K, 'The impossible profession: the doctor-priest relationship', Proceedings, *Australian Association of Gerontology*, 1974, 2:81.
60 Dekkers W J M, 'Autonomy and the lived body in cases of severe dementia', in *Ethical Foundations of Palliative Care for Alzheimer Disease*, ed RB Purtilo and *HAMJ* ten Have, Johns Hopkins University Press, Baltimore, 2004, p 115–130.
61 Lickiss JN, 'On the care of our aged', *Australian Rehabilitation Review*, 1982; (6)2:51–57.
62 Alexander L, 'Medical Science under Dictatorship', *New England Journal Medicine*, 1949, 241:39–47.
63 Brennan C, *The Verse of Christopher Brennan*, ed AR Chisholm and JJ Quinn, Angus and Robertson, Sydney, 1960.
64 Scheler M, *The Human Place in the Cosmos*, Trans MS Frings, with Introduction by E Kelly, Northwestern University Press, Evanston, 2009.

IV
ON FACING HUMAN SUFFERING
2012

An edited version is published in: In Perspectives on Human Suffering, ed J Malpas and N Lickiss, Springer, Dordrecht, 2012, pp 245–260.

Why stare at the sun? Why stare down the Gorgon? Why stare down or gaze at human suffering? Irvin Yalom would insist that staring at death is a means to face death-related anxiety (which takes on so many guises) and reduces fear of death.[1] And we humans may fear suffering rather more than we fear death. Yet suffering is an intrinsic part of the human condition: we are both contingent and fragile – we need not be, and will not be forever, and we are aware of this: this may be not only the marks of our humanity, but also our suffering as a universal feature of our condition, yet particularized in each person. Suffering rooted in this intrinsic contingency, fragility and awareness of it (and interpretations of it all) has influenced the human record since the beginning: art, writings, philosophy, and the earliest traces of medicine. Mary Rawlinson, in our own times, offered a philosophical analysis concerning human suffering – what sort of phenomenon is it? She noted that 'a tradition extending from Plato to [Immanuel] Kant through Christian Platonism proves inappropriate for the treatment of suffering insofar as it fails to locate suffering with respect to the purposive activity of the human subject, identifying it instead with distance or alienation from an ideal order.'[2] Maybe all that we can know or understand about human suffering has been said or written, but there appears an imperative in every age, and our times, to enter into an exploratory relationship with it; especially is this true for physicians, since the relief of suffering is the traditional goal of medical practice. This essay explores some dimensions of human suffering as encountered especially in the course of clinical practice, and the ponderings engendered by such personal encounters. Persons, suffering persons in their particularity, are the unseen presence in this writing.

The issue of suffering and its relief is central to the medical tradition. Early Greco-Roman philosophers wrestled with human distress and suffering, and how to deal with it, usually by more adequate knowledge, but it is noteworthy, as [Martha] Nussbaum points out,[3] that the philosophers often used medical metaphors or analogy, when discussing philosophy's potential to relieve suffering; for example, Epicurus in Greece (341–271 BCE) wrote: 'Empty is that philosopher's argument by which no human suffering is therapeutically treated. For just as there is no use for a medical art that does not cast out the sicknesses of bodies, so too there is no use in philosophy, unless it casts out the suffering of the soul.' The analogy is expressed in Rome somewhat later by Cicero (106–43 BCE): 'There is, I assure you, a medical art for the soul. It is philosophy, whose aid need not be sought, as in bodily diseases, from outside ourselves. We must endeavour with all our resources and all our strength to become capable of doctoring ourselves.'

Early medical traditions are documented by medical historians such as [Henry] Sigerist[4,5] – notable is the ancient Greek tradition which has been critical for Western medicine.[6,7] Michael Kearney, in his recent studies of healing, has emphasized the dual traditions of Hippocratic Medicine (which flourished in 5C BCE) with its stress on the understanding and treating of disease wherever possible, and the later Asklepian cult (which flourished 500 BCE to 500 CE), with its focus on healing the whole person especially when cure was no longer possible.[8] [Michael] Kearney contrasts the two streams of activity (see Table 1 derived from Kearney), but it needs to be noted that the Hippocratic tradition also recognized that there was a time when what we would call 'comfort care' should prevail. Recently there have been significant conceptual advances relevant to suffering in a medical context, although writing by practicing clinicians is sparse. Physicians in clinical practice have the personal role in society to relieve human suffering amenable to medical measures, to be present to it, to share it, not to talk or write about it. Writing about matters such as human dignity is challenging but not painful. Articulating words about human suffering may evoke, for a physician, complex emotions, memories, personal pain, regret, maybe the reliving of close-to-the-brink experiences embedded deep in memory, even the opening up of personal fracture lines, or mild aversive responses to 'mere' writing so central to the professional lives of others. Yet the strange, particular perspective of the relatively inarticulate physician may be a necessary ingredient of an interdisciplinary amalgam concerning human suffering.

HIPPOCRATIC TRADITION	ASKLEPIAN HEALING
Draws on objective evidence	Draws on subjective evidence
Calls for clinical objectivity	Calls for clinical subjectivity
Treats pain and lessens suffering by intervening from without	Concerned with healing from within
Works as *opus contra naturam*	Works with nature
Primary training involves knowledge and skills	Primary training involves self knowledge
Hippocrates b 560 BCE	Asklepios – Greek God of Healing

Table 1: Hippocratic tradition and Asklepian Healing
[after Michael Kearney, A Place of Healing (Oxford: Oxford University Press, 2000)]

Historians paint the backdrop to clinical perspectives. Sigerist, already mentioned, noted that: 'medical theories always represent one aspect of the general civilization of a period, and in order to understand them fully, we must be familiar with other manifestations of that civilization, its philosophy, literature, art, music'.[9] It is therefore not surprising that Porter, as his final contribution to medical history has raised the question of how the soul or spirit, or psyche indeed, can be understood in contemporary culture:[10] the implications of such conceptions not only for life and suffering, but also human death, are considerable. [Thomas] Sydenham (1624–1689), sometimes styled the British Hippocrates, could write: 'How my soul, which I look on to be an immortal Being in me, that is the Principle of thinking, should extinguish with my Body, I cannot in any reasonable way of thinking conceive';[11] such may not ground a medical consensus in twenty-first century, or figure in the writings of clinicians on human suffering, however such matters find place in late night musings.

In 2003, [N] Cherny contributed a review of the problem of human suffering in the Third Edition of the prestigious *Oxford Textbook of Palliative Medicine*.[12] The review mentioned that, on the basis of a consideration of the extensive clinical and psychosocial research undertaken with cancer patients, Cherny and colleagues defined suffering as 'an aversive experience characterized by the perception of personal distress that is generated by adverse factors that undermine quality of life'.[13] Others have sought to offer definitions from other perspectives.

Eric Cassell has contributed much to the medical literature on human suffering. In a landmark paper,[14] Cassell differentiated 'suffering' from 'distress' – and introduced an operational definition of suffering as 'a sense of impending personal disintegration'. Cassell's portrayal of the perception of suffering may be rendered in common parlance as 'a sense of being about to go to pieces'. An unpublished research project undertaken in Sydney in the 1990s, indicated that patients could readily recognize whether or not they had, in the course of a serious illness, ever felt 'about to go to pieces', and if so what were the circumstances. It was clear that such an experience was readily identifiable, and that the trigger for such a feeling could arise in one or more of several personal fields: loss of a relationship with persons, place, things, role, cultural matters – or concerning only the self (for example, perception of loss of some aspect of dignity, intrapersonal conflict, realization of guilt). The language of breakage was often used – such and such event 'broke my spirit'. Maybe the event was so fraught that speech failed – a possible trigger for fracture, as Shakespeare noted: 'Give sorrow words: the grief that does not speak/Whispers the o'er fraught heart, and bids it break'.[15] It was clear over decades of practice that the trigger for intense suffering could also be the witnessing of the suffering of another, or the memory of the suffering of another, a memory often prompted by another event: compassion is surely a manifestation of our radical connectedness.

Pain is recognized as a source of distress; it may or may not, on Cassell's model, be associated with of suffering. [Richard] Chapman and [Jonathan] Gavrin considered both pain and suffering, including the neurological bases of each, and noting the current range of definitions of suffering[16] – they preferred to define suffering as 'a complex negative affective and cognitive state characterized by a perceived threat to the integrity of the self, perceived helplessness in the face of that threat, and exhaustion of psychosocial and personal resources for coping'.

Although suffering is quintessentially subjective, research related to suffering in health care contexts is undertaken, despite some concern that such research is not justified or possible.[17] The research undertaken on all continents has to take into account the primacy of the subjective in the face of a regrettable tendency to objectify that which is intrinsically subjective (and less easily quantifiable), with qualitative studies the most usual approach. [S] Daneault and colleagues, in studies of patients experiencing cancer, concluded that the core dimensions of suffering are: i) feeling subjected to violence, ii) being deprived and/or overwhelmed, and c) living in apprehension.[18] Janice Morse and colleagues from Edmonton have in the last decade further enriched understanding on the basis of extensive research relating to persons in very distressing situations, notably differentiating a phase of endurance and then a phase of emotional release: in the first phase, 'holding' techniques (not touch or comfort) are needed to help the person to endure, whilst in the second, comforting and empathic techniques including touch, are appropriate.[19] On Cassell's model (as well as in practice) the distinction may be relevant to prevent a distressed person from reaching breaking point. Such considerations point to the complexity of human suffering, and the need to conceptualise it as clearly as possible.

Suffering is an inevitable companion in the lives of most clinicians in many disciplines: their perceptions, their interpretations and their responses are all worthy of consideration. The focus here is medical for pragmatic reasons; nursing literature is rich in relevant matters. Distress and, at times, suffering will be part of the life of a conscientious physician, because of a) the witnessing of great suffering, b) experiencing the inevitable failure of treatments to control disease and to relieve all distress, c) being present at, or bearing, the death of patients, and d) noting personal failings, including errors of judgment, in the exercise of high levels of responsibility, and e) increasing awareness of the limits of what one may bear noting with T. S. Eliot that 'Man cannot bear too much reality'.[20]

How is the place of suffering in the human condition understood by doctors? How do contemporary physicians, junior doctors, medical students view human suffering? Or an individual who is suffering? Apart from acute matters, possibly obvious at a glance, and fortunately open to a well-recognized and available remedy, and immediate action mandated – the delight of junior doctors, there is need to consider what meaning is given to the scene. In the presence of a person who is grossly distressed, and almost certainly suffering or clearly distraught, maybe even dying thus, how does the physician conceptualize or interpret this situation? Or simply respond? It is well known (and well-remembered by some of us) that a rapid exit either physically or emotionally is a common response. It is rare to find a physician who can truly 'stare down the sun', and stay with the suffering person whilst seeking how best to alleviate the distress, yet this is what is mandated. It is tempting to suggest that doctors may sometimes act like the friends of Job with suggestions of blame, of information withheld, or uncommonly even of a masked theodicy, but in the end there may be a wise matter-of-fact-ness (maybe accompanied, despite the appearance of almost mandated traditional medical equanimity, by distress and disquiet because of profound compassion), that such is the case. As a consequence, the colleagues of doctors, especially nurses, bear a large proportion of the clinical burden of suffering – staying there, present, when the busy doctor is drawn away by other duties, sometimes conveniently – but the patient may be the one most bereft of succour.

Physicians speak little of this. [R] Shaerer, reporting on the response of French family doctors to patient deaths wrote:

> Human suffering does not amount to a physical or moral pain or a difficulty. Suffering is something like crossing a desert; it is an experience in which a person will experience evil, and yet at the same time, will be led to discover the deepest meaning of one's own life. This is true of the suffering of a doctor.[21]

[Irvin] Yalom would recognize the experience Shaerer describes as an 'awakening' experience, which may move the doctor from an 'everyday' mode to a more 'existential' mode of living, concerned, not with *how* but *that* things are (including oneself). Nevertheless, most physicians would reject notions (often associated with traditional religions) that 'suffering is good for you', whilst recognizing that human response to extreme suffering can reveal nobility and potential for growth beyond expectations, even in themselves. The well-known 'tears on the staircase' of junior doctors may be matched by the tears of very experienced consultants experiencing, in the raw, the tragedy and grandeur of the human condition as lived out in the suffering of individuals. It is increasingly recognized that strategies need to be in place to ensure the personal sustainability and flourishing of the physician immersed in care of distressed patients:[22] what is not certain is whether or not there is benefit to the patients cared for by doctors committed to those practices, but it is likely to be so.

Cassell has expressed regret recently that we are still failing in the West (his focus) to relieve suffering, despite decades of 'talk'.[23] At a global level the inequities are so serious, unjust, immoral, and almost beyond the comprehension of most in the West – despite readily available information – that this will not

be further considered at present. In the affluent West there is
no lack of technology, intelligence, commitment or even funds
(prescinding from issues of fair intra-national distribution), nor
of compassion; however, there is evidence of unsustainability,
despite serious warnings for decades,[24] with inadequate attention
to cost/ benefit ratio, especially from the point of view of the
patient – of relevance to the genesis and relief of suffering. The
quality of clinical decision-making, especially with respect to
severely ill patients, likely to be enmeshed in a sea of suffering,
is often questionable, despite widespread attempts to facilitate
the exercise of clinical wisdom. The rising interest in advance
directives/decisions/care plans is promising and overdue –and
yet there are complex and deep problems. How can such love of
and respect for life be balanced by the appropriate acceptance
of death? King Lear had difficulty in being allowed to die (as
noted below), as do many of our fellows (fear of which is surely
contributing to the requests for physician intervention to cause
death directly). The traditional Talmudic principle, 'Affirm life,
but do not obstruct death', says it all, but is not always heard, it
seems even in centres of excellence. Sensitive understanding is
called for – and the deficiencies of medical respect for life in the
past, even in the twentieth century may weigh heavily on the
medical mind.

What is at the root of all of this? Cassell offers a twenty
first century analysis:

> I believe that there are two things that continue to hold
> back an appreciation of suffering and its relief. The first
> is a continuing failure to accord subjective knowledge
> and subjectivity the same status as objective knowledge
> and objectivity. The second is an increasing denial of
> the inevitable uncertainties in medicine and a quest for
> certainty'.[25]

It can be contended that the problems in contemporary medicine are in fact philosophical – with conceptual bases unable to sustain the weight of current practice. Inadequate understanding of human suffering is surely playing a part, but the difficulty may rest on deeper deficiencies. The phenomenon of medical burnout in the West, and now being reported in Japan (termed 'catastrophic collapse of morale') would alone suggest that something is seriously lacking at a profound level, recently discussed by Cole and Carlin.[26] These authors stress that 'there are no quick fixes for the suffering of physicians, just as there are no quick fixes for the suffering of patients,' and insist that medicine needs to be 'rehumanized'. They conclude their analysis with the telling words: 'humanizing medicine depends in no small part on recovering the humanity of physicians'. How should this be conceived?

Is it worth asking again, what does medical practice require to relieve suffering more effectively, if that be its goal? Why do medical practitioners, sometimes in the highest places, fail to comprehend the calculus of human suffering, or be paralysed by being present as witness to suffering? What does an individual physician need to be more effective? Can any matters be specified (or learned or taught)? There are many possible approaches to an examination of why contemporary medical practitioners in affluent Western contexts is, in the eyes of many, frequently failing in the core business of relieving human suffering. Phenomenological or sociological modes of enquiry with new dimensions of research? More detailed historical analysis? Or a renewed search for meaning – in case the 'terrible beauty' of the recent past may point out the need for a new Enlightenment, built on surer foundations?

Central is the need for a more adequate concept of person, and of the processes of personal development, as the foundation for much of the rest, for suffering is an essentially subjective personal reality. Jacob Needleman, some decades ago, in a discourse (New York Academy of Sciences) concerning mortality noted that, 'what medicine lacks is any fundamental notion of the nature of man and any remotely adequate understanding of that to which we refer as a person'.[27] Cassell, in the preface to the first edition of his major book appears to support such comment: 'The job of the twenty first century is the discovery of the person – finding the sources of illness and suffering within the person, and with that knowledge developing methods for their relief, while at the same time revealing the power within the person as the nineteenth and twentieth centuries have revealed the power of the body'.[28] It may also be true that the vast experience of physicians of persons in limit situations should be harnessed by thinkers to enrich our understanding of the human. A reconsideration of what we mean by 'person', and the closely related matter of the processes of personal development, may serve as a point of departure.

Ancient writers wrote much of the human predicament, and ways of consolation, though with little attempt to analyze the person. The writer of the drama of Job portrayed threats to personal integrity, but the drama was focused on other matters than exploring personhood. Renaissance writers glorified human dignity, highlighting the status of the human in the universe. Shakespeare was innovative in that Shakespearian dramas explored human interiority, portraying often the conversation of persons with themselves,[29] the changes wrought by this intrapersonal dialogue foreshadowed some contemporary philosophical thought. But, over the last century or so, for divers reasons, including dramatic changes in health care possibilities, there has been much relevant writing on the nature of personhood, some emphasizing that 'person' is a concept which extends beyond the confines of the individual. Several examples from North America may be noted.

Henry James wrote, in a rather dated and quaint way of stressing the complexity of person (from 1892), with a focus on the relationship of 'possession': 'A man's me is the sum total of all that he can call his, not only his body and his mind, but his clothes and his house, his wife and his children, his ancestors and his friends, his reputation and his works, his lands and his horses, his yacht and his bank account.'[30] Whitman expressed it otherwise: 'I am not contained between my hat and my boots',[31] inviting further thought. Charles Taylor, as philosopher, stressed cognate points, though moving between the terms 'self' and 'person':

> I am a self only in relation to certain interlocutors: in relation to those conversation partners who were essential to my achieving self-definition. A self exists only within 'webs of interlocution'. To ask what a person is, in abstraction, from his or her self-interpretations, is to ask a fundamentally misguided question. We are only selves insofar as we move in a certain space of questions, as we seek and find orientation to the good.[32]

Cassell, in the course of his deliberations on human suffering already mentioned, sketched the areas in personal 'topography' which may engender suffering. He listed those parts which constitute 'person': roles, relationships, actions, behaviours, as well as a body, dreams and a transcendent dimension – 'a life of the spirit, however expressed or known'. But Cassell stressed that persons cannot be reduced to their parts. He noted further that:

> ... all the aspects of personhood – the lived past, the family's lived past, culture and society, roles, the instrumental dimension, associations and relationships, the body, the unconscious mind, the political being, the secret life, the perceived future, and the transcendent being – dimension – are susceptible to damage and loss.[33]

This portrayal of human complexity is in the tradition of a relational concept of 'person'. The observations of the unpublished research of Best, McCosker and Lickiss, already mentioned, was clearly in accord with Cassell's 'topography' of persons.

From my own perspectives, I have found useful a cognate, schematic, ecological model of a person, stressing that 'person' is a relational reality, a web as it were, of relationships in a dynamic whole: stressing that relationships constitute, rather than add to, personhood. We are, as it were, webs – constituted by interrelating realities, and constantly in flux. From an ecological point of view a person is a relational reality with respect to the present life situation, but also to the personal past (what is done and also experienced), not only the facts regarding the past but how the past is interpreted and incorporated into the present. The inheritance (biological and cultural) of a person provides the platform, as it were, on which the personal history has been constructed and interpreted, and must continue to influence the present. Intrapersonal dialogue fits readily into this schema. The way out of what might otherwise be conceived as a closed system appears to be offered by the vector of hope. In clinical practice over decades it became clear that what a patient hoped for was difficult (sometimes painful) to articulate – and also unpredictable. It will be noted on this model, that all elements are in dynamic relationship articulated in action, apparent or not to the observer; the personal process is complex and each person is unique.

We know what may cause breakage – the shattering of a fragile web. But what holds these notional elements together? The issue of coherence invites deeper exploration. In order to consider further, and at another level of enquiry, what is a/the principle of coherence, or even what it can be named, it may be wise to return to our earliest human sources.

The earliest Hebrew scriptures give a powerful (mythical) portrayal of the formation of man and woman (Genesis), attracting continuing profound analysis.[34] Two components are delineated – dust of the earth (*nephesh*) and breath from elsewhere (breath/spirit – *ruah*), and these together form a living man; woman, being constituted as the same as man, also has these two components – and is radically connected with man, as he with her. Death, for both man and woman, is seen as the loss of whatever is from elsewhere (spirit), allowing what came from the earth to disintegrate and return to earth. Philosophers have tried to codify these profound human realities. But is remains our human experience surely that there is in us that which is of the material universe, and something other – which we may call by the generic name, 'spirit' which during our lifetime defies entropy. The principle or source of personal coherence, whereby the complex relationships which constitute as persons (as well as our material components) are held together, may surely be radically 'spirit', or bear this name. Spirit, the form of the material, may also serve as that which binds the whole as one. Such considerations are redolent of the remarks of Sydenham, already mentioned – it may be that a radical humanism needs far more focus on human origins as a means of better conceptualizing human capacities as well as the shattering that is possible in the realization of human possibility.

This statement does not take away the problem – but merely gives a name in response to a question. The shape of what Shakespeare portrayed as the inner self must surely relate to this principle. This concept does not address the notion that the form may endure on dissolution of the material – maybe emphemerality is of its essence, maybe not: this matter is not at issue at this juncture (although it is clear what position Sydenham held). Shakespeare's King Lear offers one of the most poignant portrayals in literature of human death as the time to yield up that which is the principle of coherence, or rather to allow it to be yielded up:

> EDGAR: He faints. My Lord ! My lord!
> LEAR: Break, heart, I prithee break.
> EDGAR: Look up, my lord!
> KENT: Vex not his ghost: O let him pass! He hateth much
>   That would upon the rack of this rough world
>   Stretch him out longer.'[35]

Whether the principle of coherence, which may be named 'spirit', is powerful enough to prevent personal disintegration under extreme onslaught – or in fact, cannot assist the centre to hold even under what might to other persons be minor provocation, may require an examination of the effect, not only of physical threats to survival, but also of all the constitutive relationships (other persons, place, past, culture, personal history) on the inner/interior life; we could postulate two way dynamic. But how the material affects or effects change in what is non-material appears beyond (my) present analysis, and has been a challenge to philosophers in the past. Maybe it is worth noting that there are examples of material reality appearing changed from within. Was Shakespeare hinting at something like this when offering what [Harold] Bloom calls 'self-overhearing' as a means for core (interior) personal change? The question remains however at another level – what determines or at least influences the shape of one's core or spirit? Of one's capacity not to yield to forces which threaten personal disintegration? Does a continuing awareness (despite all) of a Pattern inhering in Being prove to be a bulwark against personal disintegration? Psychologists, neurophysiologists, philosophers, theologians – all may address such questions: others of us may simply describe events, and sometimes experience them.

Reference should be made to the seminal concepts of [Aaron] Antonovsky concerning a 'sense of coherence' based on extensive sociological research. He wrote that: 'The sense of coherence[36] explicitly and unequivocally is a generalized, long-lasting way of seeing the world and one's life in it … It is … a crucial element in the basic personality structure of an individual and in the ambience of a subculture, culture or historical period.' He related social networks to the 'sense of coherence', and expressed the view that 'social supports enhance the ability of the individual to obtain meaningful information, or in my terms, enhance the sense of coherence'. Such a concept is in accord with the stress on person as a relational reality. In his later writing Antonovsky outlined how the sense of coherence develops over the life span and laid the foundations for decades of research on these themes.[37]

Personal change does occur. [Erik] Erikson, in a series of writings in the last quarter of the twentieth century, portrayed a way of considering personal development over a lifetime, and his concepts have stood the test of time.[38] Erikson (from a psychoanalytic perspective) stressed the role of psychosocial crises, occurring at various stages throughout life, as triggers for choice of a path in the face of two distinct options. He saw personal growth as taking place by negotiation of developmental tasks through the resolution of crises. The growing human person is continually faced by options, each life stage being characterized by its own options which, whilst they confront one through life, do come to ascendancy in a given stage. For example, the favourable outcome of infancy is an attitude of basic trust rather than basic distrust, and on this basis the child goes on to be faced with the next choice – that of autonomy or fear of decision. Where the life process is characterized by the embracing of favourable options, the personality becomes characterized by trust, reasonable autonomy, initiative, capacity for effort, a sense of identity (to be and share oneself) rather than confusion, capacity for intimate personal relationships rather than isolation, fruitfulness rather than stagnation, and finally a sense of wholeness of life (what Erikson calls integrity) rather than despair. In the course of the negotiation of these developmental tasks personal relationships are inevitably involved. Change is driven from the interior, but (as in the case of a growing orchid) ingredients of the environment are also critical. Actions leave marks. Life cycles, as Erikson called them, are interlocked, cog-wheeled, as it were, welding the human community into a matrix in continuous flux. It may be worth noting that the interlocking 'cogs' in the wheel differ necessarily from each other, whilst in intimate connection. Some persons will be grappling with fear, weakness, loss, even despair, whilst others are in the bloom of happiness, impelled by love and realistic hope, and dreams. But the connections between all sustain all, and form the human pattern.

Despair, on Erikson's model is one of the two options in the last phase of life – at any age: the favourable option being rather the development of a sense of wholeness (which Erikson calls 'integrity') being at one with one's place and time, and life pattern. Authentic living with frailty or dying, as authentic living, is surely embedded not in falsehood but in truth. Certainly no lie can be justified to separate a person from his or her own truth – depriving him or her of becoming what is possible. The matter of the personal significance of the last phase of life, at any age, needs far more focus: failure to appreciate it may be a potent source of deep distress. Cassell stressed that a goal of medicine is the relief of suffering (and the obverse of that notion is surely the facilitation of human flourishing in no matter what circumstances) by assisting the subject cohere (helping the 'centre to hold') – a precious service indeed, not within the capacity of all physicians, but respected by all.

The shape of the final task needs to be understood in general terms by those in contact with patients approaching death – at any age. Such patients may well vacillate between wholeness and despair, before the way is clear. They may long to express their internal states, explore the threat of despair through dialogue with others – but to participate in such dialogue is so very difficult for the interlocutor – and to reach out towards what wholeness is possible, to round out the symphony of one's life. If it is surely the task of each person to explore the limits of one's possibilities (which involve in the end the going out from oneself, as the highest exercise of autonomy) then it is surely the task of a doctor to free patients from obstacles (such as pain) to such an exploration. Furthermore, no person should die in iatrogenic despair. No person should die with the dominant perception of self as a 'therapeutic failure', nor disillusioned after being sustained by unrealistic hope, recognized as such even by the physician engendering it, conceiving it as an act of compassion. The physician, whilst emphasizing a realistic range of possibilities as a way of indicating prognosis, should assist the patient to centre hope not on what will in the end probably fail in a situation of eventually fatal illness (such as anti-disease therapies), but what should not fail – the commitment to care, the relief of pain, and in the intrinsic value of the patient as a unique irreplaceable subject of existence. These matters call for much pondering if we are not to add to the despair of those living with complex chronic diseases or dying in 'high tech' contexts – or anywhere.

On the basis of such considerations, are there ways of looking again at our approach to the relief of suffering in clinical contexts? It may be possible to categorize the various generic means for relief of suffering (of relevance to medicine) simply as follows:

1. Ameliorate a definable 'cause' of suffering, or trigger which is precipitating the sense of being 'about to go to pieces.'
2. Strengthen the principle of coherence.

Amelioration of an identified contributory factor implies that there has been a diligent search to identify whether or not the patient is suffering, what has been the trigger, and what this patient usually (historically) does if coherence is so threatened. The story told of the past, as well as the present, the narrative, will give a guide also to the patient's capacity for withholding major threats to cohesion, and may give clues also to explanations for change in that capacity, for good or ill. All gives a portrait of what the patient is suffering (literally 'undergoing'), and how best to assist. Sometimes the telling is the beginning of a sense of recovery ('I feel better now') without any removal of the 'trigger' – a pointer to the subtlety both of the dynamic of suffering, and the processes of human reconstruction. Recovery from a state of suffering should not be thought of as a process of adaptation to circumstances, but of personal growth, of the realization of new possibilities – a manner of thinking which needs to be central in the conceptualization and practice of clinical psychology.

Removal of factors threatening personal cohesion is the stuff of much medical practice, especially (but not only) in the field of palliative medicine, whether practiced in the general health system or in very specialized contexts. Pain, a feature of cancer for some patients – whether due to disease or its treatment, is relievable (even if not wholly removed) in most instances, applying contemporary principles – yet cancer-related pain is still problematic, globally and locally – for various reasons. Relief of other major symptoms is also usually possible. But no level of symptom relief can obviate all suffering – for suffering is not intrinsically medical but personal. What is sometimes called existential suffering may remain – with overwhelming grief in the face of losses or coherence unable to be restored. In such circumstances it is strengthening of the principle of coherence which offers the only possibility. Restoration of personal integrity in the face of irremediable stressors, remains the human task – and the means are not new. Interpersonal solidarity remains the lynch pin.

There are frequently, in ordinary everyday life, not only in the horrors of war, circumstances in which it is not possible to remove the stressor, but a need to help persons to endure. The work of Morse, already mentioned, warning of the need for holding techniques, not touch, until the stressor is gone, and emotions can be given full rein, is of critical importance, yet may be hard to remember in the rush of emotion felt by those responding to disaster (in an emergency department or earthquake). Attending to persons trapped in rubble in natural disasters, while rescue efforts are being made, or even failing, are also examples. Such careful research and reflection is critical and reflects in a practical and teachable way what has been long known.

The maintenance or restoration of a sense of coherence will require different means in diverse circumstances, but normally rests in the restoration of relationships, in the place of fracture. The relationships to be restored may be:

- intrapersonal – re-engagement with a self-thought lost, by removal of horrendous pain, or refreshing sleep, or release from constraint, or interior renewal, and rebirth of hope,
- interpersonal, involving the agency of another person, whether stranger or not, as simply a proximate human

('lending strength'), or involving a pre-existing significant but broken relationship (one sees this in forgiveness/reconciliation as well as a reunion, through collocation or telephone or vision),

- with place as critical to identity – for example, returning home,
- through restoration of something else central to sense of self or self-worth – a capacity or an object,
- through acknowledgement, once again, of lost or disparaged spiritual tradition, history or cultural affinity,
- through discovery or construction of meaning in the face of incomprehension or absurdity.

This restoration – wrought through changes in any of these domains, is close to a recovery of human dignity, but with a critical additional notion. Human dignity may be present in the midst of suffering, since fundamentally radical human dignity is best regarded as intrinsic and not lost even by damage to relationships constitutive of the person: the trace of what is there suffices to make human dignity present – even though not readily perceived by the person or beholder, if unmindful that dignity is in the order of being, not attributes, nor merely possibility. The relationships between human dignity and human suffering are subtle, but recent philosophical discussion has stressed that the aesthetic dimension of life needs to be kept in focus: 'the ongoing moral challenge in the face of pain and suffering is to ensure that our various expressions of the beautiful life continue to preserve and enhance the dignity we all share'.[39] Moreover, it has been said by a professor of anatomy, 'it is the task of medicine is to emancipate man's interior splendour',[40] and this may be never more poignant than in the face of human suffering. And the nature of that splendour may remain a riddle for the mind. All this is matter for reflection – and the stuff of radical humanism indeed. It will be noted that there is considerable affinity between such notions and the philosophical frame of Rawlinson.

Human suffering is uniquely personal – the universal is particularized in each individual. Communitarian suffering is radically personal and individual, though unquantifiable. Can one compute the total sum of the human suffering(s) of two World Wars, of the Shoah, of Hiroshima, of the Ruanda massacre, of recent tsunamis or earthquakes, of any natural disaster? It makes little sense to try to think in such ways. What is true is that every community is made up of persons, that the experience of each is unique, that the suffering of each is unique, however strong the attempts by tyrants or torturers to depersonalize (and usually by attacking precisely the relationships which are constitutive of the person), and however common are the external factors directed at breaking the spirit. And it is necessary but painful to recognize also that physicians have been the source of deliberately intended unspeakable human suffering – and in our own times: the Nazi doctors were not alone in this betrayal but their place has been an unforgettable blight on the history of medicine. Alexander, observer at the Nuremberg trials tried to analyze the roots of the egregious moral collapse of some of the most eminent German medical academic leaders, and pinned the beginning on a 'shift in attitude to the non-rehabilitatable sick'– a caution for our own times and forever.[41]

Reflection on the human condition is difficult, and especially in the context of contemporary medical practice, and articulating such reflections even more difficult, at least for those outside the humanities and the arts. Medical practitioners may have largely drawn back from reflection, lest such be a distraction from the pursuit of the biological basis of disease and the means to 'conquer' it, and to continue to bear the onerous burdens of practice. But a tipping point may be close. Reflection is essential, and this reflection may need to go back to ancient portrayals of the human, to Genesis, to the Greeks, to the high philosophers of the middle ages (including Maimonides and Aquinas), to the renaissance thinkers, to Shakespeare, to the struggling enlightenment philosophers, to those seeking to salvage Western thought after the catastrophes of the twentieth century, to the scientists bringing new perspectives, to non-Western traditions, and to those working to explore and harness new ideas concerning the human and the human good.

Medicine surely cannot be considered any longer as merely a natural science, nor medical practice merely the application of empirical science or technology. Illness (the subjective experience of a deficit of well-being, which may be codified into a 'disease') is a critical part of a human life, to be considered and alleviated in the perspective of that person's whole life, even glimpsed for just a few moments in time, to assist the 'centre to hold'. It could be that there needs to be a renewed focus on the thought of [Wilhelm] Dilthey, the nineteenth century German philosopher, in his careful analysis of the basis of the 'human sciences', as he pointed out the limits of the methodology and philosophical basis of the 'natural sciences'[42,43] – it would appear that there could be value in the recognition of medical science as a 'human science' in Dilthey's terms, or at the very least to be considered as a bridge between the human sciences and the natural sciences; it may be truly the synthesis of these, if adequately understood. Foucault would surely agree.[44]

At the very least, the significance of the historical and the subjective, and the dimensions of human values and experience (and narratives concerning these things) may begin to gain a status equal to quantifiable objective biological tests as tools for diagnosis and of evaluation of the worth of clinical intervention. Nothing less may be necessary to begin to relieve some of the regrettable suffering being experienced by persons in halls of clinical excellence, even where there is a perceived (but maybe inadequately conceived) commitment to the human good, as well as by so many of the human community, everywhere.

The obligation to care for each other is not rooted in law or in contract, but, as Levinas has so stressed in our time, but is rooted in the call of the other in need.[45] [Franz] Kafka reminded us in the early twentieth century: 'You can hold yourself back from the sufferings of the world; this is something you are free to do and is in accord with your nature, but precisely the holding back is the only suffering that you might be able to avoid'.[46] Such counsel has to be more poignant in the already troubled twenty-first century. Not to care is not a human option, and for a physician, betrayal.

References

1. I. Yalom, *Staring at the Sun: Overcoming the Dread of Death* (Melbourne: Scribe, 2008).
2. M Rawlinson, The sense of suffering, *The Journal of Medicine and Philosophy* 11(1986) 39–62.
3. M C Nussbaum, *Therapy of Desire: Theory and Practice in Hellenistic Ethics* (Princeton: Princeton University Press, 1994).
4. H E Sigerist, *History of Medicine. Vol 1. Primitive and Archaic Medicine* New York: Oxford University Press, 1951), H E Sigerist.
5. *History of Medicine. Vol II Early Greek, Hindu, and Persian Medicine* (New York: Oxford University Press, 1987).
6. L I Conrad, M Neve, V Nutton, R Porter, A Wear, *The Western Medical Tradition* (Cambridge: Cambridge University Press, Cambridge 1995).
7. R Porter R, *The Greatest Benefit to Mankind: A Medical History of Humanity.* Norton, New York, 1997.
8. M Kearney, *A Place of Healing: Working with Suffering and Dying.* Oxford University Press, Oxford. 2000.

9 H E Sigerist, *History of Medicine Vol 1 Primitive and Archaic Medicine*. (New York: Oxford University Press, 1951) p11.
10 R. Porter, *Flesh in the Age of Reason* (London: Norton, 2003).
11 Sydenham in Porter, 2003, op. cit. p 28.
12 N Cherny, N Coyle, and KM Foley, Suffering in the advanced cancer patient: a definition and taxonomy, *Journal of Palliative Care* (1994)10:57–70.
13 N Cherny, N Coyle, and KM Foley, Suffering in the advanced cancer patient: a definition and taxonomy, *Journal of Palliative Care* (1994)10:57–70.
14 E Cassell, The nature of suffering and the goals of medicine, *New England Journal of Medicine*, 306 (1982), 639–645.
15 W Shakespeare, *Macbeth*, Act IV, Scene 3.
16 R Chapman and J Gavrin, Suffering and its relationship to pain, *Journal of Palliative Care* (1993) 9:5–13.
17 A W Frank, Can we research suffering? *Qualitative Health Research* (2001)11: 353–62.
18 S Daneault, V Lussier and S Mongeau et al. The Nature of Suffering and its Relief in the terminally ill: a qualitative study. *J Palliative Care* (2004)20(1):7–11.
19 J M Morse, Towards a praxis theory of suffering, *Adv Nursing Sci* (2001)24:47–59.
20 T S Eliot, Four Quartets 1. Burnt Norton, *Collected poems 1909–1935*, Harcourt Brace, New York, 1936.
21 R Schaerer, Suffering of the doctor linked with the death of patients. *Palliative Medicine* (1993)7(suppl 1):27–37.
22 D E Meier, AL Back, and RS Morrison, The inner life of physicians and the care of the seriously ill, *Journal American Medical Association* (2001)286:3007–3014.
23 E Cassell, *The nature of suffering and the goals of medicine* 2nd edit (Oxford: Oxford University Press, 2004) 37–40.
24 A C Enthoven, Cutting cost without cutting the quality of care (Shattuck Lecture). *New England Journal Medicine* 1978. 298:1229–1238.
25 E Cassell, *The Nature of Suffering and the goals of Medicine*, 2nd Edition (Oxford: Oxford University Press, 2004). p. xii.
26 TR Cole, N Carlin, The suffering of physicians, *The Lancet*, 374 (2009), 1414–1415.
27 J Needleman, The perception of mortality, *Annals New York Academy of Sciences* 164 (1969: pp. 733–738.
28 E Cassell, *The Nature of Suffering and the Goals of Medicine*, 1st Edition (Oxford, Oxford University Press, 1991) p. x.

29 H Bloom, *Shakespeare: The Invention of the Human* (New York: Riverhead Books, 1998), p. xvii.
30 H James, quoted in Becker E, *The Birth and Death of Meaning: an Interdisciplinary Perspective on the Problem of Man*, 2nd edition (Harmondsworth, Penguin Books, 1971) p. 43.
31 W Whitman, Song of Myself, in W Whitman, *Leaves of Grass*, 189–1892 edition (Philadelphia: David McKay, 1891).
32 C Taylor, *Sources of the Self: the Making of Modern Identity* (Cambridge: Harvard University Press, 1989) p 36.
33 E Cassell, The nature of suffering and the goals of medicine, *New England Journal of Medicine*, 306 (1982), p 643.
34 A G Zornberg, *The Beginning of Desire: Reflections on Genesis* (New York: Double Day,1995) p.14.
35 Shakespeare. *King Lear* Act V, Scene iii.
36 A Antonovsky, *Health, Stress and Coping.* 1979 (San Francisco, Jossey Bass,1979).
37 A Antonovsky, *Unravelling the Mystery of Health: How People Manage Stress and Stay Well* (San Francisco: Jossey Bass,1988) pp. 89–127.
38 E Erikson, Identity and the Life Cycle, *Psychological Issues Monograph* (New York: International Universities Press,1968), and E Erikson, *The Life Cycle Completed: a Review* (New York: Norton, 1982).
39 D Pullman, Human dignity and the ethics and aesthetics of pain and suffering, *Theoretical Medicine*, 23 (2002) p. 75–94.
40 K Mortimer, The impossible profession: the doctor-priest relationship. *Proc Aust Assoc Gerontol* (1974) 2:81–82.
41 L Alexander, Medical science under dictatorship, *New England Journal of Medicine* 241(1949) pp. 39–47.
42 W Dilthey, *Introduction to the Human Sciences* (1923), trans RJ Betanzos, (Detroit: Wayne State University Press, p. 19).
43 H P Rickman (ed and translator). *W Dilthey: selected writings*, Cambridge. Cambridge University Press. 1988.
44 M Foucault, *Birth of the Clinic*. Trans A M Sheridan Smith (London: Tavistock, 1973).
45 S Hand (ed), *The Levinas Reader* (Oxford: Blackwell,1989.)pp. 75–87.
46 F Kafka, *The Collected Aphorisms*, no 103 (Oct 1917–Feb 1918), Penguin Classics, 1994.

8

Palliative Medicine as a Clinical Science

I

Symptoms – The Patient as Subject
1986

Based on lecture, Conference at Mt Olivet Hospital, Brisbane, 1986.

> 'Who are we? Where do we come from? Where are we going? What are we waiting for? What awaits us?' ... Such questions, with which Ernst Bloch opened his monumental work, *The Principle of Hope*,[1] set the scene for an interrogation concerning some aspects of current medical practice.

i

There are grounds for considering that nothing less than a paradigm shift is necessary and even underway concerning medical science and praxis: in [Thomas] Kuhn's term the old paradigms are outworn.[2] Kuhn, in examining the context and manner in which new scientific paradigms emerge, makes some comments germane to the present consideration.

> In the development of any science, the first received paradigm is usually felt to account quite successfully for most of the observations and experiments easily accessible to that science's practitioners. Further development, therefore, ordinarily calls for the construction of elaborate equipment, the development of an esoteric vocabulary and skills, and a refinement of concepts that increasingly lessons their resemblance to their usual common sense prototypes. That professionalization leads, on the one hand, to an immense restriction of the scientist's vision and to a considerable resistance to paradigm change.

Kuhn further points out the value of resistance to change: 'By ensuring that the paradigm will not be too easily surrendered, resistance guarantees that scientists will not be too lightly distracted and that the anomalies that lead to paradigm change will penetrate existing knowledge to the core.'

What are the main features of the contemporary paradigm of western medical science and practice? Under the influence of the dramatic advances in understanding of pathophysiological mechanisms, in diagnostic methodology, and in therapeutics of all modalities, the contemporary medical student and doctor are taught to take a medical history from which to extract the clues to the most likely diagnosis, to confirm that diagnosis by relevant investigations, and to reverse the identified pathological process by all reasonable means: the vast data base available concerning each patient ensures that in the majority of cases (at least in hospital) it is possible to know and monitor 'what is going on' – to use a commonly heard expression implying laudable accuracy, and to find relevant simple (or heroic) measures aiming to increase the chances of curing or controlling the disease – whether it be cancer, heart disease or end stage liver disease ... and so on. A rational approach indeed.

Yet there is widespread discontent about health care – not merely because of the cost escalation but because somehow the medical system appears alien to what is most profoundly human. Our people fear it, and often do not want to be readmitted to our most prestigious institutions, however promising the results of costly and complex medical treatment ... and others fear powerlessness, loss of autonomy in the face of it all. Doctors and other health professionals often delay unduly seeking medical assistance for themselves – or refuse treatment altogether, even treatment they may have advocated for others. The discontent is widespread, and that is quite apart from the disquiet of health administrators concerned with lack of efforts or results relevant to prevention, or cost containment.

A paradigm shift occurs, on Kuhn's model, through the introduction and survival of vigorous new ideas, rather than by the deliberate approximation of the paradigm to some already defined final goal. We may not know quite where we want to go, but we may well examine contemporary currents of ideas which need to be given a chance to contribute to the processes of development of medical praxis. The technological revolution of the twentieth century has profoundly shaped medical practice – but medical practice has developed largely in isolation from the wisest philosophical currents of the same period. Medicine and the humanities seem far apart.

In reflecting on medical practice, in search of significant new perspectives, several options are open: a) re-examine the past, for the history of ideas and practice in medicine will illuminate the dynamics of the processes of change; b) note carefully the analyses of clinical decision-making, hopefully assisting the emergence of more rational decisions (if sound basic premises are accepted); and c) re-examine clinical practice from the perspective of the community as a whole, with extrinsic restraints on resources, etc. to encourage certain desired patterns of practice.

A further approach to this problem is to examine the adequacy of and redefine the anthropological basis of contemporary medical practice. What view of humanness prevails? Has medical practice taken into account and into its heart the personalist philosophies which have marked the twentieth century, as well as the awakening of the spiritual dimension of the human person, possibly best expressed by [Victor] Frankl's celebrated remark (after surviving Auschwitz) that the twentieth century has known not only the evils of the gas chambers but also the fact that men and women entered them with the Lord's prayer or the Shema Yisrael on their lips? Exploration along these lines to garner the wisdom of the ages and the most profound contemporary understanding concerning humanness – what it means to be human, would be a major undertaking, even with respect to the relationship of anthropology to medical practice. Yet some comments may not be valueless in the present groping for a new paradigm for *human* medicine.

ii

The human patient-as-subject

The human person has been the object of close scrutiny and study, and the fruits have been a prolific growth in the various sciences – biological sciences, clinical sciences, and the social sciences. Psychiatry has explored the bases of abnormal mental states and behaviours. But the human person as subject, that is as a thinking and feeling entity and centre for agency, may not yet have received adequate consideration with respect to 'ordinary' medical practice. Yet the praxis of medicine, the application of medical science demands an adequate view of the patient as subject.

[Richard] McCormick has recently drawn attention to matters of relevance.[3] The second Vatican Council asserted that: 'the moral aspect of any procedure ... must be determined by objective standards which are based in the nature of the person and the person's acts'. The official commentary on this wording noted two things: that in the expression there is formulated a general principle that applies to all human actions, and that the choice of this expression means that 'human activity must be judged insofar as it refers to the human person integrally and adequately considered.' No adequate consideration of man can maybe ever be made solely by another human, or even humans acting in concert throughout the ages, but it is open to each person to contribute in a small way to whatever conceptual construct is possible. The present contribution (by a medico, not philosopher) is merely a small contribution.

a) The human person-as-subject is situated in a context.
The human person may be thought of as situated at the centre of a complex environment (material, personal) with which he or she is in constant (dialectic) interaction – with each interaction changing the composite as time passes. Some persons within this environment or personal field are of high significance, and interaction with such persons is so crucial that the existential well-being of the person as *person* is dramatically changed by any changes in that inter-relationship. The person may, as we say, 'go to pieces'.

Further, the present pattern of interaction is preceded by a personal history, lived through by that particular person with his or her unique mix of biological and cultural inheritance. The present, whilst not a mere product of the past, is in continuity via that person (whatever else is different) with the past and is influenced by it.

Such an ecological view of the human person, incorporating adequately the temporal dimension, gives a richness to the notions of the situated human subject. The implications for medical practice include: i) an adequate understanding of the processes of bereavement and grieving as the self resynthesises the field of significant others; ii) recognition of the disastrous effects of cultural withdrawal as experienced by patients, for example, from tropical islands (or indigenous Country), sent to major referral centres for demanding treatment – no matter how kind (and 'culturally competent') the receiving staff; and iii) the priority to be given to personal interaction when time consuming or isolating investigations or treatment are being considered in the light of the yield to be reasonably expected.

b) The human person-as-subject is constantly 'in process'.

There has been considerable clarification in this (twentieth) century of the processes of human personal development throughout the life stages: the early twentieth century stress on the paramount effects of the experience of very early life have opened out to a richer concept of human personal development and unfolding, with potential for dramatic change even in the very last phase of life.

[Erik] Erikson's corpus of writing and teaching still serves as a useful conceptual frame.[4] He stressed that lifelong personal development occurs through stages, by resolution of crises, in the context of social relationships, and that the successful negotiation of the developmental tasks of each stage of life is a necessary prerequisite for satisfactory progression to the next task. When the life process is characterised by the embracing of favourable options the personality becomes characterised by trust, reasonable autonomy, initiative, capacity for effort, a sense of stagnation, and finally a sense of integrity or wholeness of life rather than despair.

Illness of any significance is in some sense a crisis, a developmental node with its own tasks: the person needs the time, space, privacy, access to significant persons, and opportunity for decision-making appropriate to the developmental stage. Persons in the last phase of life, at any age, faced with a developmental task of the achievement of a sense of wholeness rather than despair, are in very great need. At a point when it is clear that hope cannot be anchored in success in personal projects, cure of disease, or even in other persons (for any reason), then the question 'In what may I hope?' involves the testing of one's inner compacities and perspectives (as [Ernest] Bloch noted). Maybe hope is then anchored in a yearning for integrity in the forgiven self after all, as all that is left within the context at least of mortality: a radical humanism. Judeo-Christian traditions have taught that the search for wholeness in the self is in fact in accord with the notion the human person is called to express the image of God more and more clearly, and that this is of the fullness of human life. The human person then, in this frame, is called to hope within an ultimate dialogue with hope in the self anchored finally beyond the self. But there are many images of human possibility, each profoundly influenced by cultural traditions: the richness of this diversity may be inadequately appreciated.

c) The human subject is a knowing entity.

The cognitive aspects of human subjectivity have considerable implications for medical science. 'History taking', that task learned so early in clinical education, is a communication exercise designed to elicit relevant information which can point towards a diagnosis – as well as, in passing, to help the doctor learn what is essential concerning the patient's past and present personal context. However the perceptions of the patient ('symptoms') are not mere pointers to what may be wrong ; the perceptions of the human subject in whom a significant disease process is present have other scientific values.

   i Symptoms, as [Alvan] Feinstein stressed, in relation to cancer[5] are tools for understanding the chronometry and extent of a disease process (at least in neoplasms), and hence usefully aid in defining prognosis with or without intervention, and accordingly may influence recommendations and decisions concerning intervention.

   ii Symptoms are significant in evaluation of interventions aimed at alleviating them, whether or not measures of a disease process are used. Trials in some areas of clinical science, for example, rheumatology, have recognised the significance of symptoms as measures of success. In cancer trials aimed at arrest or control, not cure (and many trials are in the former category) symptom relief (a subjective measure of success) should be paramount.

   iii The human subject is the one to order the priorities for symptom control, in accord with his or her hierarchy of perceived problems.[6]

d) The human subject as agent or 'actor'.

The human person not only *knows* but can *intend,* can move out of from the self into intention and into action, which in turn integrates the self.[7] The human being is both the actor and the subject, and has experience of being both. The human subject can in fact endure what is suffered, can remain (however stripped) as a knowing, willing entity just as gold endures the crucible, but more so as the experiencing self. Even in utter passivity when something 'happens' to the subject there is still the possibility of freely creating the shape of the response to that happening: the human person is not only the agent of their acting but creator of it.

Action reflects and reveals the subject as well as integrates: the human person as actor is expressing the shape of the self. [Ludwig] Wittgenstein, who so influenced twentieth century philosophy, would warn here against the model of an interior self and an exterior self ... in a sense we are what we say and do, we do not merely express a hidden reality. Knowing, willing, are capacities of the human subject, capacities which need opportunities for continuous realisation. (Thinking, as a capacity, may need further thought.)

The implications of even the above brief mention of some ideas have relationship to the concept of autonomy which has crept into contemporary medicine. For example, Grimley Evans postulates the 'preservation of autonomy' as a goal for the care system of the elderly.[8]

Autonomy, which focusses on the power of the human self to formulate and follow principles of action, has been a central notion in western moral philosophy in the nineteenth and twentieth centuries. Recent re-interpretation[9] of Immanuel Kant's account of autonomy assists us to move away from the interpretation that leads to the turning of 'autonomy' into a moral self-sufficiency that strangers need to deal with one another, and instead move into a commitment to dwell in a shared moral world. Kant, according to [P] Rossi, did recognise a relationship between autonomy and a world that exhibits human mutuality and interdependence.

Such an enriched notion of autonomy needs to be taken into account in reflection on medical practice. How, in circumstances of relative or actual weakness, can the human person-as-patient. express his or her autonomy. Or recover it?

III
Autonomy focussed care

Formulation of an approach to medical practice based on the patient-as-subject who is situated, who is in the process of personal development, perceives/understands/comprehends, and who wills/intends/acts has been given some consideration in specific care situations. The approach, which could be termed 'autonomy focussed care', may in some circumstances (notably in geriatric medicine and in the care of the dying) supplant the traditional processes of practice. Previous attempts to order medical practice in relation to a complex array of information concerning a patient have included a) the clarification of the medical problem list (active and passive) and b) the generation by the patient of an hierarchy of problems. These two approaches can be subsumed into autonomy focussed care, very simply, as follows:

1 Ascertain the patient's priorities for action: 'What are the things you most want to be able to *do* but cannot because of a health problem?' (The answer is unpredictable!)
2 Ascertain the *obstacles* and from this, construct the *patient's* list of problems, perceived as obstacles to desired action.
3 On the basis of closer questioning, history taking of each problem, clinical examination and, if essential, appropriate investigations, make an etiological diagnosis of each.
4 Devise a management plan for each of these problems.

5   Evaluate progress in the alleviation of these 'obstacles' *and* the achievement of the desired actions.

Some of these concepts are already in place, but the relevance of this approach to the measurement of 'response' in therapeutic trials in conditions such as ineradicable cancer may be obvious – but rarely adopted. Objective criteria of success, such as tumour regression (however measured) need to be supplemented by subjective criteria for success of treatment however challenging the methodology required to measure the subjective.

Obviously there are limitations, most notably in respect to preventive medicine; nevertheless, the potential is considerable for not only giving well-based personal satisfaction to our patients, but also for more rational allocation of resources. If personal integration and development of patients were facilitated by wiser clinical action, the benefits to the community would be multiplied.

IV
The patient-as-subject dies eventually

Diverse concepts of human dying and death have been the hallmark of humanity throughout recorded history, and these concepts find expression in art, literature and various other forms of human activity. The concept held of human death must influence medical practice and some articulation of this relationship may be of value. For it may be that the act of looking at the phenomenon of human death and clarifying one's perspective may assist in shaping the goals and processes of medical practice.

1) If death is seen as utter defeat or even an 'unjustifiable violation' (as Simon de Beauvoir styled her mother's death), clinical practice is a battleground with the doctor (with

other staff, of course) as protagonist/knight ... until the end, and regretting the end as defeat; 'we did our best but ...'. Such may indeed be the case, and a strong pro-life thrust is essential for medical practice and its practitioners. But there is need for a strong life-affirming thrust to recognise the fittingness of human death as a quiet dignified folding of the tent – or unfolding indeed of a flower – when the time has come, at any age. And to strive to achieve such a death for each patient, everywhere and always.

2) If death is seen as a culmination of life lived out as a mystery of exchange[10] in which human interaction is always exchange, never merely giving and receiving, then what of the medical care system, especially as the patient approaches the apex of the exchange, the moment of death when he or she utterly surrenders the self to others, and the doctor as companion along the way is both receiver and giver?

   Medical practice is a classic example of hyperactivity with more and more action (work) with less and less opportunity for reflection: reflection not merely on the need to clarify objectives to avoid what Tolstoy called 'mindless labour', but also in the realities of human exchange within which clinical activity is embedded.

3) If human death is conceived as a rite of passage, a passover, a breaking out from a cocoon, a moment of birth (as in several traditions), then medical activity is properly seen as a small part of a drama, with the patient in the centre, and all of us present to an event beyond our understanding. Some religious tradition has even perceived dying as the going forth of the person into an encounter with God as bearing a bridal character. If such concepts are dear to the patient and family, reverence should mark the conduct of

all: there is need for gentleness, awe and silence. Such is fitting in any case.

If there is awareness that the human subject is dependent on another not only for origin but for continuing in being, then the richness of human autonomy is not lost but heightened – for it is open ended with surrender to what is beyond the self as its highest expression. And we are all dependent on what is beyond the self: none is radically self-sufficient.

For in the end, the human person as subject is transcendent, transcending context, transcending time, place, even the closest human ties, even transcending the self, made in the end for communion with the whole. It is not unfitting to quote in this hallowed place a prayer composed by Jesuit Teilhard de Chardin (as quoted by McCormick):

> When the signs of age begin to mark my body(and still more when they touch my mind); when the ill that is to diminish me or carry me off strikes from without or is born within me, when the painful moment comes in which I suddenly awake to the fact that I am ill or growing old; and above all that last moment when I feel I am losing hold of myself and am absolutely passive within the hands of the great unknown forces that have formed me; in all those dark moments, O God, grant that I may understand that it is you (provided only my faith is strong enough) who are painfully parting the fibres of my being in order to penetrate to the very marrow of my substance and bear me away within yourself.

[Albert] Einstein has said that it is given to every man to set the direction of his striving. These words have been concerned with redirecting the striving characteristic of the medical profession so that we may care more surely for the real needs of our fellows, in so far as in us lies, nothing more and nothing less.

REFERENCES

1 Bloch E, *The Principle of Hope* (1938–47), translated by Neville Plaice, Stephen Plaice and Paul Knight, Oxford, Blackwell, 1986.
2 Kuhn TS,
3 McCormick RA, Health and medicine in the Catholic Tradition, New York, Crossroad, 1984., 2nd edit, Chicago, University of Chicago, 1970.
4 Erikson EH, *Childhood and Society*, Revised edition, Harmondsworth, Penguin and Hogarth Press, 1965.
5 Feinstein AR, *Clinical Judgment*, Baltimore, Williams and Wilkins, 1967.
6 Lickiss JN, 'Dying from cancer: what are the questions?', *Australian Family Physician*, 1979; 8: 991–1003.
7 Wojtyla K, *The Acting Person*, Translated by Andrzej Potoki, London, Reidel, Dordrecht, 1979.
8 Evans JG, 'Prevention of age-associated loss of autonomy: epidemiological approaches', *J Chronic Disease*, 1984; 37: 353–63.
9 Rossi P, 'The foundation of the philosophical concept of autonomy by Kant and its historical consequences', *Concilium*, 1984; 172/2: 3–8.
10 Haughton R, *The passionate God*, London, Darton, Longman and Todd, 1981.

II
Palliative Care in a Modern Society: Giving Structure to Compassion
1993

Presentation at International Medical Symposium (Almeida Commemoration Symposium) Ohita, Japan, 1993, as one of two Western doctors invited to Japan to celebrate the coming of Western thought, 400 years previously.
Published in International Medical Journal
December 1995, vol 2, number 4, pp 259–262.

Abstract

Japanese people are aware of the increasing needs for care of those in the last phase of life. In the context of discussion concerning the anniversary of the coming of western ideas to Japan (400 years ago), the opportunity was taken to offer concepts of palliative care which give structure to the compassion felt by Japanese people for those in need of care.

Introduction

It is a rare privilege to be able to participate in a medical symposium commemorating the first contact of Japan with the West (including western medicine) four hundred and fifty years ago, and to contribute to the dialogue between East and West in the context of palliative care.

Japanese people are well aware of the possibility of cancer pain relief: this widespread expectation has been achieved by the effects of Dr. F. Takeda (Director WHO Collaborating Centre for Cancer Pain Relief and Quality of

Life, Saitama.), with the assistance of extensive coverage of the issue by the educational division of Japan's Television Authority (NHKY).[1]

The word "hospice" is also familiar because of recent TV programs. The challenge of making available palliative care in a sustainable fashion to those in need, in a nation of 180 million people with rapidly increasing percentages of elderly citizens is of much concern to senior health administrators and clinicians.

It appears wise to focus first on the perspective of the World Health Organization.

i

Global Perspective[2]

Palliative Care has been defined by World Health Organization:

> Palliative Care is the active total care of patients whose disease is not responsive to curative treatment.
>
> Control of pain, of other symptoms, and of psychological, social and spiritual problems is paramount. The goal of palliative care is achievement of the best possible quality of life for patients and their families. Many aspects of palliative care are also applicable earlier in the course of the illness, in conjunction with anticancer treatment.
>
> Palliative care:
> - affirms life and regards dying as a normal process;
> - neither hastens nor postpones death;
> - provides relief from pain and other distressing symptoms;
> - integrates the psychological and spiritual aspects of patient care;
> - offers a support system to help patients live as actively as possible until death;

- offers a support system to help the family cope during the patient's illness and in their own bereavement.

  Radiotherapy, chemotherapy and surgery have a place in palliative care, provided that the symptomatic benefits of treatment clearly outweigh the disadvantages. Investigative procedures are kept to a minimum.'[3]

The World Health Organisation statement is made in relation to cancer but is clearly applicable to the other diseases: there is a clear trend for the principles of palliative care in cancer to be recognized as valid in relation to patients with other incurable and progressive diseases such as AIDS [1993], not only in the terminal phase but earlier in the course of the disease: palliative care embodies the principles and practice which evolved within the hospice movement, and gives opportunities for further development of the core ideas. Palliative care includes terminal care but is much broader in scope: palliative care may be needed concurrently with therapy directed towards control of the disease process and should not be regarded as commencing when all else has failed. Palliative care includes the concept of rehabilitation: physical, emotional and spiritual – such rehabilitation is not dependent on cure or even control of the underlying disease process.

Programs of palliative care stress that illness should not be regarded as an isolated aberration in physiology but considered in terms of the suffering that it causes and the impact it has on patients' families. The "unit of care" is thus the family rather than the patient alone. This setting is regarded as most important; inquiries from the family are encouraged and the family's active participation in care is expected.

The World Health organisation stresses the need for adequate resources for palliative care – at least equal to all the resources available for anticancer treatment in a developed country, and the major part of all cancer resources in a developing nation.

ii

Palliative Care Implies Two Elements: Palliation and Care

Good palliative care, in all contexts, requires clear goals, precise strategies and adequate resources.

The goal is surely that each person in his/her total context (including family/friends) in accord with his/her unique personal priorities and personal philosophy, may be free, despite incurable disease, to live in dignity and harmony (free of pain and other distressing symptoms), and when appropriate, prepare peacefully to die.

There is now abundant literature on the science as well as the art of palliative care with a recent landmark textbook[4] as well as monographs and journals devoted to the subject. It is to be noted that although nurses and other professionals have essential and well defined roles, doctors have a major responsibility and challenge, in view not only of their clinical knowledge and skills but also of their privileged situation in relation to patients in countries like Japan, where medical care is so strikingly hospital based.

Palliation involves the application of modern concepts of palliative medicine and nursing – including:

a) attention to appropriate decision-making regarding the choice between various treatment options by a frank discussion with a well informed patient (and usually family members),

b) good symptom relief (including pain relief) which is usually possibly not only during anti-disease treatment (e.g. surgery, radiotherapy or chemotherapy) but also when such treatment is not appropriate and better replaced by competent symptomatic measures, and finally when a patient is actually dying, and

c) careful personal and family support including care of the family, during the period of bereavement after the death of the patient.

The place of care and the organisation of care, as well as the persons (professional and others) involved, depend on the circumstances of the patient and the complexity of the problems being caused by the progressive disease. Cultural factors must influence all these matters but some comments based on the Australian experience may be useful:

> Care at home amidst the family is preferred if possible by many patients – and requires a commitment by the family doctor to continue to be involved with the patient and to visit the patient at home; nursing assistance for the family may be needed, and often assistance also with other matters such as housework. The family doctor and/or community nurse may need the assistance of a medical consultant (in palliative medicine) and/or a nursing consultant (in palliative nursing) to assist with specific problems. It is important that there be good communication between the family doctors and the palliative medicine or pain consultants.
>
> Care in a specialist palliative care unit may be needed, for a few days to review all aspects of care and improve symptom relief, or to give the family a rest or because the problems of home care have become too great. A core of expert nurses and doctors with deep understanding of palliative care is essential in such a palliative care unit. Other health professionals such as a social worker, a bereavement counselor, a physiotherapist, an occupational therapist and well trained volunteers may all have an important place.

Palliative care of hospital patients must not be neglected – patients in general hospitals or cancer centres under the care of specialists have much need of good palliative care. Many patients in hospital are very ill, often incurably so, and suffer much with unrelieved symptoms and personal distress. Many patients actually die in hospital, especially in so-called advanced nations, despite all efforts to facilitate home care.
It is increasingly clear that palliative care for patients in hospitals has been much neglected. A hospital should take pride in –
- good palliation
- good care

with respect to such patients – and quality assurance programs of major hospitals and cancer centres should include evaluation of palliation (e.g. pain relief) and care (as judged by patient and family).

The overall integration of palliative care in home, hospital or special unit requires a creative approach to administration: with the emphasis on continuity of care as an individual patient moves within the health care system requiring, from time to time, involvement with general hospital, special unit and home care.

Considerable attention has been given in all parts of Australia to palliative care in all of these various situations[5] especially care in specialized units (hospices or palliative care within major hospitals is getting increasing emphasis. Integration of palliative care in hospital, home and palliative care units/hospices is now a matter of policy in New South Wales as articulated in recent statements.[6] The Central Sydney Palliative Care Service based on Royal Prince Alfred Hospital is already familiar to senior Japanese health administrators. Brief comments follow, as requested: Further detail is available elsewhere.[7]

iii
Royal Prince Alfred Hospital (RPAH), is a large teaching hospital (800 beds) of the University of Sydney

In 1982, it was decided that palliative care should be given more attention by means of a palliative care service offering medical and nursing consultations within the hospital and after a careful start in 1982, a restructuring of the service occurred in 1985, and included the appointment of a senior staff specialist as full time Director, the linking of RPAH with the long established palliative care unit (owned by the Anglican Church) at Eversleigh Hospital, Petersham, 4 km from RPAH and the establishment of a community service.

The Central Sydney Palliative Care Service based on Royal Prince Alfred Hospital integrates hospital, inpatient unit and community palliative care by means of a common core of medical staff (3 senior, 5 junior) in partnership with nurses, in three locations: hospital, inpatient unit and community. (Figure l) This service is financed by the Central Sydney Area Health Service, with some assistance from the Federal Government.

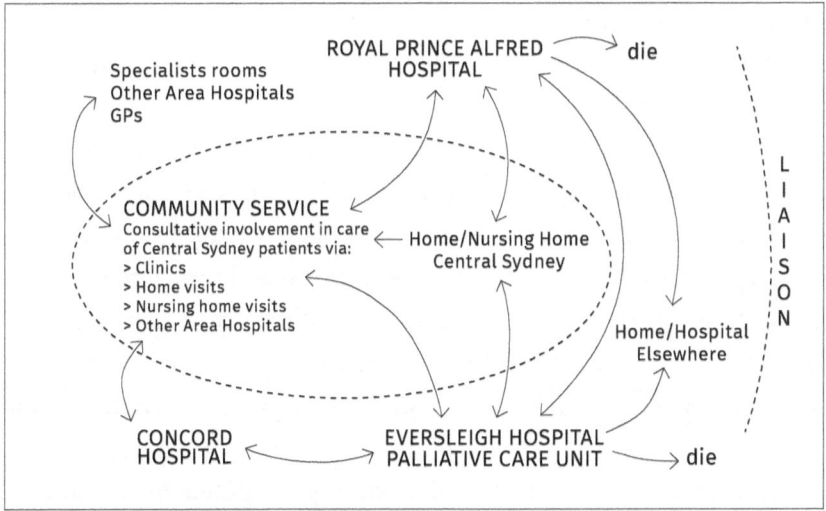

Figure 1: Central Sydney Palliative Care Service

There is an increase each year in the numbers of patients referred by both specialists and family doctors. Over 1000 new patients will be formally referred in 1993 by doctors (almost ⅔ hospital specialists and ⅓ family doctors) for medical consultation. Patients come from a wide range of ethnic and cultural backgrounds reflecting the multicultural characteristics of modern Australia.

Initially most referrals were for pain relief but there has been a change in the reasons for referral, with requests for advice and involvement in total medical management becoming more common (including consultation on ethical matters). Almost every specialist unit in Royal Prince Alfred Hospital consults our doctors, and also the emergency department. In addition, nurses consult independently our consultants in palliative nursing within the hospital and community. Nurses are given much responsibility, once competence is achieved by specific education and training in technical aspects of palliative nursing and family care. Most patients referred have cancer but a significant number of patients have other conditions, with AIDS patients steadily increasing in number.

Most patients are seen first in the wards at RPAH but others are seen first in nursing homes, in small hospitals and especially in the patient's own home. Some of the patients are in the last few months or weeks of life but approximately one third are alive a year later. Many patients get back to useful activity and in the majority good symptom relief is achieved. Some referred patients (the minority) need at some time to be admitted for review or for intensive palliative care to the inpatient unit (35 beds) at Eversleigh Hospital, Petersham: about half of those admitted are discharged home or to a nursing home, and about half of them die usually very peacefully in the unit. Approximately 60 (sometimes more) patients are admitted to Eversleigh Hospital each month – a high level of activity for a small unit.

There is evidence that the palliative care service has, since 1985, influenced medical practice within RPAH especially with respect to cancer pain relief: the patterns of drug use demonstrate a clear shift towards the use of oral morphine instead of less useful opioid drugs, with respect to the opioid component of cancer pain therapy.[7]

All staff involved in the care of very ill patients especially those who are dying, need adequate support. Palliative care is person intensive, not machine intensive, and the professional-as-person is irreplaceable and priceless as well as a fragile instrument of care. The patients and their families need professional assistance but are also, themselves, teachers and sources of inspiration. There are restrictions on our resources – WHO recommends much higher proportion of funds should be available for palliative care than are currently allotted in most countries and Australia is no exception.

It is to be stressed again, that there are many patterns for organization of palliative care in Australia – and even a wide variation in concepts of care and the application of core principles. Royal Prince Alfred Hospital clearly has emphasized the medical component of palliative care (and postgraduate medical training) and the concept that palliative care is to be available in all situations irrespective of contexts. Each hospital and each community has its own strengths and weaknesses and much depends on the expertise available in relation to palliative medicine and palliative nursing and also, indeed pastoral care – as well as the commitment of health and administrators and political leaders to improve the care of the very ill.

iv
The Patient as Guest

Ideas evolve during time – and ideas have adventures and a life of their own once articulated and objectified. Over the centuries there has been a development discernible in the use of the word "hospice". In the Middle Ages in Western Europe a hospice was a place of rest for pilgrims and later a place for the care of the sick and very ill. People in those days often died. The hospice as "place" remained the dominant notion well into the 1970s. The "place" which was the hospice (such as St Christopher's Hospice, London) embodied also a hospice "philosophy" and "processes" of care but St Christopher's still is very much a place. In USA in late 70s hospice programs became prominent, often community based without specifically designated beds.

In Australia all these concepts are present – and although the word hospice is less used, the reality which is palliative care continues to evolve with less emphasis on place, and more on process and even relationship.

Is it possible that the person who is charged with the responsibility for a consultation in palliative medicine, palliative nursing or for comprehensive palliative care may (himself or herself) become the place of rest for a needy patient? Can the concept of hospice be now focussed in a responsible person, with the patient as guest?[8]

It is said that a society may be judged by its response to the needs of its weakest members. Japan is already demonstrating profound concern for the care of all those in need of palliative care, and awareness of the ethical imperative to incorporate palliative care within the existing health system.

The need may be not so much for new institutions, nor even many special inpatient units, but a grasp of the new knowledge, and a new attitude in the mind and heart of every doctor and nurse, practicing in hospitals or in the community – in all the nations of the world. There is need to make every place where such patients find themselves a safe place to be very vulnerable, a safe place be in pain because pain relief and care as well as respect will be there ... especially at home.

Palliative care in the hospital or community is characterized by competence and courtesy, as Cicely Saunders, the British founder of the hospice movement stresses. It is above all an exercise of appropriate competent courteous hospitality, with the patient with advanced incurable disease not the obedient servant or client of the doctor and nurse or even merely their partner but their honored guest, however vulnerable, maybe in a strange land.

In a country like Japan, if the patient towards the close of life may be regarded (at home or in hospital) as the honoured guest of the family and of the health system, the community will be much blessed. In this way, palliative care may give new structure to the compassion, deep within the Japanese people, for all human life.

References

1. Takeda F. Japan: Status of cancer pain and palliative care. *J Pain Symp Manage*, 1993:8:425–6.
2. Stjernswaard J. Palliative medicine – a global perspective. In: Doyle D, Hanks G W H, MacDonald N, eds. *Oxford Textbook of Palliative Medicine*, Oxford Med Publications, 1993:805–15.
3. WHO Expert Committee, Cancer pain relief and palliative care, World Health Organisation, Geneva, 1990.
4. Doyle D, Hanks GWH and MacDonald N. *Oxford Textbook of Palliative Medicine*, Oxford Med Publications, 1993.
5. Lickiss J N. Australia: Status of cancer pain and palliative care, *J Pain Symp Manage*, 1993;8:388–96.
6. Report of the NSW Health Palliative Care Working Party, NSW Department of Health, June 1993.
7. Lickiss J N, Glare PA, Turner K, et al. *Palliative care in Central Sydney: The Royal Prince Alfred Hospital as Catalyst and Integrator*, J Pall Care, 1993; 9:3–42.
8. Saunders C. Foreword. in: Doyle D, Hanks G W H, MacDonald N, eds. Oxford Textbook of Palliative Medicine, Oxford Publications, 1993:vviii.

III
Palliative Medicine at the Edge? Questions Worth Asking?
2004–2006

Substance of presentations in Sydney, Boston (Harvard Medical School), Kuala Lumpur, Hangzhou and Tehran:

i   Valedictory address at the conclusion of full-time clinical service at Royal Prince Alfred Hospital, Sydney 2005 (Palliative medicine at the edge?);

ii   Lecture given in the 'Etherdome' at Massachusetts General Hospital, Harvard Medical School, 2007 ('Palliative medicine in retrospect and prospect – palliative medicine at the edge?);

iii   Keynote address, Annual Scientific Meeting, Malaysia Cancer Society, September, 2005. (Approaching clinical decision-making in the care of patients with eventually fatal illness);

iv   Also at Hangzhou and Tehran.

It is said that Gertrude Stein, the savant, when dying in mid-twentieth century was asked, 'Gertrude, what is the answer?' She is said to have replied (as her last words), 'What is the question?' The quality of science (or of a person) may, in the end, be judged, not by the answers furnished, but by the questions shaped ... After nearly twenty years in full time consultancy in palliative medicine (and over a decade before that in oncology practice), spent mainly in teaching hospitals,[1,2] one may be entitled to begin to formulate questions worth asking.

Palliative medicine as a clinical discipline involves participation in clinical decision-making and clinical science regarding especially relief of symptoms and distress (based on adequate understanding not only of the state of the disease pathology and pathophysiology – afflicting the patient, but also the capacity to communicate with the patient as subject – a person with agency); there are particular responsibilities for the care of a patient approaching to death. Palliative medicine, because of its focus on the patient as subject – a perspective which may specify palliative medicine among the clinical sciences,[3] requires comprehension of the relational dimensions of human existence – mandating care and concern for the significant others (notably family) who are involved in the life and/or care of a patient with advanced progressive disease with the horizon, so to speak, in view.[4]

There are many questions which need to be formulated and explored regarding the field of symptomatology despite notable advances especially in the last 40 years, with much of the accumulated knowledge codified in major textbooks – though far more is or has been known than has ever been written. Despite distinguished writing and practice in the field less may be understood of the relief of suffering or human 'limit' situations of distress: we remain maybe at the edge of understanding existential distress, as at the rim of a fire. Indeed, the understanding of humanness may be better explicated in literature – and the arts – than in medical writings or teaching. Nevertheless, with the present focus on medical lore, questions may be worth raising on some aspects of palliative medicine in relation especially to the whole of medical, especially cancer, practice. For the moment I consider the following (interrelated) questions:

1. How may we recognise and curtail flat-of-the-curve medicine?
2. Should we reframe our clinical decision-making?

3   What are some educational implications of such considerations?

4   Is palliative medicine at the 'edge'?

Flat of the curve medicine

In the prestigious Shattuck lecture of 1978, [Alain] Enthoven raised the challenge of 'curtailing flat-of-the-curve medicine'.[5] The basic concept is familiar in the world of industry and commerce. 'As one input is applied to a production process in successively larger amounts, the resulting increases in output will each be successively smaller. The marginal return – i.e. the increase in output associated with a unit increase in output – may even become zero or negative'. The basic concept of flat-of-the-curve medicine is easy to grasp and its dangers are obvious. However, beyond the apparent simplicity of the concept, there are issues of note when we seek to explore it in a health care context.

How should we measure costs? What costs are relevant? dollars? energy costs? distress? time lost? of patient? of family/friends/carers? of community? Who pays or shares these various costs is an issue in itself – raising questions of self-responsibility, co-responsibility, and even the question so hard to hear, 'Who is my neighbour?' – and 'Where are the limits to care?'

Costs are hard to measure, so is benefit. What do we mean by benefit? And in whose eyes? – those of patient, family/friends/carers, community? Unidimensional views of benefit such as survival time, in some circumstances, are seriously inadequate, as is being increasingly realised by oncologists (as well as patients). Clearly the notion of quality of life brings a second dimension into some outcome studies, but even the vexed and hard to measure notion of quality of life may not suffice to measure benefit, even if the measure strives to take into account the patient's unique perspective, and the dynamic nature of illness. For a patient is not an isolated monad, but a *person* existing in and in a way partly at least constituted by a web of relationships. No man is an island – good or harm has a communitarian dimension, just as a web is affected by change in one node in the whole and recent research is beginning to address this issue.[6]

There is a case for examining closely the trajectory for every patient – to recognise the nodes for decision-making, to articulate the decisions made, and to assess ideally in prospect (or at least in retrospect) the 'costs' and the 'benefit' which ensue (or ensued) from the course of action taken. Such trajectories invite scrutiny for patients with serious, probably eventually fatal diseases such as chronic neurological conditions, eventually fatal cardiac disease, progressive and irreversible renal disease, as well as neoplastic diseases, but a focus on cancer is reasonable for present purposes.

In cancer medicine there are many situations where flat-of-the-curve practice may occur. At least in such definable circumstances there is a strong case for extreme care in decision-making such that the possibility of 'benefit', the reasonableness of the 'costs' in relation to the hoped for 'benefit', and the possibility of harm are all carefully considered. There is a case for preparation of a carer impact statement with respect to a choice, for example, of a further trial of chemotherapy. It is not that no attention to cost/benefit has been paid (the notion is commonplace): it is rather that these considerations need to be more adequate and fearlessly incorporated into everyday thinking and into hospital and health service as well as the whole culture (including the media).

In a major acute hospital, and in a major cancer centre there are significant research implications of such notions – even as part of a program to incorporate such dimensions into the clinical thought-world.

There appears to be, for example, a case for descriptive, prospective studies of all patients treated in the centre who are: a) noted to be of low performance status, for example, in bed most of the day or b) requiring admission to hospital for symptom relief. There appears need to clarify the subsequent course of such patients in terms of realistic parameters – survival time, days in hospital or clinics or in investigative facilities (implying not only utilisation of health care services but also loss of time for patient and family), quality of symptom relief (on a daily basis), and well-being of carer/family/friends (hard to measure), expenditure (irrespective of source of payment), circumstances surrounding death, well-being of carer/family/friends during the year(s) after death. Obviously many of these matters have been much researched throughout the whole illness trajectory, but issues may need to be placed in the frame of cost benefit/analysis to give a richer perspective.

There appears also a case for flagging patients in either of the above groups (either noted to have poor 'performance status' by conventional measures, or admitted anywhere for symptom relief) for formal review and clarification regarding matters such as:

a   What are current goals and objectives of any anticancer treatment – are these clear to patient and family, carers, as well as the treating clinicians ('the team')?

b   What are the current symptoms (in priority order established by *patient*) and their relief?

c   What problems are likely to arise in the near future? – and are carers, including the family doctor, as well as the patient reasonably informed about these?

d   Is the care system identified in place and well supported?

e   Is there clarity of follow up arrangements and procedures to be followed in emergency?
f   Are the personal objectives of the patient understood by both doctor responsible for treatment and others close to patient?
g   Are advance care directives in place (and accessible; preferably with the patient at all times)? and/or a person with enduring power of attorney identified? There may or may not be a formalised advance care plan or advance directives in place – but the clarity of understanding and the recognition of the need for respect is the key element.

There are other matters worth investigating – notably, the consideration of a hospital (or a cancer centre) not as a fragmented collection of units of activity but as a cohesive whole, a therapeutic community. Integrated patient care will not occur unless the components of that care are seamlessly integrated. The history of hospitals indicates clearly an evolution from a place of safety ('hospitality') for travellers (especially pilgrims) on dangerous medieval roads, to a place to which the sick came (and often died), to a place where those expected to die could find care, to (by twentieth century) an institution where cure of many conditions, and control of many other diseases, became a realistic possibility. Those who were approaching death were always recognised as a burden in society, but whether or not the burden could be borne gracefully or reluctantly depended on many factors and not only virtue: in some nomadic societies the dying had to be abandoned. Harshness could prevail in public policy: even in colonial Australia in mid-nineteenth century there were limits in some hospitals about how many 'moribunds' could be accepted. By mid-twentieth century, in parallel with advances in medical knowledge and practice, there crept in some other problems – a tendency to neglect those who were not amenable to therapeutic success (and especially the dying), and some articulation of fear in society (of medical advances) by such notable persons as [Peter] Medawar[7] and [Ian] Kennedy in the BBC Reith Lectures of 1980.[8] Despite many signs of increased societal sensitivity to neglect and cruelty there is continuing fear of neglect – or over aggressive anti-disease treatment (even prolonging life) without concomitant care. Increasingly complex treatment may yield increasingly complex consequences calling for (in vain) dramatically enhanced care.

By the late twentieth century the dangers became explicit of the possibility of hospitals becoming places only for interventions and not for care. [Guenter] Risse in the course of the major recent history of hospitals declared: 'as traditional monuments to human empathy and benevolence, hospitals must remain houses of healing'.[9] A personal visit to Auschwitz in 2002 prompted for me an increased awareness of the danger of efficiency, if ever a goal in itself and not a strategy: a pattern to be watched for in contemporary hospitals.[10]

Clearly there is room for new thinking, for reflection, despite (and because of) intense preoccupation with earnest endeavours to improve cancer treatment: the people should not be afraid.

It is to be kept in mind that decisions made early in an illness trajectory may have significant influence on the quality of the last phase of life and the manner of dying: moral responsibility for unnecessary suffering related to unwise decision-making is not abrogated by transfer of a patient to another facility. In part, for this reason, local study is needed not to test hypotheses or to generate comparative studies, but to document/audit the circumstances of dying with regard to all patients dying in a particular hospital or cancer centre, or in another residential facility, or at home. The *patient-centred* audit (linking information from several locations) should include documentation of all critical clinical decisions made in the course of the illness, as well as the prevalence of symptoms and quality of symptom relief in the days preceding death, some external measures of apparent loss of dignity,[11] and the quality of support of significant others. Assessment also should include state of significant carer and/or next of kin at some months (maybe 3, 6 and 12 months) after the death. Information from such a study should give indication of matters needing improvement: furthermore, as Popper emphasised, knowledge is advanced by recognising error.[12]

Even while waiting for an audit to be organised there is the possibility of immediately introducing on each ward or unit of a major hospital (or other facility or service) a simple 'bad outcome' audit to be undertaken regarding every admission occurring in that precinct, constructing a list of a few outcomes to be avoided wherever possible. Such an approach has been undertaken for over 15 years in Royal Prince Alfred Hospital within the palliative care service – as an intrinsic (10–15 minutes) part of the weekly unit meeting. An honest audit for any recognised bad outcomes in undertaken in a 'no fault' atmosphere – any contributing factors are mentioned, and a correction to procedures or some other action may be rapidly undertaken. The list of bad outcomes sought for may be varied as new matters come to attention, and existing matters appear to be less relevant, hopefully not now occurring! This simple methodology – which assumes that, on the whole, all goes well, is highly efficient and effective and able to be transported to other locations.[13] The influence of this clinical perspective may subtly, and over time, influence the larger culture of a major hospital.[14,15]

Reframing our decision-making?

There is widespread concern about the quality of *care* within hospitals especially as the emphasis has shifted with increasing possibilities of treatment/life prolongation, and with the focus shifting to economic considerations; persons, our friends, may *fear* hospital admission. But place must be found for care. Patients living with cancer, going through sometimes stressful treatments and investigations with often periods of uncertainty concerning even survival for the next few months ... and the multitude of losses consequent upon the diagnosis of a serious condition: such patients need care, not merely treatment.
It is obvious. Yet, [JP] Kassirer in an editorial concerning managed care in the USA, pointed to essential changes in our understanding.

> No matter who provides the care ... it will never be complete unless those responsible for it seek a far deeper understanding of the patient's social, economic, and ecological contexts than we do now.[16]

It is significant that Kassirer does not point to the need for economic manipulations or new clinical research but growth in understanding the 'soft' dimensions of medical practice – the social, economic and ecological contexts of patients.
It is legitimate to recognise that we are deficient in such understanding and the implications are evident to the wise. Shift is needed.

There is abundant research on clinical decision-making, and various models of it. In principle, most would agree that beneficence (doing good) is the goal, seeking the patient's perception of the good in the light of his/her personal objectives and priorities regarding life prolongation, comfort etc. and the development of strategies to achieve that good at least inconvenience (to all), within the limits of the resources available. It may be useful to try to situate a difficult interpersonal activity within a wider context – as a small contribution to what may be termed 'clinical ethics' (recognising as I do the vast old and recent published resources concerning this matter).

It may help to consider rapid clinical decision-making process in a wider context. It may be useful as an ecological view of the processes involved. On the table as it were, are the objective and verifiable facts (legal and medical) – in the 'air' are the values. In the centre of all of this there is the need to make a decision. In the culture(s) within which the decision makers and the patient and significant others are embedded, are values and concepts of profound significance: liberty, the significance of last phase of life, human dignity, human possibility etc. and each of these requires consideration. It may well be that there is divergence with respect to the weight given to (or ranking of) such values or concepts by different protagonists in this drama. Prolongation of life even by a day or two, or a week or two, when dying, may be regarded as a manifestation of respect for the significance of the last phase of life – or may be regarded by others as an unwise objective (even if achievable).

Shakespeare clearly recognised divergence of views: Edgar pleads with King Lear (close to death) 'Look up my Lord' ... but the Duke of Kent counters with the memorable words:

> O, let him pass! he hates him,
> That would upon the rack of this rough world
> Stretch him out longer.[17]

Others may consider autonomy – attention to the whispered wish of the patient (to whom?) should be the only and final arbiter as to whether an attempt should be made to gain another two days or two weeks of life ...

In this complex context there is the need to make a decision, not to linger in indecision – unless circumstances mandate a pause. One can conceive that decision-making involves a balance between competing pressures/demands of autonomy, beneficence, non-maleficence and justice (individual and social). Furthermore the processes of decision-making need to respect not only the patient but family/friends/carers and professionals, as well as the cultural context(s). The implications of the various realistic therapeutic options need to be systematically considered, until the positive and negative consequences of each become far more clear – a movement towards desirable ethical transparency. The abundant (superabundant) literature in medical ethics delineates various traditions, for example, 'deontological (or command) ethics', 'principle based ethics' and 'virtue ethics'.

Clinical wisdom is required to discern where the best decision lies on the balance of probabilities (as in a civil court) rather than beyond reasonable doubt (as in a criminal matter). Such wisdom requires, in the decision-maker(s), true virtue – integrity honed by interiorisation of ethical principles and the habit of right action. The fundamental principles, the infrastructure as it were, of clinical decision-making must indeed be internalised so that in a fraught situation the sound ethical instinct may prevail, with the good of the patient-as-person embedded in society the ultimate guiding light, the dominant impetus. The implications for education and training – and continuous lifelong learning – are compelling. The approach outlined above may bring together principle based ethics and virtue ethics – or at least take further the discussion.

The comments of Kassirer have already been noted here, but central to the concern about care and decision-making there is lurking another issue – the need for far more adequate understanding of the personal. Jacob Needleman, a generation ago, articulated to New York Academy of Sciences, very explicitly the critical need of medicine to have a more adequate anthropological basis: 'What medicine lacks is any fundamental notion of the nature of man and any remotely adequate understanding of that to which we refer as a person'.[18] Attempts since that time to enrich medicine by concepts articulated in the humanities are to be recognised as not optional or marginal but core activities with potential to contribute to the recovering of the central thrust of medicine in society as well as in individual lives.

The schema seeking to contextualise decision-making requires a complementary approach to contextualise a person. Philosophers have stressed that we as persons are situated, have histories, have hopes (a way out of a closed system), and in a profound sense are persons only in relation ... We are not isolated nomads in a definable place and time and personal network (or web), but may be best thought of as *constituted* by these realities. Our inheritance (biological and cultural) inheres in our whole, as does our relation with the cosmos/all that is (however named) ... Persons are not static: not a closed ecological system: hope, however articulated, may integrate, give direction to, currently fragmented existence, and lead out into new possibilities.

Furthermore, persons evolve, change, develop over time. Some conceptual frame for personal development needs to inform the practice of human medicine.

There have been myriad attempts down the ages to illuminate the personal including the manner in which persons change over time – for better or worse. Shakespeare profoundly enriched our understanding in so many ways – countless images of personal development inhabit his plays.[19]

Psychological portrayals of the stages of personal development laid down half a century ago by Erik Erikson may still be the most useful for physicians seeking richer understanding [20,21] despite a plethora of other conceptualisations.

Erikson saw human growth as taking place by negotiation of developmental tasks through the resolution of crisis. The growing human being is continually faced by options, each life stage being characterized by its own options, which, while they confront one throughout life, do come to a point of ascendancy in a given stage. Erikson's analysis of personal growth is sensitive indeed in its consideration of the developmental task of the elderly and, by analogy, to those of any age approaching death. He conceives that task as the development of a sense of wholeness of integrity.

The shape of this last task needs to be understood by those in contact with patients who are approaching death. Patients may well vacillate between wholeness and despair and need to be supported gently. They may long and need to try to express their internal states, explore the threat of despair and through dialogue with significant others reach out again towards the wholeness, which is possible.

Carers (professional and non-professional) of persons in the final phase of life need to have some awareness of the complexity of personal development, not only because of the patterns to be respected in the patient, but also because of the possible difference between the developmental tasks of the patient (fluctuating may be between despair and a sense of wholeness) and that of carer (who may be struggling with intimacy versus isolation as may be expected of a young carer).

Dying remains the last phase of human growth and personal development but death is a new frontier, expressing utterly our bodiliness. Walt Whitman famously noted, 'I am not contained between my hat and my boots' – yet the fact of embodiment is central – and the difference between a living body, with a person continuing to exist within its web, and a dead body (an object deserving of respect, capable of evoking emotion, yet not acting, except as a passive physical object) remains a mystery which has enthralled philosophers and the common man throughout the ages ... [Richard] Dawkins may declare that ... 'There is no spirit-driven life force, no throbbing, heaving, pullulating, protoplasmic mystic jelly. Life is just bytes and bytes and bytes of digital information.'[22] But physicians (and others) near a person at the moment of death are aware of the withdrawal of some influence (given many names throughout the ages) integrating the processes which resist the return to entropy: some may speak of a 'person departing'. One remains (appropriately) in awe at the change.

The *facts* to be noted in the course of decision-making, (the objective 'platform' on which we stand) are easier to establish – but need to be precisely noted, especially in situations fraught with high emotional intensity, 'chaos', and divergence of opinions regarding the most desired or most feared outcomes. The relevant law in any situation must always be kept in mind and accepted usually as binding (though carefully interpreted without ideological 'spin'): there needs to be clear understanding of the differences between legal constraints and guidelines ... And also the difference between legality and morality. It is wise to be afraid of a doctor whose actions are constrained only by the bounds of legality.

Evidence-based medicine –
its place in the schema of clinical decision-making?

Part of the fact base is available documented medical evidence with respect to any aspect of the therapeutic options being considered ... for example, what is the probability that an intervention being considered is likely to be effective in this patient, here and now?

Several points need to be made in view of the prominence of evidence based medicine (EBM) in the minds, publications, if not clinical practice of contemporary doctors at least in the west:

> Medical evidence is concerned with precise questions which can only be one segment of the overall tapestry in the frame of complex decision making in such a case as outlined above.
>
> Evidence is taken note of, but is not identical with a therapeutic decision nor is it to be equated with clinical wisdom.
>
> EBM has contributed richly to the recent progress in the therapeutics – and has notably reduced many hazards, saved lives and morbidity by demonstrating that favoured treatments are harmful – and so on – with a rich literature significance readily available. All serious scholars recognise the need to use EBM as part of a decision-making context.

However, there are serious limitations to evidence based medicine as currently widely understood – and taught/learned in the course of medical education, and these limitations need further examination.

First, the nature of the randomisation process necessarily excludes from consideration many of the factors which make us human – and the *experience* of disease (illness) is a human reality. Contemporary approaches to evaluation of evidence, to enumeration of quality of life and other (laudable) attempts to express, to objectify, to quantitate matters of human complexity rooted in subjectivity and/or in subtle relationships may be in need of a new style of thinking: Feinstein's wise words over a long period, and especially at the close of his career, need to be heeded.[23,24]

Whilst EBM exponents do stress the need to take into account other factors when applying 'evidence', it is necessary to emphasise that the trials which give rise to class 1 evidence (the prize, recognised as such by students and junior medical staff) do not take these into account at all. In fact lower levels of evidence – series of cases, anecdotal evidence, even the point of view of experienced clinicians may give 'evidence' which is far closer to the clinical wisdom so crucial in a complex situation. It seems dangerous to rank such forms of evidence as inferior – where in fact they may be far more useful.

Second, a profound reductionism is afoot in the selection of information to be used in the derivation of 'evidence'. Simply put:

a   not all that is known (or relevant) is written,
b   not all that is written is written in European languages,
c   not all that is written even in those languages is retrievable by Cochrane methodology.

It is facile to regard the universe of information utilised by enterprises like the Cochrane Collaboration as commensurate with relevant information/knowledge/understanding.

Third, Karl Popper, whose influence on scientific thinking has been so powerful, despite some recent reappraisal and controversy, stressed that knowledge is advanced by looking for and understanding observations which do not fit in the current hypotheses – rather than doing experimental studies aimed at confirming it. Popper stressed the logical asymmetry here, and urged to exploit it. One arresting negative finding may be the clue to a leap of understanding: basking in the warmth of several confirmatory studies may be less useful. A clinical diagnoses is indeed an hypothesis, and this approach can be very useful in clarifying the correct diagnosis among a list of possibilities. 'What investigation could prove the preferred diagnosis wrong?' is a question worth asking quickly whilst at the same time carefully noting opportunities of confirmation.

The weaknesses of meta-analyses have been outlined by others – but it remains that the search for confirmation and the exclusion of results of trials found to be very far away from the majority ignores Popper's warning. In fact, such 'deviant' trials deserve a high level of scrutiny – and may hold clues to a leap in knowledge.

Despite the human complexity of clinical situations, and the limitations of EBM, senior clinicians must make decisions or there may be clinical paralysis – felt keenly by other clinicians (doctors, nurses, other health professionals) as well as family/friends, and the patient in the centre. Sometimes there is no option but to wait for clarity on one or other point at issue in the complex tapestry ... but this reason should be specified as the explanation for delaying the decision. So, despite the complexity we must make decisions, recognising that it may be on the 'balance of probabilities' as in civil actions, rather than 'beyond reasonable doubt,' (as in criminal courts) and recognising that autonomy is one, just one, of the principles at stake, for each 'principle' needs careful consideration.

There is need to recognise compassionately that if it is true that, as suggested above, decisions will need to be made, with the best wisdom available, on the balance of probabilities, then error will always be possible. The litigation climate makes error feared – and a dramatic change in community understanding of these matters (as well as good communication, and exercise of integrity) may well assist. The people may well understand, and appreciate the opportunity for the deepening of the grasp on the complexity of clinical decision-making.

There needs to be cultural shift away from the glorification of autonomy as the sole guiding principle of decision making in complex situations – and many are addressing this issue. Notable points worthy of consideration include of course a re-examination of what really is meant by informed consent ...

Which information? And what do we mean by consent? The Nuremburg Code of 1947 which in the face of the horrors of the moral collapse of the medical profession in the 30s and early 40s stimulated the concept of informed consent,[25] did so for the sake of the patient, not as a shield for doctors against litigation – and it is the patient's need which must prevail in the current discussions concerning informed consent.

The implications for carers of proposed options may need further focus. The problem of carers and their need for support are currently in focus in many jurisdictions. But should there be a 'carer impact statement' prepared, albeit briefly, of each of the seriously considered options prior to making the final decision of what appears wisest to do, 'on the balance of probabilities'? Even attempts to prolong life by a few days by various means, even at the request of relatives ('Do everything possible, doctor') may need quite explicit (and documented) carer impact analysis. It is to be noted also that the fear of unwanted life prolongation looms large in the psyche of many patients: the decision-making in the face of such a fear expressed to a compassionate doctor calls for decision-making of the highest skills and integrity as well as well-honed clinical competence.

It has already been stressed that if it is true that our very personhood involves relationships, the time has surely come to recognise that the autonomy (self-directedness) of the patient cannot even be considered without taking into account the existence, influence of and impact on those relationships ... and a large literature has focus on these matters. Indeed, every action in the course of medical practice has an ethical dimension, because it is intrinsically involving interpersonal interaction in some measure; even the reading of a radiological image, or the interpretation of a biochemical test, are fundamentally related to persons (and for example, require respect for confidentiality). Practical everyday ethics in the course of medical practice involving those approaching death requires far more focus than simply concern with decision-making, but the comments above may contribute at least to enhancement of discussion (and maybe research). Recent writing is noted, for example, by Welie[26] and Gillon.[27]

Educational Implications

Education, especially of ourselves, our students, and community may be essential to support our attempts to curtail flat-of-the-curve medicine and to reframe our ethics so that decision-making is seen as appropriately contextualised.

Education is a complex undertaking. The word 'education' derives from the Latin *educere* (to lead out) and *educare* (to nourish). We are to be led out (and to lead students out) from where we are, to where we are not – as into a desert – but in the process we (and they) need nourishment.

Education, the 'leading out' and 'nourishment', involves interpersonal communications, *par excellence* – in the form of words, non-verbal communications, and the sharing of experience. The education may be considered to occur in the space between persons (where so much happens) and requires space and time. Medical education involves not only the imparting of information or concepts but also the fostering of the development of persons. The mind crowded with too much information may impede intellectual growth; the day too crowded or programmed too tightly may lack the chance for a personal 'pause' which appears so essential for the exercise of wisdom especially in fraught situations. The compressed, intense contemporary experience of medical education and postgraduate training must contemplate the need for space and time for reflecting so that the ethical instinct may emerge to ensure that the moral collapse of doctors under extreme stress is at least made far less likely.

The educational process involved in learning to be a physician, especially with significant involvement in the care of patients with probably eventually fatal disease, should involve opportunities for sensing the deeper self, and glimpsing not only the possibilities of others but one's own possibilities ... in the course of growing through the adult developmental stages as outlined so cogently by Erik Erikson.[28] Clinical encounters involve persons at different life stages, facing different developmental tasks – and therefore crises – the junior doctor in his/her 20s in the course of developing a life partnership must have a psychological orientation different from a person in the 5th decade embedded in major business decisions, or from a person facing evidence of the fragility of old age with concurrent losses (and gains) ... and yet a conceptual frame of a person such as mentioned above, may assist in grounding ideas and emotions – even in the midst of chaos. I was reminded once by visiting Japanese dignitaries (in the midst of a chaotic clinical day) that it may be in the midst of chaos, not order, that new ideas are born.

There is need for fundamental optimism with regard to human possibility – which has been articulated in many traditions with greater or lesser associations with identifiable spiritual roots. As one grows older, the core messages of such diverse strains of human constructs may merge in one's mind, with some diminishing of differences and deeper contentment with similar formulations of these matters. In a secular society there is a rich tapestry of views, and a search for common depths in the midst of diversity of surface appearances (including language) may prove enriching: authors such as [Peter] van Ness offer food for thought:

> Briefly stated, the spiritual aspect of human existence is hypothesized to have an outer and an inner complexion. Facing outward, human existence is spiritual insofar as

one engages reality as a maximally inclusive whole and makes the cosmos an intentional object of thought and feeling. Facing inward, life has a spiritual dimension to the extent that it is apprehended as a project of people's most enduring and vital selves and is structured by experiences of sudden self-transformation and subsequent gradual development. These two formulations should not be rigidly separated. Their integration can be highlighted by expressing them in a more dramatic idiom: 'Toti se inserens mundo' (Plunging oneself into the totality of the world). In other words, the spiritual dimension of life is the embodied task of realising one's truest self in the context of reality apprehended as a cosmic totality. It is the quest for attaining an optimal relationship between what one truly is and everything that is; it is a quest that can be furthered by adopting appropriate spiritual practices and by participating in relevant communal rituals.[29]

Stress has been laid recently on the need for recognition of and the fostering of the inner life of physicians – as well as the recognition of the shape of distress experienced by physicians at the death of patients:

> There is a last point to make about the doctor's suffering: suffering cannot be restricted to a list of feelings, causes, reactions and coping strategies ... Human suffering does not amount to a physical or moral pain or to a difficulty. Suffering is something like crossing a sea, traversing a mountain or a desert; it is an experience, painful indeed, in which the person will become more oneself and will discover oneself; it is an experience in which a person will experience evil, and yet, at the same time, will be led to discover and express the deepest meaning of one's life. This is true also for the suffering of the doctor.[30]

There is a case for the customary non-recognition (or non-articulation) of loss experiences to be recognised as 'disenfranchised grief'[31] with the potential for serious consequences in well-being of the physician concerned. Psychological distress, or burnout of oncologists is well documented – is this, in part at least, related to failure to grieve? It is conceivable that not only is well-being seriously impaired but the capacity for wise decision-making may be compromised. At least there is room for thought about these matters: the issues are so profound that empirical research is unlikely to be useful.

There are other notions, some philosophical, which may be of assistance as the task of education is pondered. Michel Foucault in his consideration of some aspects of medical practice commented:

> What counts in the things said by men is not so much what they may have thought or the extent to which these things represent their thoughts, as that which systematizes them from the outset, thus making them thereafter endlessly accessible to new discourses and open to the task of transforming them.[32]

What can be the underlying themes now of medical discourse? What can be the underlying passion, which will energise the life work of physician, now in such a manner that effort is truly sustainable and outcomes optimal? Students, and junior doctors in training in the sharing of experience do feel the passion, the integrating themes, the passion (or lack of it), and in private, sometimes long afterwards, may speak of it. Many integrating ideas are possible. Philosophers may be said to have a passion for wisdom ... What of physicians? What are our passions? Each must find his or her own – it may be 'to maximise the good of all' (classic utilitarianism), 'to minimise the harm of the worst (like the black spot approach to reducing traffic accidents), or on the application of EBM always and everywhere, or on advancing knowledge or at the exercise of wonder: the author was, at 21, while changing culture nutrients at midnight in a deserted medical school, in near ecstasy at the sight of beating heart cells in tissue culture. O the wonder of it!

But, could our passion be focussed on the recognition of the *dignity* of every individual encountered in whatever circumstances, and its restoration or enhancement? The passion for the dignity of Everyman. If the last is taken as an integrating passion (and there are grounds for doing so at an individual and community level), there is mandated an exploration and articulation of the concept of human dignity now, in several disciplines.[33] The diverse concepts of human dignity currently abroad (sometimes seen to be in competition) appear to be the residues of strands of thought which became apparent and gained ascendency in differing times and places (and with different nuances) in the course of human history. *Dignitas*, worthiness, was initially vested in civic (or ecclesiastical) status conferred by an accepted process (heredity, custom, election, decree etc). Later, the focus appears to be found in the excellence of the human as such, not necessarily tied to station.

Later again dignity appears to be tied to the exercise of autonomy – insistence on self-rule, the claiming of perceived rights – with [John Stuart] Mill (on liberty) spelling out that restraint should not be for one's own good, but justified if one's action might harm another[34] (and this, by implication may extend to others – the community). However, one perspective on human dignity would insist on the relational dimensions ... not only with regard for avoiding harm to the other or doing good (however perceived), but reaching, even stretching out to the other (even to an absolute other however conceived) even as to a 'matching' fragment – dignity expressed in process, and situated in connectedness.

Medical practice is an engagement with the human condition, often in limit situations. Each of the dimensions of human dignity alluded to above impinge on it: bringing light, and raising matters for debate. The facilitation (for each person encountered) of living (and dying) with dignity by medical practitioners, lawyers, philosophers, politicians, teachers, writers, parents, friends, combatants ... that is, by all of us, requires attention not only to respect due to status, confirmed by position, but by the fact of common humanity, provision of opportunity for the exercise of autonomy (as participant-in-community), and the recognition of the critical need for relationships, and exercise of the search for and/or response to, and rest in an other, others, or an absolute other.

The implication for medical practice of such ideas require further articulation: recent attempts to focus on some aspects of human dignity in practice and/or to take the discussion further are noted, and thoughtful research is available concerning some Western contexts of patient care, leading to recommendations worthy of notice.[35,36]

Integrating themes or passions for the professional life of physicians – require not only the formulation of goals/objectives/points of focus – but also some principles for action in complex situations when the patient is nearing the time of death. It may be of assistance to note traditional Jewish principles articulated memorably (for this physician) by a Boston haematologist in Sydney in the mid 90s, namely '*Affirm life, but do not obstruct death*'.

But what does it mean for a physician to *affirm life*? Surely to offer unfailing respect, measures to improve quality of life (by wise decisions, good relief of symptoms, and support for patient and family), and careful efforts to prolong life, if the patient wishes, at acceptable 'cost', if resources utilised would not compromise the care of others. The foregoing indicates the complexity of each of these considerations.

What does it mean *not to obstruct death*? There is the obligation to 'diagnose dying' (and there are criteria known to experienced clinicians such as converging organ failure, psychological signs of withdrawal – possibly heralding much intra psychic activity – we cannot know), to improve the quality of dying if the patient's priority problems are amenable to solution, to cease or refrain from measures aimed at prolongation of life, to care for all concerned especially those closest to the patient ... There is much more which could be and has been said about the care of those actually dying, but the principle of 'not obstructing death' may be useful addition and deserve further articulation. The diagnosis of potential or actual death obstruction is a matter justifying a place in medical education throughout life.

The overall perspective is that clinical practice, appropriately practiced, should be not the cause of fear or constraint, but an agent of liberation – freeing a person to become what he/she can be, and do what is most in accord with his/her possibilities. Kingsley Mortimer, then (1974) a Professor of Anatomy in New Zealand, offered memorable and thought-provoking words which may be worthy of documentation: 'It is the task of medicine to emancipate man's interior splendour':[37] we can surely disregard the sexist language!

Is palliative medicine at the edge?
After all, is palliative medicine at the edge? The edge is a place of danger: one can fall off, and uncertainty – there may be little one can do to ensure that the edge does not crumble, and constraint – which way to proceed from an edge? The options are limited.

However, the edge may also be a growing point. If the task of formulating a much more adequate philosophical anthropology is undertaken, preferably from within the situation of medical practice or at least in organic association – rather than from outside the medical context – then the edge may truly be a growing point, a point of departure for a new, enriched, radical humanism capable of incorporating not only the content of traditional humanism (which may have in some part failed us) but also the transcendent dimension of human personhood. These are heady thoughts but the possibility is there. Historical and philosophical studies of death such as those of [Philippe] Aries [38] and [Jeff] Malpas and [Robert] Solomon [39] could be much enriched by an anthropology which rings true to clinicians who have walked the wards of hospitals, faced the chaos of mass disaster, tiptoed in the presence of the silent (often) distress of the aged and fragile – and lived with life and death daily in its myriad forms, steeped daily in the vagaries of the human condition, forced to ponder on the nature of hope as well as despair – and maybe, like Dr Rieux at the end of [Albert] Camus' *La Peste* concluding that after all, there is more good in men than matters to despise.

There is more to say about an edge! The edge may be the edge of an umbrella under which many diverse entities – even clinical specialities – may shelter. Palliative medicine is practiced (in one way or another, at varying degrees of excellence and specialisation) by a large array of clinicians. Many physicians are involved in the care of patients who have incurable, progressive and probably, if not certainly, eventually fatal illness. Palliative medicine, as a branch of clinical science, does not begin when all other clinical science has failed to cure the patient! Palliative medicine is relevant wherever there are difficult decisions to be made, symptoms to be relieved, distress to be addressed – as part of care. Just as palliative medicine is relevant to the practice of many kinds of doctors, so is palliative care the province of many kinds of professionals: nurses, physicians, social workers, family members, and volunteers. These two fields may usefully overlap in specialist palliative care services, so valuable for patients with complex needs.

Such specialist services may be evident, and well developed in some places and institutions but not at all in others. Sometimes specialist level palliative medicine would be of much value – just as (analogously) competence in specialist cardiology may be at times highly relevant, but basic palliative medicine should be part of the kit of every doctor. Hopefully there will be persons who have special competence to assist colleagues in situations of exceptional difficulty – and there is justification everywhere for efforts to ensure that such help is available somehow to all those in need – a global objective, a long way off from achievement despite enormous advances since the mid twentieth century in both developed and less industrialised countries. At the very least, even if cancer services are grossly limited, relief of major symptoms such as pain should be ensured; a pressing moral, clinical and political imperative.

But is palliative medicine at the edge? There is a further (painful) consideration arising from some of the above considerations. *If society may be judged by attitude to the weak, palliative medicine is not the edge of medicine but its centre.*

The history of medicine in the twentieth century is fraught. Why did some European doctors in mid-20C betray the people? Much has been documented concerning the appalling actions of elite members of the medical profession in Nazi Germany. The early twentieth century was characterised by a fascination with eugenics – in USA, UK as well as Germany, with compulsory sterilization practiced and accepted. In Germany this fascination was combined in the early 30s with the idea of purifying the race and relieving the fraught economic situation by the removal of burdensome persons: the burdensome included the handicapped, mentally ill, feeble aged, and disabled children. And this was carried out through euthanasia programs in several hospitals in Germany several years before the commencement of the war. [Leo] Alexander, one of two medical witnesses at the Nuremburg trial of 24 doctors, wrote a lengthy account (which should be required reading of every doctor). He expressed his view of the genesis of the moral collapse which occurred:

> The beginnings at first were merely a subtle shift in emphasis in the basic attitude of the physicians. It started with the acceptance of the attitude, that there is such a thing as life not worthy to be lived. This attitude in its early stages concerned itself merely with severely and chronically sick. Gradually the sphere of those to be included in this category was enlarged to encompass the socially unproductive, the ideologically unwanted, the racially unwanted and finally all non-Germans. But it is important to realise the infinitely small wedged-in lever from which this entire trend of mind received its impetus was the attitude toward the non-rehabilitable sick ...[40]

We know the eventual consequences and (especially we doctors) must never forget. The search for human perfection may be Faustian if not pursued with both wisdom and integrity – and apprehension. We must recognise the first hints of a 'shift in attitude' toward the vulnerable.

So, in any health system, in any hospital, in any cancer centre, in the mind of any clinician, palliative medicine may need to be in the centre, not at the edge. And a test of the quality of that health system or institution – or physician – may be whether or not palliative medicine is recognised as central.

We live (in some ways) in dark times. Harshness is apparent the world over – and dominates the news, The late Kenneth Clark, in 1969, in his considerations of civilization expressed concern (quoting Yeats) that the 'centre may not hold'.

> Things fall apart; the centre cannot hold;
> Mere anarchy is loosed upon the world,
> The blood-dimmed tide is loosed, and everywhere
> The ceremony of innocence is drowned;
> The best lack all convictions, while the worst
> Are full of passionate intensity.[41]

Clark noted that 'we can destroy ourselves by cynicism and disillusion, just as effectively as by bombs'.[42] But we need to hope in ourselves, too. Human persons, though able to be vitiated, are radically good – as is the reality in which we are embedded. This goodness may be manifested in the sheer goodness and radical kindness of doctors to every person found to be in need, even and especially to strangers; and this not only in far countries in heroic services but in emergency departments, intensive care units, and clinics – everywhere. Goodness is abroad.

Recognition that palliative medicine is central – even to society – may permit the rediscovery or strengthening of the role of physicians not only as upright citizens, but as healers (not destroyers), leaders ('at midnight confident of the dawn 'as Ernst Bloch wrote somewhere) and advocates of the weak – always.[43]

The recovery of the core dimensions of clinical practice may lead physicians to revitalise even the centre of civilization, even in a dark night. It would be in accord with the finest formulation of the task of medicine. The centre may hold.

References

1. Lickiss JN, Wiltshire J, Glare PA, Chye R, 'Central Sydney Palliative Care Service: potential and limitations of an integrated palliative care service based in a metropolitan teaching hospital', *Ann Acad Med Singapore* 1994; 23:264–270.
2. Turner K, Lickiss JN, 'Postgraduate training in palliative medicine: the experience of the Sydney Institute of Palliative Medicine', *Pall Med* 1997; 11:389–394.
3. Lickiss JN, *Symptoms and science: implications of the patient as subject*. Lecture, Mount Olivet Hospital Brisbane, 1986.
4. Christakis NA, 'Social networks and collateral health effects', *British Medical Journal*, 2004;329:184–185.
5. Enthoven AC, 'Cutting Cost without Cutting the Quality of Care', Shattock Lecture. *N Engl J Med*, 1978; 298.
6. Christakis NA, Lamont EB, 'Extent and Determinants of Error in Doctors' Prognoses for Terminally Ill Patients: Prospective Cohort Study', *BMJ* 320:469–473, 2000.
7. Medawar PD, *The Threat and the Glory*, Harper Collins Publishers, 1990.
8. Kennedy I, *Unmasking Medicine*, London, George Allen & Unwin, 1981, based upon The Reith Lectures, 'Unmasking Medicine', pub. *The Listener*, Nov to Dec 1980.
9. Risse GB, *Mending Bodies, Saving Souls A History of Hospitals*, Oxford University Press, 1999.
10. Lickiss JN, 'Late lessons from Auschwitz – Is there anything more to learn for the twenty-first century?' [letter], *Journal of Medical Ethics* 2001; 27:137–8.
11. Turner K, Chye R, Aggarwal G, Philip J, Skeels A, Lickiss JN, 'Dignity in dying: a preliminary study of patients in the last three days of life'. *J Palliat Care* 12:2 1996; 7–13.
12. Popper K, *Conjectures and Refutations: The Growth of Scientific Knowledge*, Routledge, London, 1989.
13. Glare PA, Lickiss JN, 'Quality assurance in palliative care', *Med J Aust* 1992; 157:572.
14. Lickiss JN, Glare PA, Turner K, et al, 'Palliative care in Central Sydney: The Royal Prince Alfred Hospital as catalyst and integrator', *J Pal Care*, 1993; 9:33–42.
15. Glare PA, Virik KA, Aggarwal G, Clark KL, Pickstock SE, Lickiss JN, 'The interface between palliative medicine and specialists in acute-care hospitals: boundaries, bridges and challenges', *Med J Aust*, 2003; 15:179 (6 Suppl):S29–31.
16. Kassirer JP, 'Is managed care here to stay?' [editorial], *N Engl J Med* 1997; 336:1013–1014, 1229–1238.

17 Shakespeare W. *King Lear* Act V.
18 Needleman J, 'The perception of mortality', *Annals New York Academy of Sciences*, 1969; 164:733–738.
19 Bloom H, *Shakespeare: The Invention of the Human*, Riverhead Books, 1998.
20 Erikson J, *Childhood and Society*, Norton And Company, 1994.
21 Erikson J, *Psychological Issues*: Stages of Psychosocial Development.
22 Dawkins R, *The Selfish Gene*, Oxford University Press, 2nd ed, edition 1, 1990.
23 Feinstein AR, 'Clinical Judgement Revisited: The Distraction of Quantitative Models', *Ann Intern Med*, 1994;120:799–805.
24 Feinstein AR, 'Meta-Analysis: Statistical Alchemy for the twenty-first century', *Clin Epidemiol* 48; 1:71–79.
25 The Nuremberg Code (1947) In: Mitscherlich A, Mielke F, *Doctors of infamy: the story of the Nazi medical crimes*, New York, Schuman, 1949: xxiii–xxv.
26 Welie JVM, *In the face of suffering: The Philosophical-Anthropological Foundations of Clinical Ethics*, Creighton University Press, Omaha, Nebraska, 1998.
27 Gillon R (ed), *Principles of Health Care: Ethics*. John Wiley, Chichester, 1995; and Gillett G, 'Euthanasia: letting die and the pause', *J Med Ethics*, 1988:14(2):61–68.
28 Erikson J., *Childhood and Society*, Norton and Company, 1994.
29 Van Ness P, *Spirituality and the secular quest*, SCM Press London, 1996.
30 R Schaerer, 'Suffering of the doctor linked with the death of patients'. *Palliative Medicine* 1993:7 (suppl 1):27–37.
31 Doka JK, *Disenfranchised Grief: New Directions, Challenges, and Strategies for Practice*, Research Press (IL) (March 1, 2002), or *Disenfranchised Grief: Recognizing Hidden Sorrow*, Lexington Books, (August 1, 1989).
32 Foucault, M, *The Birth of the Clinic: an Archaeology of Medical Perception*. (AM Sheridan Smith, trans.), New York, Vintage Books, 1975.
33 Malpas J and Lickiss, N (eds), *Perspectives on human dignity*, Springer, Dordtrecht, 2007.
34 Mill JS, *On Liberty*, Harvard Classics, Volume 25. Copyright 1909 P.F. Collier & Son 1860.
35 Chochinov HM, Hack T, Hassard T, Kristjanson L, McClement S, Harlos M, 'Dignity in the terminally ill; a cross sectional cohort study', *Lancet* 2002;360:2026–2030.
36 Street A, Kissane D, 'Constructions of dignity in end-of-life care', *Journal of Palliative Care* 2001; 17:93–101.

37 Mortimer KE, 'The impossible profession: The Doctor/Priest relationship' *Proc Aust Assoc Geront* 2(2) p 81–2, 1974.
38 Aries P, *The hour of our death*. Oxford Univ Press (T); Reissue edition 1, 1991; and Aries P. *The Hour of our death*, Tr H Weaver, Knopf, 1981.
39 Malpas J and Solomon R, *Death and Philosophy*, Routledge, 1998.
40 Alexander L, 'Medical Science Under Dictatorship', *New England Journal Medicine*, 1949; 241:39–47.
41 Clark K, *Civilization*. A personal view. British Broadcasting Corporation, London, 1969.
42 Kirby, MD, 'The Rights of the living and the Rights of the dying', *Medical Journal of Australia*, Mar 1980, 1: 252–255.
43 Lickiss JN, 'On the care of aged persons: privilege and responsibility', *Australian Rehabilitation Review*, 1982; 2(6):51–57.

9
LATE MUSINGS

I
ART, PERSONAL CARE AND THE JEWISH TRADITION
2016

*Comments at the Opening of the
Exhibition of five Jewish Artists, Reflections on Care –
Comber Street Studio, Paddington, 22 May 2016.*

The opening of an art exhibition is a significant moment: the gaze of others may rest for the first time on what is mainly closed to view – expressions of the core of self. A juxtaposition of art and the care of those in crisis or persons with probably eventually fatal illness often close to death, and the Jewish tradition? How to think of this association? Is there a synergy? What is common to all? Surely all are rooted in the personal. And the juxtaposition of all three offers the opportunity to explore newly illuminated dimensions of human being. Three major traditions are represented here! Three traditions, as it were, in conversation. A glance at each may be useful.

1
Art

We know that *homo sapiens* has lived for around 150 000 years, but that there was a creative explosion around 30,000 years ago – leaving us traces of art on rocks, found notably in France and Spain, with images usually of animals deep in almost inaccessible caves. There has been much debate concerning the meaning of the images and of the arduous processes involved in painting them.[1,2] Current thought is that the paintings on these ancient rocks are not merely portrayals of everyday life such as hunting scenes but relate to a symbolic universe, and expression of a spiritual dimension of human *being*. Ritual such as associated with Shamanism may well have been involved in the process of creating this extraordinary art; it is relevant that an eminent anthropologist such as Roy Rappaport (1926–1997) wrote of the critical role of such strands in the development of humanity (as distinct from the evolution of the human – a biological phenomenon). Rappaport wrote in his final book, in 1999, about 'the nature of humanity, a species that lives, and can only live, in terms of the meanings it must construct in a world devoid of intrinsic meaning but subject to physical law.'[3]

There is art of great antiquity also in Australia – maybe over 25,000 years old, even older than the rock art in Europe. It is notable that not only animals but humanlike figures are to be seen – eg. the Gwion paintings of the Kimberley or the mysterious Wangina figures: to be in the presence of such art is a powerful experience. There is little doubt that, similarly, these paintings belong to the symbolic universe and manifest the spiritual dimension of the first Australians. There is an explosion of interest in this treasure trove.

So, art has always expressed and continues to express complex dimensions of humanness, and also contributes to the development, even healing of persons: art may indeed be therapy! But there is another perspective: with respect to human flourishing art is not means but end. Furthermore each person is at core an artist – responsible for the shaping of the self as a work of art, whether flawed or refined ... So, we are person-makers, not only by making children but by making that which we become. And each is unique – and each has a song to sing.

See echoes of this notion in the poets, such as W.B. Yeats:

> An aged man is but a paltry thing,
> A tattered coat upon a stick, unless
> Soul clap its hands and sing, and louder sing
> For every tatter in his mortal dress.[4]

Harold Bloom (1930–2019), renowned literary critic, after enduring nearly fatal illness, wrote in his memoir of the experience, 'at the gates of death I did not seek an interlocutor' – poetry sustained him.[5] Tellingly (for our theme) he next published an anthology of favourite poetry entitled tellingly, *Till I End My Song*.[6]

The person as artist, as creator of the self, may be, especially in extremis, of special relevance in the context of this exhibition – and there are many limit situations in which people may urgently need care. It is because the song may 'falter' – but is not yet finished (whether in the midst of life or at its close), that personal care (incorporating appropriate professional skills) may be needed, either in crisis intervention or prolonged and definitive care, to shape the self, in order to become what he or she (alone) may be: a personal partnership indeed, a sacred trust.

2
The Jewish tradition
The Jewish tradition goes back several millennia. The Hebrew scriptures, even in the earliest form (very different from the present versions) reflect a long oral tradition in Mesopotamia

basically concerning the human condition, and our perceptions of all reality. We find in these rich sources the portrayal of the human person as composite – with affinity with the earth ('dust') and also with transcendence (beyond the dust), as essentially social, as responsible (for self, the earth, other persons – including strangers), and as mortal. And pervading all is the concept that man is image of God (however 'God' be understood – 'I am who I am' – of the being of being, ultimate reality); the meaning of which concept may imply especially the human as maker/creative/benevolent. 'Be ye holy as I am holy'.

Furthermore there is the haunting theme in the Hebrew scriptures (celebrated at Passover) of the possibility of being freed from slavery, of liberation, of being able to go out into a new place, of human possibility for newness.

The theme of the appropriate conduct towards strangers is not only justice but also 'kindness' – and this is mentioned again and again in the Hebrew scriptures – to be noted. The kindness of strangers to strangers is at the core of contemporary crisis care and palliative care – if not in civil society.[7]

3
Personal care

Humans are social beings. Persons have cared for persons from the beginning of human emergence – if only for biological reasons! We cannot be born or survive without the care of other persons, and nor should we try to cope with frailty. Artists down the ages have repeatedly portrayed persons caring for other persons in all sorts of circumstances, including the bodies of persons after their death. Indeed, one of the earliest marks of humanness has been the detection of complex burial rituals – care of the body of persons after death (whether to benefit the dead or the living). Lake Mungo in NSW was the site for the finding of a body in 1974, buried at least 30,000 years ago, sprinkled with ochre which had been carried many miles.

Wherefore the obligation to care for another – even a stranger? The philosophical basis for the duty of care is, according to Levinas (twentieth century Jewish philosopher), not law, not contract, but the call of the other.[8]

There is another dimension. Not only do we need other persons to care for our basic biological needs: we cannot grow and flourish optimally as persons except through interpersonal interaction – even the conversation with oneself has the properties of dialogue: there is a rich and long Jewish philosophical tradition concerning these concepts – Martin Buber (1878–1965) may be the name best known. No man is an island. A person is intrinsically relational, incomplete and stunted in permanent total isolation from other persons (*pace* hermits). It may take a lifetime to appreciate fully this profound truth: we need each other in order to be who we may become, not merely to survive. To become transparent, instead of opaque to others may be very costly: crisis or grave illness may force this transformation: carers need to be sensitive to the cost.

Personal care is the place of the personal *par excellence*. Crisis management demands understanding of the opportunity for growth inherent in crisis (Erikson is still maybe the most useful theorist – noted below) as well as the processes for supporting persons in crisis. Palliative care involves not only precise understanding of illness, symptoms and relevant therapy, but also a perspective on the whole of life trajectory of persons.

The UK Hospice Movement that became so obvious in the mid-twentieth century must have been influenced by the effect on the medical community in UK of the fact that British medical students participated in the liberation of Belsen concentration camp in 1945. Cicely Saunders (1918–2005) (a doctor by the 60s) may have embodied the protest against such violations of power, inflicting gross human indignities and neglect of the dying (an obvious link between the Jewish tradition and personal care). The burgeoning of palliative care in twenty-first century Australia may be a protest, not against formal neglect of the frail and dying in an affluent society, but against the relentless trend towards depersonalisation in the search for efficiency – virtually all commercial cost-saving measures (even in education) involve reduction in significant personal interactions. I go on record as noting that a late lesson from Auschwitz may be the danger of efficiency as an end in itself, instead of a means to human flourishing: I make no apology. Robots can perform tasks, but cannot *care*. Persons in crises and in the midst of frailty and suffering, especially when approaching death need *care*.

There may be another point worth making, another dimension to the protest. Not only is there steady erosion of the opportunities for personal interaction, but also erosion of some aspects of privacy! Persons are unique, not merely consumers worth counting, profiling, observing, cultivating, even placating – so that they may be commodified for gain, a means to another and lesser end instead of an end – as the Kantian tradition urged. There are subtle dangers in this loss of privacy. There is room to protest by ensuring that a person is recognised as unique, so that he she may be truly valued as an end not a means. A patient in need of palliative care is a patient, not a customer.

Our concern for privacy of those in need of care should extend to spiritual privacy. There was a vogue for developing a scale regarding spiritual health – of measuring even that most private of aspects of the self – that which is the well-

spring of personal life, that which may express the person's
sense of meaning and relations, not only with persons,
places, things, the past as remembered, inheritance – roots
in culture, hopes/dreams and with oneself, but also the
relation with all-that-is, with transcendence whether or not
called 'God' or expressed in treasured ritual. This is sacred
ground. Once again, it is a poet who gives expression to
such notions: this time Christopher Brennan (1870–1932), a
Professor of German and Comparative Literature (University
of Sydney), whose life crashed around him – and he walked
the hills of the Bondi area, sometimes in despair. He includes
in the Epilogue of his 1913 edition of his poems a moving
image from 1897 of his personal core – and its supports and
articulations of relationships including that with a beloved
woman and with God:

> Deep in my hidden country stands a peak,
> and none hath known its name
> and none, save I, hath even skill to seek:
> thence my wild spirit came.
> Thither I turn, when the day's garish world
> Too long hath vexed my sight,
> And bare my limbs where the great winds are whirl'd
> And life's undreaded might.
> ...
> The gift of self is self's most sacred right;
> only where none hath trod,
> only upon my most secret starry height
> I abdicate to God.[9]

Sacred ground indeed. And no carer should seek to explore
it – or tread on it unless unshod and explicitly invited.

So, what links all three of these traditions (art, the Jewish
tradition, and personal care)? Surely, the focus on the *personal* –

even the crisis of the personal. But there may be need to explore further about what we mean by the personal; not all would wish such exploration and it can be left aside.

Jacob Needleman (1934–2022) a philosopher, in 1969, in a communication to the New York Academy of Sciences wrote: 'What medicine lacks is any fundamental notion as to the nature of man and any remotely adequate understanding of that to which we refer as person'.[10]

The shape of the final task of personhood needs to be understood by those in contact with patients approaching death – at any age. Such patients may well vacillate between wholeness and despair, before the way is clear. They may long to express their internal states, explore the threat of despair through dialogue with others – but to participate in such dialogue is so very difficult for the interlocutor – and to reach out towards what wholeness is possible, to round out the symphony of one's life. If it is surely the task of each person to explore the limits of one's possibilities (which involve in the end the going out from oneself, as the highest exercise of autonomy) then it is surely the task of a doctor to free patients from obstacles (such as pain) to such an exploration. Eric Cassell (1928–2021) stressed that a goal of medicine is the relief of suffering – and the obverse of that notion is surely the facilitation of human flourishing in no matter what circumstances – by assisting the subject cohere – helping the 'centre to hold': a precious service indeed, not within the capacity of many physicians.

No person should die in despair. The physician – and all involved in palliative care, whilst emphasizing a realistic range of possibilities as a way of indicating prognosis, should assist the patient to centre hope not on what will in the end probably fail in a situation of eventually fatal illness (such as anti-disease therapies), but on what should not fail – the commitment to care, the relief of pain, and in the intrinsic value of the patient as a unique irreplaceable subject of existence. These matters call for much pondering if we are not to add to the despair of those living with complex chronic diseases or dying in 'high tech' contexts – or anywhere. No person should die with the dominant perception of self as a 'therapeutic failure', nor disillusioned after being sustained by unrealistic hope, recognized as such even by those (especially a physician) engendering it, conceiving it as an act of compassion. Despair, on Erikson's model is one of the two options in the last phase of life – at any age: the favourable option being rather the development of a sense of wholeness (which Erikson calls 'integrity') being at one with one's place and time, and life pattern. Authentic living with frailty or dying, as authentic living, is surely embedded not in falsehood but in truth. Certainly no lie can be justified to separate a person from his or her own truth – depriving him or her of becoming what is possible. The matter of the personal significance of the last phase of life, at any age, needs far more focus.

In conclusion, we as persons at an exhibition are gifted with a glimpse of precious art today. Maybe we could recall one patient's response to such an experience. John Keats born in London 1795 (when Sydney was hardly born) developed tuberculosis from which he died in Rome in 1821. But in the last words of his 'Ode on a Grecian Urn' (after describing its artistic features) he gave us the memorable (and well-remembered) words:

> Beauty is truth, truth beauty – that is all
> Ye know on earth, and all ye need to know.[11]

Maybe in looking at the paintings in this exhibition – and the thoughtful captions supplied by the artists, we may ponder again on those words, and wonder still.

REFERENCES

1. Lewis-Williams D., *The Mind in the Cave: Consciousness and the Origins of Art*, Thames and Hudson, London, 2004.
2. Whiteley D., *Cave Paintings and the Human Spirit*, Prometheus Books, Amherst, 2008.
3. Rappaport Roy A., *Ritual and the Making of Humanity*, Cambridge University Press, Cambridge, 1999.
4. Yeats WB., *Journey to Byzantium*.
5. Bloom H., *Where Shall Wisdom be Found?* Penguin Putnam, NY, 2004.
6. Bloom H., *Till I end my Song: A Gathering of Last Poems*. Harper Collins, New York, 2012.
7. Sacks J., *To Heal a Fractured World: the Ethics of Responsibility*. Schoken Books, New York, 2005, p 97–112.
8. Manderson D., *Proximity, Levinas, and the Soul of Law*, McGill-Queens University Press, Montreal, 2007.
9. Brennan CB., *Poems 1913*, Philip and Son, Sydney 1914. Facsimile edition 1972, University of Sydney.
10. Needleman J., 'The perception of mortality', *Annals of the New York Academy of Sciences*, 164 (1969), pp 733–738.
11. Keats J., *Ode on a Grecian Urn*.

II
LIVING IN THE DECADE FOR DYING
2017

> To everything there is a season, and a time to every purpose under heaven; a time to be born, and a time to die; a time to plant, and a time to pluck up that which is planted ... A time to keep silence, and a time to speak.
> —*Ecclesiastes* 3

Is the time come for me to try to articulate some of the traces of the years?

Maybe, maybe.

Montaigne said of such an undertaking:

> It is a thorny undertaking, and more so than it seems, to follow a movement so wandering as that of our mind, to penetrate the opaque depths of its innermost folds, to pick out and immobilize the innumerable flutterings that agitate it.

Many have mused about the interior colloquy within the self, and there is reason for caution. David Hume, in his *Treatise on Human Nature* talked of those who think to find in themselves some perception of a self:

> But setting aside some metaphysicians of this kind, I may venture to affirm of the rest of mankind, that they are nothing but a bundle or collection of different perceptions, which succeed each other with an inconceivable rapidity and are in a perpetual flux and movement.

The explorations articulated here reflect a state of mind at a particular point in time and space: a thought (or a bundle of thoughts) is held there and given the form of an essay, without reference to the other pieces grouped here. Like a sea anemone sitting on a rock has many elements each with its many parts exploring the scenery, engaging with its own portion of sea water, sifting for nutrition – so have I lived, just exploring, not thinking of a defined end but responding to the striving within, which seventeenth century philosopher Baruch Spinoza called '*conatus*'. Each essay has its own unity – none was written with an eye either to publication or to companions, rather as a means of exploring a new terrain which I now realise others may encounter one day.

Written over the years by a changing (ageing and growing) person, there is some continuity here, and therefore repetition: but hopefully, even over a few years, there is some evolution of thought, reflecting growth in *awareness.*

Old age should be, truly, *a celebration of awareness* – if the onset of sometimes almost blinding clarity can be borne with equanimity, and if one can also bear also the clarity – augmented restlessness which is a mark of agency and sign of continuing life.

Living in the 'Decade for Dying':
the years of living dangerously

A rather close-to-the-bone remark made at recent Grand Rounds concerning distressing outcomes in two elderly patients stirred me significantly: 'After all, in Australia, the decade in which in which deaths commonly occur is 75–85 years … This is the decade for dying.' This set me to muse: what is it to *live* in the decade for dying? By the time I had reached home, ideas were taking shape and were laid down in the following few days. Of course one hears echoes in the poets, such as WB Yeats:

> An aged man is but a paltry thing,
> A tattered coat upon a stick, unless

> Soul clap its hands and sing, and louder sing
> For every tatter in his mortal dress[1]

But what *does it mean* to *live* in the 'decade for dying'? Is there anything worth thinking about, or saying? Is it wholly self-indulgent consideration for one embedded in a privileged context where probable death has been several times averted by Western medical interventions *and* the kindness of strangers, in a world scarred by violence and inequity, the consciousness of which is made almost unbearable by one's present powerlessness? Such pressure of mind does not usually issue in logical and ordered prose, nor in usefulness. Maybe in the circularity or, better, spiral structure of such ponderings there is something to articulate.

First of all, there is an imperative to view the life of each person as one whole, recognising phases which, although merging into one another, may be roughly delineated, especially retrospectively: it is increasingly evident as one ages, that, as a wise one remarked, one lives life forwards but understands it backwards.

Developmental psychologist Eric Erikson guided us to think of life stages as marked by tasks involving choice between clear alternatives.[2] He sensitively conceived the developmental task of the elderly and, by analogy, to those of any age approaching death as the development of a sense of wholeness or integrity. In late adulthood the choice is to have [what he calls] 'integrity', that is a sense of wholeness, or to despair, and his analysis is singularly appropriate for clinicians:

> Only he who in some way has taken care of things and people and has adapted himself to the triumphs and disappointments of being, by necessity, the originator of others and the generator of things and ideas – only he

> may gradually grow the fruit of [...] integrity. It is the acceptance of one's own and only life cycle and of the people who have become significant to it as something that had to be [...] an acceptance of the fact that one's life is one's own responsibility. It is a sense of comradeship with men and women of distant times and of different pursuits, who have created orders and objects and sayings conveying human dignity and love.

And of despair:

> [T]he lack or loss of this accrued ego integration is signified by despair and an often unconscious fear of death: the one and only life cycle is not accepted as the ultimate of life. Despair expresses the feeling that the time is short, too short for the attempt to start another life and to try out alternative roads to integrity.[3]

The role of life events (including onset of illness or even frailty) in prompting leaps in personal development may need far deeper appreciation. Physicians may be often, unwittingly, players in a complex (intrapersonal and interpersonal) personal drama, with subtle influence on the outcome. Personal evolution then is complex, and much of it hidden, yet some elements may be manifest.

Edward Said's book *On Late Style* was written in the last phase of his life, exploring styles of musical composition[4] – [Ludwig van] Beethoven especially came into focus:

> Beethoven's late works exude a new sense of private striving and instability. The masterpieces of Beethoven's final decade are late and the extent that they are beyond their own time, ahead of it in terms of daring and startling newness, later than it in that they describe a return or homecoming to realms forgotten or left behind by the relentless advancement of history.

Said emphasised the diversity of late style, which he thought as sometimes defiant, incongruous, tumultuous, even subversive, with the theme of death undermining, and, strangely, elevating their uses of language and the aesthetic. One is left with the overall impression of 'late style' radiating a new and radical freedom.

It would be worthwhile to carry this theme further than the arts: to study the modes of *thought* in the late writings of notable thinkers in medicine, for example. Decades of clinical life built on extraordinarily privileged education should surely yield such creative thinking, albeit hard to discern in the less heard voices of the old. Evolving over a lifetime, even if in quasi exile from the rush of things (or because of it) one becomes aware not only of increased freedom of thought but also of the limitations of one's knowing and understanding.

We are aware also of the fact that as ageing clinicians taught by our patients (and our failures and successes) we have a store of human experience which may illumine the common search of all scholarly disciplines for understanding not only the natural world, but, within it, the human person, and the place of persons as connected with all nature.

We are singularly aware of the interconnectedness of the material web and of the web of thought in which we are individually embedded. Our intuition may find resonance in the thought of 17C philosopher [Baruch] Spinoza, notably articulated by Australian philosopher Genevieve Lloyd,[5] because we have *experienced* what Spinoza discerned: that the essence of a living thing is *conatus*, that is, its 'striving to continue in being'. We have experienced in ourselves this striving: we know the compulsion to be true to our *vocation* and to respond to the call of those in need of us. We have seen the striving in a weak newborn baby or a patient emerging into life again after being near death. And we have witnessed the striving cease.

One becomes aware of new challenges as the decades roll by. In old age there are both *losses and gains*, and onerous personal *tasks*. There is work to do and time is at a premium, energy may be diminishing, and the unexpected is also bound to intervene.

Losses and gains attend every life: they etch the emerging pattern. Losses are particularly poignant in late life and often obvious: losses of roles, of persons (by death, displacement, dementia), of things, of place, of memory, of personal capacity – and maybe of dreams? Adverse life events are frequent. Grief is a subtext: the elderly are deeply bereaved and therefore constantly remaking patterns of thinking, doing, and relating, remaking the self. These are matters not much spoken of, yet central in the dialogue with the self.

There are more subtle losses in every human trajectory which may be particularly poignant in old age, when awareness may be heightened by deep reflection. As [Genevieve] Lloyd writes:

> Our separation from things in space can have deep emotional effects but it does not have the unthinkability of the lost past or the indeterminate future, the strangeness of a present which did not exist, the mind – stopping absence of what did exist, which we try ineffectually to map onto the more comfortable and comforting images of spatial presence and absence.[6]

Gains are also many and subtle, leading to shifts in perspectives. For example, we may find an increased freedom regarding choice of action even in the midst of complex difficulties. According to Lloyd, Spinoza offered an alternative concept to that currently prevailing regarding freedom, traceable to [René] Descartes whose philosophy influenced the world of thought in which we have lived and practiced:

> In Descartes's treatment of freedom, an inherently free will forces back ever further the limits of what must be accepted as beyond human control. The prevailing imagery is of border skirmishes [...] Spinoza offers instead a vision of freedom as the joyful acceptance of what must be ... [F]reedom derives from the active engagement of the mind with necessity, an engagement that flows from the understanding of the truth.[7]

We know also the refreshing freedom of thought fostered by richness of experience: increased understanding as distinct from information or knowledge, and even wisdom; increased awareness both of human frailty and human possibility for good as well as harm; heightened awareness of self, others, world, All-That-Is, and of the long human heritage, of the human malaise at the root of the galaxy of social problems in affluent societies – problems embodied in persons who have impinged on our professional lives: suicide, violence, addiction, despair, demeaning poverty, rejection. We have been witnesses to it all. After so many winters, there is also awareness of the signs of spring and of hope – even in dark times and in the most unlikely places.

Perceptions of the subtleties of, say, conversations or political or moral complexities may be painfully powerful, as may be the poignancy of powerlessness, and the eventual acceptance of the fact of uselessness. Just because elderly persons, even clinicians, may not volunteer judgements or comments, it is not to be assumed that issues are unperceived (or even possible solutions not glimpsed). Reticence may be the fruit of experience, and an expression of wisdom; it may also arise from the felt need to prioritise activities calling for the expenditure of energy, for the tasks are onerous and life is very busy and the pressure of time is palpable.

Losses and gains may intermingle, but concurrently, as in other phases of life, there is personal work to be done. *Tasks* in late life are many and use up time and energy, and some are specific to life stage. The shape of the late-life tasks need to be understood by those in contact with patients late in life, who may well vacillate between wholeness and despair and need to be supported gently. They may long and need to try to express their internal states, explore the threat of despair and through dialogue with significant others, reach out again towards the wholeness which is possible.

Late-phase-of-life tasks particularly concern *closure*, with respect to persons, place, things, and aspirations, often involving reconciliation (even with oneself) or reformulation. Closure is never complete, any more than achievements may be complete. The awareness of incompleteness may be a component of anticipatory grief. [Franz] Kafka, who knew a lot about the vagaries of life, mused in his diaries about the last days of Moses, denied the chance to cross over into the land for which over forty years, he had sought to prepare his people:

> He is on the track of Canaan all his life; it is incredible that he should see the land only when on the verge of death. The dying vision of it can only be intended to illustrate how incomplete a moment is human life, incomplete because a life like this could last forever and still be nothing but a moment. Moses failed to enter Canaan not because his life is too short but because it is a human life.[8]

No comment would be adequate.

Exploration is the second task. Obviously (but is it obvious?) activities of closure do not preclude the making of plans for undertaking something *new*.

Again, poets have set the scene. For example, T.S. Eliot (who surely could have included women):

> Old men ought to be explorers
> Here or there does not matter
> We must be still and still moving
> Into another intensity …[9]

What is this exploring?

There is a new terrain, and new experiences for body and mind and spirit. There are new perceptions of personal identity. The learning curve is steep but critical, particularly for doctors, after sometimes decades of work, not to be able to care for others in the old ways, not to 'fix problems' as usual, not to be needed by the hospital or practice day after day, night after night, not even to have the protection against commitment 'I might be on call' – but to be an ordinary citizen needing help of others, even the kindness of strangers. And to be grateful to be one of this different community now, even the community of those living dangerously, precariously, knowingly close to the edge, but *living* still.

New possibilities are there to be glimpsed, new sources of pain and joy, new appreciation of the kindness of strangers, new places where beauty is found, new ideas to be considered and connected with old insights, new framings of hope, new respect for the fabric of human diversity, new synthesis of personal philosophy – one's search for meaning has a new urgency and shuns glib answers, and a new response to the haunting questions: who and where am I now? Who is my neighbour? What can I be for you? The particular becomes more precious, as does the present moment. One realises at last that meaning is in the exploring not the finding. Maybe, above all, there is new awareness of the possibility of (and need for) freedom, even in the face of necessity, and the need for respect for one's personal freedom and priorities by those who compassionately seek to care.

Umberto Eco cautions at the end of his novel, *Foucault's Pendulum*:

> Where have I read that at the end, when life's surface upon surface, has become completely encrusted with experience, you know everything, the secret, the power, and the glory, why you were born, why you are dying, and how it all could have been different? You are wise. But the greatest wisdom, at that moment, is knowing that your wisdom is too late. You understand everything when there is no longer anything to understand.[10]

But we need not be so pessimistic!

The third task? Preparing for the act of dying.

Death of a person is the closing of a human life, not an unthinkable happening, even if a surprise. It may be a welcome friend, a conclusion to striving: German philosopher Ernst Bloch called dying the 'master test of our journeyman years'.[11] Or maybe it is the last phase of the symphony I am writing – the last touches to the sculpture I am making, for which I am wholly responsible. Each one of us humans is an artist, shaping oneself, come what may; the creative task is to shape one's life according to whatever pattern one has in mind, recognising that it is not what happens but the responses to what happens which are the creative tools. One is responsible for what one becomes, surely far more than for one achieves. But once the horizon of life is being glimpsed, the task of preparing for one's own dying is a major personal task.

Preparing for the time when I will, as a person, no longer be 'here', no longer 'placed' – I am passing away. The body dies and remains in place, but the person passes away, and what is there in that bed is rightly called 'remains'. The old folk phrases are tellingly precise. In a sense, Spinoza's articulation of the individual person as part of the whole (that to him is Nature) enriches one's grasp of life and illumines human death, which, in the acceptance of radical personal transience may be not only the spur to seize the day but also the root of contentment. Emily Dickinson depicted dying as 'a wild night and a new road'. Maybe, indeed.

So, human life remains complex to its close. French philosopher Michel Foucault, reflecting on the 'archaeology' of aspects of medical practice commented:

> What counts in the things said by men is not so much what they may have thought or the extent to which these things represent their thoughts, as that which systematizes them from the outset, thus making them thereafter endlessly accessible to new discourses and open to the task of transforming them.[12]

American philosopher Jacob Needleman remarked that, 'what medicine lacks is any fundamental notion of the nature of man and any remotely adequate understanding of that to which we refer as a person'.[13] At the centre of thoughts about the care of those living in the twilight, robust concepts not only of the nuances of living in the dangerous years, but also of 'person' need to underpin all cogitations and action and, of course, policies.

The philosophical tradition concerning [the notion of] 'person', though rich,[14] may be relatively inaccessible to busy clinicians. A relational or ecological view may offer a foothold for thinking. Just as a spider's web *is* the complexus of filaments, a person may be thought of as not *supplemented* by but *constituted* by relationships with persons, place, things, memory, inheritance – biological and cultural, hope and aspirations, and with All-That-Is (however conceived and named). In this perspective, relations *constitute* the person. They are not add-ons, and the rupture of any one of them may lead to perturbation or even disintegration of the whole. This notion is in accord with Eric Cassell's definition of suffering as a sense of impending personal disintegration.[15,16]

The concept of person as constituted by a web of relationships brings new life into the exigencies of personal care, and make impossible travesties of health care which, for example, exclude desired significant others or patient's priorities from the field of focus in clinical decision-making.

As we age and may even be on the receiving end of care we understand more clearly than ever, that it is imperative to weigh the cost and benefit from the patient's perspective of any intervention – including (especially) drugs, investigations, or clinic visits. Clinicians need surely to be aware of probable, possible and unexpected consequences to the patient as person (including all constitutive relations – with self, other persons, place, culture, including personal ritual). Experience or tales of cognitive deterioration or other drug side effects contribute to the calculus of fear inchoate in the consciousness of the old and frail.

Only the competent patient can really measure benefit, and evaluate any intervention. It is good that this principle is being increasingly recognised. It is also logical, and kind, to keep clinical contact (days in hospital, clinics, investigations, drugs) to a minimum so that *life* is not submerged or worse, wasted. There is need also to recognise the limitations of 'evidence' in distillations such as guidelines or protocols; specifically blurring the individual differences between persons (even differences in patterns of co-morbidity as well as priorities for action and goals) and radical uniqueness of each person in all his or her complexity.

Considerations of such matters highlight the need for *privacy*. In health services there is not only depersonalisation (a tendency shared with society) in the interests of efficiency, but also erosion of some aspects of privacy by those intent on doing good. The trend to teams, with all their benefits, risks not only exhaustion of the patient by sapping of energy and time but also invasion of personal privacy.

Concern for privacy of those in need of care should extend to spiritual privacy. There was a vogue for developing a scale regarding spiritual health, the health of the *spirit* – that which is the well-spring of personal life, that which may express the person's sense of meaning and relations, not only with persons, places, things, the past as remembered, inheritance – roots in culture, hopes/dreams and with oneself, but also relation with All-That-Is, with transcendence, whether or not called 'God' or expressed in treasured ritual. This *is* sacred ground, and no carer should seek to explore it, or tread on it unless unshod and explicitly invited.

It may be that admirable modern contemporary clinicians (even seniors) sometimes lack an adequate perception of the ageing person's view of personal being and trajectory in the 'decade for dying' and capacity for the exercise of responsibility in the context of freedom, even in freedom exercised in finally surrendering one's self to another in trust. There is room for quiet thought, and at least, acceptance of the fact of a chasm in understanding, and continuing search for a bridge.

Living in the 'decade for dying' is indeed a time for living dangerously, with losses and gains, with increasing agenda of tasks, all against a backdrop not only of the experience of time pressure and powerlessness (even frailty), but also of increasing awareness of the complexity of oneself and other persons as simply nodes of concurrence of interconnecting strands in a vast web, each one flawed, yet striving like all living things, to continue in being and (as Pindar urged long ago) to 'exhaust the limits of the possible'. And all of this, somehow, in new radical freedom.

REFERENCES

1. Yeats W.B., *Byzantium*.
2. Erikson E.H., 1965, *Childhood and Society*, 2nd Edition. Penguin Books, Harmondsworth.
3. Erikson E.H., 1959, 'Identity and the Life Cycle', *Psychological Issues*, Vol 1, No 1, New York.
4. Said E., *On Late Style*, Bloomsbury, London, 2006.
5. Lloyd G., *Spinoza and the Ethics*, Routledge, Abingdon, 1996.
6. Lloyd G., *Being in Time: Selves and Narrators in Philosophy and Literature*, Routledge, London, 1993, p13.
7. Lloyd G., *Providence Lost*, Harvard University Press, Cambridge Mass, 2008, p200 ff.
8. Kafka F., *Diaries 1914–1923*, trans M Greenberg and H Arendt, Quoted in A.G. Zornberg, *Moses: A Human Life*. Yale University Press, New Haven, 2016, p192.
9. Eliot T.S., 'East Coker' – from *The Four Quartets*.
10. Eco U., *Foucault's Pendulum*, Vintage Publishing, London, 1989.
11. Bloch E., Karl Marx, Death and the Apocalypse in *Man on His Own: Essays on the Philosophy of Religion*, trans by E.B. Ashton. Herder and Herder, New York, 1970, p47.
12. Foucault M., *The Birth of the Clinic: The Archaeology of Medical Perception*, trans. Sheridan Smith A.M., Tavistock, London, 1973.
13. Needleman J., 'The perception of mortality', *Annals New York Academy of Sciences* 164; 733–738, 1969.
14. Thomasma D.C., D.N. Weisstub and C. Herve (eds) *Personhood and Health Care*, Kluwer Dordrecht, 2001.
15. Lickiss N., 'On Facing Human Suffering', in Malpas J. and Lickiss N. (eds) *Perspectives on Human Suffering*, Springer, Dordrecht, 2012, pp 260–345.
16. Cassell E.J., 'The nature of suffering and the goals of medicine'. *New England Journal of Medicine*, 306: 639–64, 1982.

III
AFTER THE DECADE FOR DYING (75–85): WHAT NOW?
2018

In Australia the decade in which many people die is the decade between 75–85 years. An attempt has been made elsewhere to muse on the experience of *living*, not dying, in that period of life, on its tasks.[1] But what if one has outlived it this span of years after negotiating a decade of living dangerously: what now? The focus may shift from the hazards of negotiation to a poignant search for meaning: what now? Maybe it is like a yacht which has won through the hazards of an ocean race having now to find safe harbour! The issues which concern us now are not the battle with life-threatening waves – we may be getting used to such encounters – but matters far more complex: indeed, issues of ultimate concern. Even the recurring obsequies for companions and colleagues emphasise the need for scrutiny of our grasp of what is beyond the ephemeral: there is a new solitude now, and a new companionship.

Erich Auerbach (1892–1957), German philologist and literary critic, having had to escape in 1936 from Germany to Istanbul, where he then lived for eleven years, wrote a book titled *Mimesis* that helped define the discipline of comparative literature – all without the benefit of a major library. Towards the end of his magnum opus, as he struggled with his more recent past, he gave us a pointer:

> We are constantly endeavouring to give meaning and order to our lives in the past, the present, and the future, to our surroundings, the world in which we live; with

the result that our lives appear in our own conception
as total entities – which to be sure are always changing,
more or less radically, more or less rapidly, depending on
the extent to which we are obliged, inclined, and able to
assimilate the onrush of new experience.[2]

To be able to give meaning and order to our lives depends, wrote Auerbach, on how we assimilate the *onrush of new experience*. It is what happens in the future, from now on, and how we assimilate it – take it into our being – which has critical influence on our capacity to give order and meaning to our self – to have a sense of our whole.

What do I know of my future? The only certainty is that I will come to the close of my life – I will die: this is the 'known known'. The rest is unknown. Maybe there will be distress (almost certainly), and even 'suffering' – which Eric J. Cassell (1928–) distinguished from distress and defined as 'a sense of impending personal disintegration' as if my centre is not holding.[3] Maybe the context will be so difficult that I, however weakened, will need to try to remember that in my lifetime other persons, even in extreme conditions due to human malice I cannot know or imagine remained capable of heroic morality. I find it apposite to recall the words of the psychotherapist Victor Frankl (1905–1997), a survivor of Auschwitz: 'the last of human freedoms is to take an attitude in a given set of circumstances'.

Maybe there will be not suffering but frailty, and maybe losses I have not foreseen as well as those foreseen. Maybe loss of place, loved ones, comfort, cultural compatibility, beauty in forms I cherish, freedom I value (both freedom from constraints, and freedom to act), and capacities (physical and intellectual) in which my security may rest. Auerbach writes of the 'onrush' of new experience – maybe the suddenness will take me unawares. It is easy to lose heart, to be afraid. Afraid of much – but maybe notably frailty. It is not just the 'sans everything' of Shakespeare but the possibility of fragility, and the press of contingency which may induce dismay.

Frailty – the notion is worth a pause. The *Oxford Dictionary* defines 'frail' (derived from Latin 'fragilis') as liable to be broken; easily destroyed. Weak. Easily overcome. 'Frailty' is the liability to be crushed or to decay; being perishable, weak. The nuance is unmistakeable and familiar with regard to material things and persons and even concepts and perspectives which hitherto have seemed solid.

In fact, frailty is commonplace in the human condition, a facet of many lives, and not restricted to old age – but prominent of the last phase of life and advanced age. The possibility of frailty may invoke fear, not only in general, but in me, potentially facing it. And it is hard not only to face frailty oneself, but also to face frailty in another: we may *fear* weakness as well as power, both in self and in others. Fear of a frail 'other' may contribute even to deficiencies in communication and care.

There is no place in the context of frailty for what is sometimes called the 'Tarzan complex', so pervasive in our times, a time when personal power is glorified and weakness denigrated. And this, at a time of the need for imagination and the continual shaping and reshaping of possibility even in the midst of weakness. For, on the other hand, in some contexts frailty is also highly valued – consider the delicacy of porcelain, of a butterfly's wings, of a gossamer thread … sometimes the stuff of poetry. Could the frail person ever be seen as beautiful and valuable as rare porcelain? What would it take to have such a seismic cultural shift? What would it cost society (or me) to look frailty in the face? Yet the facing of not only frailty (fragility) but actual brokenness in oneself (without despairing) is a larger task, not to be accomplished alone.

In fact, frailty, the propensity for being broken, like the fact of inevitable death, provides a frame in which one's basic notions may be tested, like an alloy in fire. It is a complex evocative human reality worth careful exploration in case such consideration yields a new sense of possibility and responsibility – especially on the part of those like physicians radically committed to the human good and the furthering of human flourishing, come what may – to say nothing of the challenge for oneself. Clearly some notion of the human good – and of concomitant human flourishing must enter in to any adequate consideration, and such is the stuff of the human wisdom tradition – that which is *handed over* from generation to generation. But however human good and human flourishing are envisaged, frailty appears to be a danger to their achievement, and especially in our time.

So, late old age has many recognisable features. But *is this period essentially different from any other period of life?* – really different? It has always been the case that we cannot determine the cards dealt to play with, only how we play. It has always been the case that the task of life is to become what we may truly be. We need *wisdom*: where is wisdom to be found *now*? now, when our institutions are failing, and reflection seems stifled by the rush of things. Yet, wisdom may still be sought above all in persons, in the root notions of traditions, in art, in writings, in named disciplines, in literature, and notably in poetry. Recently, literary critic Harold Bloom (1930–2019), in a pensive mood after recovering from a near fatal cardiac illness which reduced his activity for many months, wrote, 'At the gates of death, I have recited poems to myself, but not searched for an interlocutor to engage in dialectic': for him, in his extremity, only the poetry he remembered nourished the mind and heart.[4]

He further wrote: 'We cannot all become philosophers, but we can follow the poets in their ancient quarrel with philosophy, which may be a way of life but whose study is death'.

So he sought instead the *poets* as distillers of wisdom. In the *Hebrew Scriptures*, in the drama of Job within the so-called wisdom literature, Job burst into poetry: philosophy was of little use. Nevertheless, there may still be a place for considering philosophers in our tradition – maybe a resonance will occasionally carry us through our nights, when we most need light.

Human life is beset with questions – the *Hebrew Scriptures* at the basis of much of Western civilisation spelled some of them out thus: God to Adam: 'Adam, where are you?' Cain: 'Am I my brother's keeper?' Philosophers also articulated them: for Immanuel Kant (1724–1804) philosophy could cohere around three questions: 'What can I know? What should I do? What can I hope?'[5] and Ernst Bloch (1880–1959): 'Who am I? Where did I come from? Where am I going?'[6] Kant offered, late in his career, his solutions to his three questions, but each of us must formulate an individual construct.

There is a burgeoning literature on seventeenth century philosopher, Baruch Spinoza (1632–1677), based in Amsterdam, well aware of the appalling suffering of the Jews in the Iberian Peninsula which made his family flee to Amsterdam where they joined the Jewish community. Steeped in both philosophical and rabbinical traditions, a forerunner of Enlightenment he offers rich insights apposite for our times. Spinoza was a Marrano, thus a marginal man, what Yirmiyahu Yovel (1935–2018) calls a ' multilayered' individual, welding several cultures, modes of thinking, and indeed of being.[7] Yovel perceives the Marrano as a foreshadow of the modern individual emerging later in Europe. Cast out from the Portuguese-Jewish congregation in Amsterdam as a 'heretic' (the excommunication was lifted in the last century) he remained profoundly Jewish. In the boldness of his deep-rooted thought, he questioned the transcendence of God, the divine origin of the *Hebrew Scriptures*, and individual immortality – and throughout it all he opened up far richer perspectives which could found a new and radical humanism: surely a task for our times.

Spinoza is (to me) somehow reminiscent of a contemporary physician, made in a sense marginal not by being 'cast out' but by our privileged experience of the heights and depths of humanness, and the tutelage of our patients. While we are deeply conscious of our complexity, our multilayered selves – we hide it. The bonds of physicians with one another may stem from our common struggles together at the limits of human life; we know the edge of it, its limits and possibilities, even if we do not speak about it even to close ones, for we mostly lack the language in which to dare to articulate what we know. It is of interest that Spinoza had an eminent physician as his close friend and was much respected by the German theologian Henry Oldenburg (1619–1677), a leading light in the newly established Royal Society – at a time of hostility between England and The Netherlands.

Spinoza, not only in his own person, but in what he wrote, most of which was published after his death offers insights which are useful for any stage of life, but (I think) poignantly relevant in very old age: some may be worth mention. Australian philosopher Genevieve Lloyd has made his ideas remarkably accessible.[8,9] Several of the fundamental concepts of Spinoza offer food for thought as one, even an ageing physician, explores the big questions.

1
Spinoza's concept of conatus as the essence of a living thing: the striving to continue in being

A central Spinozian concept is that of *conatus,* an old word best translated as 'striving to continue in being'. Spinoza considered the human *essence* to be *conatus.* In fact, he thought conatus was the essence not only of the human, and of all living things, but of all things. There is a vigour in his concept.

We, the very elderly have surely *experienced* what Spinoza intuited, that the essence (not property) of a living thing is its 'striving to continue in being'. We experience in ourselves the striving: we know the compulsion to be true to our human *vocation* to respond to the call of one in need of us – an imperative brought to a fine focus in the life of a clinician. And we have seen the striving in a weak new born baby or a patient emerging into life again after being near death. And we have witnessed in others the striving cease.

Conventional terms like 'life force' do not wholly express what Spinoza was articulating. Striving for me (as an ageing person) to continue in being implies the impulse to continue to try to become what I really am – there is even a note of 'ontological' authenticity here. Does this mean that I strive to continue to live even if at the increasing expense of others? Never yield to the idea that the time has come to die? American philosopher Margaret Battin (1940 –) wrote years ago of the 'challenge to our moral selves' of at least refraining from claiming expensive medical resources as we are about to die, if the resources saved could be transferred to more needy others, especially if mechanisms could be constructed to reduce global inequities in care.[10] Incidentally, the development, even publication in our journals, of policies constructed by persons at the height of their powers about when elderly or frail (at any age) persons should be given access to expensive health services, or 'treated', risks diminishing the awareness of the agency of each of us vulnerable persons – as if we ourselves did not realise the issues at stake, nor were capable of recognising when the time had come for measures to maximise our function, comfort and dignity, rather than increasingly futile efforts to reverse disease. For the vulnerable or frail, each of whom is a unique person, to be as it were, de-differentiated, homogenised, considered *en masse* as a problem in society to be solved (even if using the language of concerned compassion) is a frightening notion. For we individuals, unique persons, are already in danger of being demoralised by our apparent uselessness in society, and we, above all, realise that we are indeed a burden: a fact which cannot be denied, yet a truth which must be tempered by adequate understanding of the personal and our possibilities as community.[11]

So, striving to continue in being ordinarily implies the striving to continue to live as well as possible within whatever limits prevail. But could it be acknowledged that there may indeed be a duty to request or assent to be allowed to die (in the midst of as good a care as is reasonably affordable given the resource restraints in our context) if our being sustained is costing others too dearly? Indeed, also, there may well come a time when to continue in authentic being means to allow oneself to die, hopefully with dignity in the midst of good care, as a time of completion, even celebration, not negation of life – and (in Spinoza's terms) all as 'part of nature' now even more clearly manifest. Such a perspective on life at any adult age, but especially in old age, and acquiescence in its closing, is in *no* way supportive of notions of suicide (however 'assisted') or euthanasia (however euphemised), nor of devaluing the most weak in society as 'unworthy of life'.

2
The human person as part of nature

This notion is liberating! The image of the human as 'master' of nature is so very sad as well as dangerous and disturbing. The recognition of our place in an interconnected web of all that is, part of the fabric of nature, issues in calm. The implications are endless. Spinoza sees no *purpose* (or meaning) to be sought and found in the universe – the universe is not teleological; we, through our emergent capacities, energised in our striving, *construct* purpose and meaning: this notion is liberating indeed!

There is room also for a far more adequate notion of 'person': the philosophical tradition includes relational views, and Spinoza is a valuable contributor. He recognised that I, as a person, *essentially* interconnected in time and horizontally (so to speak), with other persons, am part of nature, part of the whole, participant in its interconnectedness, with responsibilities to care for the whole (especially but not only the most proximate) according to my capacity. I as human am not above the rest of nature, just part. Sometimes Spinoza is said to be the forerunner of 'deep ecology' – certainly the stress on interconnectedness makes for a rich view of personal being. I am what and who I am in connectivity with other persons, place, and with what other persons have done, thought and been – what I know as history, culture and remember – and maybe hope in or dream about. The relational view of a human person is central to Spinoza's concepts; he does not go further to conceive of relations as *constitutive* of 'person', but it would be of interest to discuss this concept with scholars deeply immersed in his thought.

3
Freedom in contingency

The history of freedom as an idea is complex – and cannot be even hinted at here. The focus here is kept on the individual acting person. There are ideas, emphasised currently, that freedom (like dignity) is vested in autonomy – 'self-rule'. Each of us must form some concept of the good, and accept responsibility for what we do and become, but thoughtful consideration should lead to a realisation that freedom is not merely the right to choose or control. There is a mood, at least in the West, for glorifying choice not as a means but as an end in itself (even in health care), as a central expression of autonomy; and also a tendency, in the name of autonomy, for success to be measured by the pushing away of all obstacles to individual desires, and frustration in the face of what must be, of what philosophers call 'necessity'. Such notions betray, I think, an inadequate concept of autonomy, and even if pervading the culture, require deep scrutiny. Such matters are a backdrop to living in old age and may come together critically in the making of difficult clinical decisions. In fact, the freedom which education gives is not freedom of action but freedom of thought, and these matters require pondering especially by the privileged and those in power.

Autonomy specifies the ruling of self by self and is indeed a highly esteemed value in contemporary Western culture – although there are ironic notes in the history of its exercise, even in the West. In the first century of the European colonisation of Australia, soon after convict transportation had ceased but when cruelties were persisting, notably towards the indigenous inhabitants of Australia (who had never ceded sovereignty) the English philosopher, John Stuart Mill (1806–1873), in his essay entitled *'On Liberty'* (first published in 1859) exalted individualism and non-interference by others, even for motives of beneficence:

> The principle is, that the sole end for which mankind is warranted, individually or collectively, in interfering with the liberty of action of any of their number is self-protection. That the only purpose for which power can be rightfully exercised over any member of a civilized community, against his will, is to prevent harm to others. His own good, either physical or moral, is not a sufficient warrant.

Some paragraphs later Mill further notes:

> Each is the proper guardian of his own health, whether bodily, or mental or spiritual. Mankind are greater gainers by suffering each other to live as seems good to themselves, than by compelling each to live as seems good to the rest.[12]

Clearly the health of individuals and the community presupposes and is expressed in liberty. But how free are we in the decisions we make? How diverse are our perceptions of the 'good'? And, tellingly, how truly individual are our actions in the light of an adequate (and I now consider, relational) concept of person, with implications of how we understand human dignity, and indeed human suffering, and human complexity? These questions have abiding relevance, notably the issue raised concerning whether or not one's individual actions are truly individual. I would suggest that the nature of persons in the human web is such that hardly any so-called 'individual' action fails to have social dimensions; indeed, actions sometimes spoken of as 'private' or 'individual' are intrinsically as well as extrinsically *social* – such as *how* we are born, live, suffer, or *how* we love, hate, face frailty in our old age, or die. This needs much pondering if we are to judge wisely. When should I insist on a so-called 'individual' action which is intrinsically social – with social consequences? And when is it justified for others to intervene to restrict my freedom, or privacy for the sake of my good or of others (even my family or carers) – or community? Serious questions always and all this may be hard for me to think through if my cognitive powers are waning (as is almost inevitable in very old age) – and impossible if significant dementia supervenes – as becomes increasingly possible after 'the decade for dying'.

Spinoza offered an alternative concept, far richer than currently prevailing notions, many of which are traceable to René Descartes (1596–1650). As Genevieve Lloyd (1941–) wrote:

> In Descartes' treatment of freedom, an inherently free will forces back ever further the limits of what must be accepted as beyond human control. The prevailing imagery is of border skirmishes ... Spinoza offers instead a vision of freedom as the joyful acceptance of what must be ... [F]reedom derives from the active engagement of the mind with necessity, an engagement that flows from the understanding of the truth'.[13]

Freedom understood as the 'joyful acceptance of what must be' is surely not a recipe for passivity or fatalism – nor sheer Stoicism! Spinoza is the same philosopher who highlighted the impulse inherent in all living things, *conatus* – a striving to continue in being, a long way from conventional determinism. Discussion of the nuances of Spinoza concerning personal freedom and its limitations cannot be undertaken here. Suffice to note that we need freely to accept what must be ... And how to do this if cognitively compromised? That indeed is the question, while our carers strive to diminish suffering and maintain what flourishing is possible – and to minimise threats (including pharmacological) to cognition; there are clinical imperatives in these words, and grounds for gratitude.

It was widely rumoured in his time (and written since then) that Spinoza denied 'free will': he did insist that the laws of nature cannot be broken – he denied the possibility of miracles, but he conceived that we are free within contingency. Descartes thought that freedom resided in the will, whereas Spinoza stressed our knowing. Surely, he would have agreed with Victor Frankl: 'to take an attitude in a given set of circumstances' may be a stance of the mind, rather than an exercise of will, but one must concede that the differentiation may be somewhat blurred.

This is all a far cry from the glorification of 'choice' or misunderstood autonomy. The highest expression of autonomy (and personal liberty) may indeed be the yielding of control, to surrender in trust to the kindness of strangers. It is hard to learn this! (Cain asked: Am I my brother's keeper? Cain's question still stands and the answer may be unwelcome – and there is a twist to it: we, in a profound sense, whilst being responsible selves, also may need to be keeper of 'proximate others' – and need in turn to accept one day the 'keeping', by another! Indeed, 'another may gird thee' – words also found in sacred texts.)

4

The highest exercise of human knowing

It has been mentioned that Spinoza may offer a way into a new humanism, a frame for our times: a humanism which considers the human awareness of a relation with All-That-Is, however named, and however expressed – often in ritual which might be called 'religious'. Anthropologist David Rappaport considered ritual as a critical element in the evolution of humanity – not the biological evolution of the modern human but of *humanity*.[14] Neil Gillman offers a perspective of religion and ritual which Spinoza would have I think approved, worth a lengthy quotation:

> [T]he function of religion is to discern and describe the sense of ultimate order that pervaded the universe and human experience ... The whole purpose of religion, its liturgies, rituals, and institutions, is to highlight, preserve, and concretize this experience this sense of cosmos, and to recapture it in the face of the chaos that hovers perpetually around the fringes of our lives as we live them within history.[15]

Such a perspective would be a useful antidote to the travesties of religion tearing at the fabric of our world – and is relevant in the search for a new and inclusive humanism.

Spinoza was scorned in his day as an atheist and, in my view, misunderstood even by thinkers of renown today. In fact, his concept of God is rich and deep. He sees God as not essentially transcendent, separate from material reality, but rather, as immanent in all reality. He should be labelled as a panentheist (which label implies the idea of an immanent God also overflowing, transcending the universe).[15] Thinkers continue to probe into the 'history of God'. Christian theologians rejoice in the notion of transcendence *and* immanence – with some overflow of God as the beyond in the midst. But not only Christian: rabbis traditionally recognizing immanence insisted on a nuance of overflow – 'God is the place of the world, but God's place is not the world', and, in our times, redolent notes are implicit in the writings of some theologians, including contemporary Jewish liturgical sources[16] and thinkers such as Neil Gillman (1933–2017) in his later writings.[17] The idea of God, whether or not wholly immanent, offers as Wordsworth might say – a precious place for the 'mountings of the mind' – and a grandeur for the mind to dwell on, or gaze on. Spinoza wrote that the highest activity of the human person is to gaze on God.[18] At the very least there is a focus here for the quiet or unquiet mind, in the midst (or at the waning of) the striving (*conatus*) which is the essence of life.

Is there more to say on the God question? Moses in the encounter with the burning bush (Exodus 3:15) was conscious of a deeper level of reality. The question he asked 'Who are you?' and the response may haunt the mind. I gaze in awe at the whole and know that even I am simply part of the whole. Our scientists discover more and more of the whole, even in its mathematical uniformity allowing us to land on the moon or utilise cyberspace. What a piece of work is man – as discoverer! But as a human person, radically part of the whole, even I with my emergent complexity as a person, cannot *exceed* the whole. The whole therefore must have the complexity of the personal: but 'person' is intrinsically relational. Is the whole radically relational? Does the whole *care* about that which is sustained, energised? If so, does this care ever involve contravention of cosmic law, even mathematical law, that is, the order in the universe which is to me the most evident manifestation of the unity of the whole? In other words is the Whole (which I may call 'God') ever *interventional*? I personally think not. But to gaze at the whole, of which I am a faint reflection ('image') as well as part, and because of this, have deep affinity of which I am, at some times more than other, aware: this is my glory and my peace. 'What a piece of work is man'! Indeed. And as a woman, I may not only gaze, but take it all in, interiorise it, *incorporate* it …

Can Spinoza's notion of the highest human good being to gaze on God, as immanent in all reality (and somehow more), be powerful enough to sustain one even when the 'centre seems not to be holding' (a nod to WB Yeats' *The Second Coming*)?

Is this powerful enough to sustain not only patients but also *doctors* in distress? And we doctors do know distress. But what of frailty – feared maybe by the very elderly more than the reality of approaching death? Can Spinoza illuminate the ambiguity of frailty – treasured, even revered, and yet feared? Maybe. I think so. Spinoza's enhancement of the concept of freedom within contingency, the perspective of being part of nature, complementing the steady 'gaze' on the unity within all, may help the centre hold, come what may.

And when dying? Surely the boundary between myself and the rest of nature is now yielding – the differentiation between myself and the rest of nature is diminishing. Dust to dust ... It may be appropriate to turn to another philosopher to complement the perspective of Spinoza. Ernst Bloch, a twentieth century philosopher also within the Jewish tradition, but, like Spinoza, outwardly marginally so. Bloch wrote of death as the master-test of our journeyman years, a test of our inner metaphysics. In his words:

> ... if in view of death the inner man comes wholly into the open – death serves as the master-test of our journeyman years. It tests the height we have reached, the value of our inner metapsychics; it examines its strength, its utility, durability, and suitability in mobilization ... it introduces a factor alien to the subject and thus summons us directly from the subjectively ideal sphere, from the freely suspended realm of self-definitions, to the 'cosmic' realm of danger and diffusion, and of the gathering from the bustle of this world of death in which the self finally proves itself, after all.[19]

What could this mean – 'our inner metapsychics'? Our interior intellectual architecture? The shape of our interior colloquium? Each of us has values, and principles we live by, despite our failures, and aspirations, and personal priorities. Very few may know these aspects of our individual humanness. Each of us may, in fact, live according to what medical ethicists noted as four ethical principles: beneficence (doing good), non-maleficence (not doing harm), autonomy ('self-rule') and justice (to individuals and society). The average conscientious person lives by these notions, without maybe naming them – and the way we understand and live them is profoundly influenced by the cultural context within which we live as well as our personal nurturing, education and history. The philosophical tradition has wrestled with these matters. All come to fine focus when one is not only caring for the frail, but also when living with frailty. There is a case for thinking about each of these four 'principles' in relation to frailty – both caring for the frail and enduring frailty. There may be much that is contentious in Bloch's words, including the unspoken question: does it *matter*, what or who I have, by my death, become? But there is need to ponder them.

To return (maybe with relief) to Spinoza. It may be that a recovery of Spinoza's insistence on the highest good being awareness of All-That-Is as the unifying anchor of life, however fragile, maybe the pointer to the recovery of integrity, the elusive wholeness possible for each of us unique persons, even as we approach the close of life. Is *this* 'salvation' which Spinoza mentions in the closing lines of *The Ethics*? Spiritual growth may be just this – the increasing clarity of awareness, and 'spiritual care' (that controversial element in care) simply the facilitation of just this process, mainly by ensuring a clearing and utmost personal privacy. The place is holy ground – and one (especially, but not only, a carer especially professional) should take off one's shoes.

5
The thought world and the eternity of the mind

Spinoza anchors the mind in the body. My mind is virtually the unique pattern of my thought activity and leaves its traces in the vast neuronal complexities of my brain: this is in accord with contemporary neuroscience. Spinoza saw the thought world, anchored in the material, as eternal – and on death, one's thoughts (as now) merge imperceptibly and forever into the thought world, the eternal mind. One's thinking is finished when one dies but not lost – simply part of the whole. For better or worse.

Spinoza denied the immortality of the body – or the immortality of the soul (of which he had no concept): he was a master of the philosophical tradition but clearly diverged from much of it. His position again placed him at odds with religious traditions as widely (but in my view unnecessarily) understood – and with much religious authority, then and now. Spinoza alienated many contemporaries by denying personal immortality – a central tenet of the Christian theological tradition. But he had a view concerning the eternity (not 'immortality') of the mind, a view which, to the mind of this non-philosopher, rings true, and is indeed, consoling. He considered that what we have contributed to human thought is, as it were, gathered up into the thought world which parallels the material universe – and is thereby eternal. Contemporary physicians, imbued as we are by some of the principles of the humanist tradition and contemporary possibilities for its reframing whilst retaining respect for other traditions, may find these ideas resonating with our experience as well as our aspirations.[20]

One becomes aware also of the limitations of one's knowing and understanding but also of the fact that as ageing clinicians taught by our patients (and our failures and successes) we have a store of human experience which may illumine the common search of all scholarly disciplines for understanding not only the natural world, but, within it, the human person, and the place of persons as connected with all nature. We are singularly aware of the interconnectedness of the material web and of the web of thought in which we are individually embedded and we recognise with Spinoza, the power of knowing, the power of being wholly *aware*. Is it possible that, even in very advanced age, in sight maybe of 'harbour' and as we struggle with meaning in modes not experienced since the heady days of adolescence, that some of the notions of Spinoza may assist our centre to 'hold' even in extremity, and even as we are yielding?

Spinoza closes the *Ethics* with the following words, which despite their complexity, are worth close pondering:

> An ignorant man, besides being agitated in many ways by external causes, never possessing true contentment of mind also lives as it were unaware of himself, God, and things, and as soon as he ceases to be passive, ceases to be. On the other hand, the wise man ... is scarcely moved in spirit: he is aware of himself, of God, and things by certain eternal necessity, he never ceases to be, but always possesses true contentment of mind. If the road I have shown to lead to this is very difficult, it can yet be discovered. And clearly it must be hard when it is so seldom found. For how could it be that if salvation were close at hand and could be found without difficulty it should be neglected by almost all? But all excellent things are as difficult as they are rare.[21]

Is it the case that in very old age do we need not only care in our frailty, but above all, a *clearing* – the space in which we may grow in being wholly aware? A professor of anatomy in our region wrote that it is the task of medicine to manifest man's interior splendour:[22] can one bear the unmasking, here, now? Is this the task, now?

References

1. Lickiss N., *Living in the decade for dying: the years of living dangerously*.
2. Auerbach E., *Mimesis: The Representation of Reality in Western Literature* (1942–45), Translated WR Trask, Princeton University Press, Princeton, 2003.
3. Cassell E, 'The goal of medicine the relief of suffering', *New England Journal of Medicine*, 1982, 306: 639–645.
4. Bloom H., *Where Shall Wisdom to be found?*, Riverhead Books, New York, 2005.
5. Kant I., *Critique of Pure Reason*, 1781–87.
6. Bloch E., *The Principle of Hope*, Translated by N Plaice, S Plaice and P Knight, Blackwell, Oxford, 1986, p1.
7. Yovel Y., *The Other Within. The Marranos: Split Identity and Emerging Modernity*, Princeton University Press, Princeton, 2009.
8. Lloyd G., *Part of Nature: Self-Knowledge in Spinoza's Ethics*, Cornell University Press, London, 1994.
9. Lloyd G., *Spinoza and the Ethics*, Routledge, London, 1996.
10. Battin MP., 'Global life expectancies and the duty to die', in *Is There a Duty to Die?*, eds JM Humber and RF Almeder, Humana Press, Totowa, New Jersey, 2000, pp 3–21.
11. Lickiss N., 'On facing human suffering', in *Perspectives on Human Suffering*, ed J Malpas and N Lickiss, Springer, Dordrecht, 2012, pp 245 –260. (see also 'On personal care', Barbara Leroy Memorial Lecture, NSW Palliative Care Association, 2014).
12. Mill JS., 'On Liberty' (1859) in *Utilitarianism, On Liberty, An Essay on Bentham*, by J S Mill, ed. M Warnock, Collins, 1962.
13. Lloyd G., *Providence Lost*, Harvard University Press, Cambridge Mass, 2008, p200 ff.
14. Rappaport RA., *Ritual and Religion in the Development of Humanity*, Cambridge University Press, Cambridge, 1999.
15. Gillman N., *Doing Jewish Theology*, Jewish Lights Publishing, Woodstock, Vermont, 2008, p3.
16. Plaut WG (ed), *The Torah: A Modern Commentary*, Union for Reform Judaism, New York, 2005, note 38, p 211 and 1509 (attributed to R Eliezer).
17. Gillmann N., *Believing and Its Tensions*, Jewish Lights Publishing, Woodstock, Vermont, 2013.
18. Lloyd G., *Spinoza and the Ethics*, op.cit, pp109 –131.
19. Bloch E., Karl Marx, 'Death and the Apocalypse' in *Man on His Own: Essays on the Philosophy of Religion*, trans by EB Ashton, Herder and Herder, New York, 1970, p47.
20. Dalmasio A., *Looking for Spinoza*, Vintage, London, 2004.

21 Spinoza B., *The Ethics* (1675), translated A Boyle and GHR Parkinson. Dent, London, 1989.
22 Mortimer K., 'The impossible profession: the doctor-priest relationship', *Proc Aust Assoc Gerontol* 1974 2:81–82.

IV
Spinoza and Medical Practice: Can the Philosophy of Baruch Spinoza Enrich the Thinking of Doctors?
2019

(An edited version appeared on line in Hectoen International Journal 2019)

Background
Contemporary doctors, like those who lived before us, seek to assuage the distress of our fellows by application of our competence in response to their need, seeking to relieve distress, guard or restore personal dignity and walk the walk with our fellows even as they are dying. So why the disquiet? There are facts suggesting profound disquiet, albeit well disguised: high rates of substance abuse, burnout, suicide ... and this in persons of exceptional intelligence, personal capacity, high socioeconomic status, in unquestionably 'meaningful' occupations. Why?

The literature of the great traditions is weighty with exploration of the great questions, spoken by our conspecifics, even fellow professionals ... Where are you, Adam? Am I my brother's keeper? Where do I come from? Why am I here? Where am I going? What shall I do to inherit eternal life? Or, [Immanuel] Kant's three questions: What can I know? What should I do? What can I hope? The great philosophers have searched such questions. Religious leaders have formulated various and varying responses – but we may cringe in hidden unbelief. We are limited in our knowledge of the thought world of our time, and limited (ever since adolescence) in the time we have for reading or discussing ideas which may replenish parched wells within us: we are always so busy. The urge may take over to settle for living without any overarching vision. But without vision the people perish, the prophet says, and so may I perish. Is there any way to enrich our lives, give our roots rain?

Many persons have found the thinking of the 17C philosopher Baruch Spinoza to be a source of richness: writers like Goethe, Heinrich Heine and George Eliot as well as significant philosophers like [Georg] Hegel and [Friedrich] Nietzsche. Australian philosopher Genevieve Lloyd, in her fine introduction to Spinoza, quoting the pertinent comments of French philosopher [Gilles] Deleuze, writes:

> This 'most philosophic of philosophers', commanding a highly developed, systematic and scholarly conceptual apparatus, can nonetheless be the quintessential object of an immediate, unprepared encounter, such that a non-philosopher, or even someone without formal education, can receive a sudden illumination from him, a 'flash'.[1]

His life as a Marrano, had layers of complexity not unknown to our contemporary selves (even as physicians) and thoughtfully explored by philosopher [Yirmiyahu] Yovel.[2,3] But aside from the vagaries of his life, some of his ideas may be worth pondering, despite the complexity of his thought. It is useful to be introduced by wise guides. Clinical colleague, psychiatrist Irvin Yalom, gives a sense of his life in his philosophical novel, *The Spinoza Problem*:[4] in fact one of his closest friends in Amsterdam was a physician, and he was much admired by one of the founders of the (London) Royal Society. His thought however enraged philosophers and theologians of his time – he was regarded, for a start, as an atheist and heretic; he was expelled, at 24, from the (traditional) Amsterdam synagogue. However, Spinoza is now widely regarded as one of the forerunners of the Enlightenment, and a potential light for our 21C path.

These few volumes mentioned might together offer a useful platform for doctors beginning to think about the thought of this extraordinary man. It is a rare delight to free one's mind to explore Spinoza's thought-world, despite the limits of our understanding.

What key ideas (key for us doctors) emerge? I list them, as I see them, not in any particular logical order:

1. An ecological view of all reality: we as humans are interconnected part of the whole – not master, not servant, not interpreter, just part of Nature. The human person within the whole is an emergent phenomenon: increasing complexity brings with it the possibility of increased awareness. There is order in Nature and I as a person am part of that order. I have my place in the pattern of it all.

2. Nature is not teleological – there is no 'purpose', no ultimate goal to be striven for, just the energy within all things (which Spinoza calls *conatus*, reviving an old term) impelling each thing, including each person, to continue in being.

3. The mind is grounded in the body, an idea of the body. Minds are inserted into the totality (as Lloyd puts it). The thought world, grounded in the body, is eternal. There is no personal immortality. Death is not a passage into another mode of existence, but an illustration of how I am part of Nature; as a person I cease to be, but my thoughts are incorporated into the eternal mind. Spinoza's concept of the body resonates with present medical understanding. Lloyd writes (p55), 'the human body is

thus a composite individual, a union of parts acting as a centre of communicating and communicated motion. Each individual body exerts a causal force on others. Each needs for its preservation a great many other bodies, by which it is, as it were, continually regenerated'.[5]

4. Cognition, knowledge is crucial in our personal function. Emotions are kept in check not by will (eg repression) but by thought/knowing.

5. Far from being 'Godless' Spinoza offers many almost tantalising notions concerning 'God'. God is in all, and all is contained in God. There is no concept of 'God' as transcendent, separate from Nature – 'God' is wholly immanent. There is profound unity in the whole – and this unity may be called 'God'. It is the atheist of Amsterdam who insists that the 'intellectual love of God', gazing on this wholly immanent God, this unity, in which we as part of Nature are contained, this whole as *conatus*, is the highest form of knowledge we may attain. The fact that we can gaze on God may be an inspiration and source of strength. There is no end to wonder.

6. All is determined. This immanent 'God' does not intervene to break the laws of nature – there are no 'miracles', and prayers of supplication to change nature are meaningless (save to articulate the expansive awareness of the supplicant). But freedom is to be found within contingency, within necessity. Spinoza moves away from Descartes on this matter.

> Genevieve Lloyd:
>
> In Descartes's treatment of freedom, an inherently free will forces back ever further the limits of what must be accepted as beyond human control. The prevailing imagery is of border skirmishes …

> Spinoza offers instead a vision of freedom as the
> joyful acceptance of what must be ... [F]reedom
> derives from the active engagement of the mind
> with necessity, an engagement that flows from the
> understanding of the truth'.[6]

Freedom understood as the 'joyful acceptance of what must be' is surely not a recipe for passivity or fatalism – nor sheer Stoicism! Spinoza is the same philosopher who highlighted the impulse inherent in all living things, what he called *conatus* – a striving to continue in being.

It is clear (to me) that Spinoza's notions (merely touched on) have relevance to how we live, how we think about our responsibility to realise fully what we as individual persons are or should be as simply one element in an interconnected whole, what we hope for, and how we think about dying in which we prepare to be more evidently part of the whole. Clearly we are being encouraged me to accept freely what must be, whilst at the same time striving to relieve suffering and to enhance human flourishing, all the while striving to continue in being, to become what we may be, and truly are: there is no passive acquiescence to 'fate' here, but deliberate and thoughtful dynamism.

There are pointers also about how to think about 'spiritual care' which, when mentioned, often leads busy clinicians (say, at a meeting) to glance away or be very busy. Any idea that we ourselves need 'spiritual care' is usually cast aside, not from disrespect but because the notions spelt out by some colleagues have no resonance in our thought world.

Yet the ramifications of these seminal ideas are in fact very precious, and each physician (as unique person) will appropriate, and indeed *embody* them in a distinct fashion: the mind is changed (and *pari passu*) the brain is changed by the acquisition of new concepts. I form a new synthesis, as I connect thoughts, and the new synthesis is embodied in the neuronal complexities of my brain – and I remember; neuroscientists have much to glean.[7]

In the midst of deep disquiet there is the longing in many thoughtful physicians for healing, for 'salvation', for 'redemption' – and the ideas peddled by religious institutions seem often so very alien. Can Spinoza's frame offer anything? I think, yes. My redemption may involve the deliberate and painful turning of my being so that I gaze more and more at 'God' – the Other within all that is (rather than focus on myself); religious rituals may help me undertake such a turn of my inmost being – away from narcissism, acquisitiveness and hyperactivity desiccating the soul. Religion has been critical in the *making* of humanness[8] and is best understood not as a matter of belief, but a dimension of human *being*: we ignore the symbolic universe to our peril. We spend our privileged clinical lives seeking to heal the world in the spirit of the Hebrew *Tikkun olam*:[9] we may ourselves find healing in this gaze, this awareness of the whole and one's place in it, this radical connectivity. Spinoza at the end of his masterpiece, *The Ethics*, writes of 'true contentment of mind' as the fruit of such awareness. He concludes with the following words, which could have been written for ourselves:

> If the road I have shown to lead to this is very difficult, it yet can be discovered. And clearly it must be hard when it is so seldom found. For how could it be that if salvation were close at hand and could be found without difficulty it should be neglected by almost all? But all excellent things are as difficult as they are rare.[10]

Can one say that there is a basis here in the seminal ideas of Spinoza, for a new and radical humanism? Maybe. Maybe indeed.

REFERENCES

1 Lloyd G., *Spinoza and the Ethics*, Routledge, Milton Park, 1996, p23.
2 Yovel Y., *Spinoza and Other Heretics*, Vol 1, The Marrano of Reason, Princeton University Press, Princeton, New York, 1998.
3 Yovel Y., *The Other Within: The Marranos, Split Identity and Emerging Modernity*, Princeton University Press, Princeton, 2006, p358.
4 Yalom I., *The Spinoza Problem*, Basic Books, New York, 2013.
5 Lloyd G., *Spinoza and the Ethics*, Op cit. p55.
6 Lloyd G., *Providence Lost*, Harvard University Press, Cambridge Mass, 2008, p200 ff.
7 Damasio A., *Looking for Spinoza*, Vintage, London, 2004.
8 Rappaport R., *Ritual and Religion in the Making of Humanity*, Cambridge, University Press, Cambridge, 2004.
9 Sacks J., *To Heal a Fractured World: The Ethics of Responsibility, Continuum*, New York, 2005.
10 Spinoza, B., *The Ethics*, Trans. A Boyle and GHR Parkinson, Dent, London, 1989, p223.

V

THE TASKS OF LATENESS: AN EXPLORATION OF LIVING LATE
2020

Literature and art are replete with images of later human life, such as the measured active folding up of affairs seen in the last days of the patriarchs – think of the last days of Moses and of Joseph; the anguished King Lear on the moors; words of deprivation if not ruin in the poem of Yeats *'A tattered man upon a stick*; words of rage *'against the dying of the light'*; or acquiescence to the outgoing tide. Matthew Arnold may have been writing of the tide of faith in *'On Dover Beach'* but the image may have been a metaphor for much more. Edward Said wrote a set of essays *'On Late Style'* relating particularly to ageing composers.[1] Harold Bloom has published a book of last poems *Till I End My Song*.[2] Many muse on death as the horizon looms more clearly, and it is logical to do so, just as the young muse on what to become or the dreamed-of soul mate. Literature is replete with the human rhythm, even at its fading: I cannot add to this store of riches ... Yet *Old men should be explorers*, wrote TS Eliot.[3] Is there anything worth exploring, now?

Each one of us experiences living, its moments, its phases, its light and dark, differently. I do not see late life as a time of folding up, but of exploration, truly. George Eliot warned us in *Daniel Deronda*: 'There is a great deal of unmapped country within us which would have to be taken into account in an explanation of our gusts and storms'.[4] Indeed, the terrain – that unmapped country, may differ from that of previous parts of life, but so do the tools, and so do the tasks which beckon, and the questions which fascinate.

1
A note on exploration

What does the terrain look like? Well, it is, for a start, uneven, rough, mountainous, with a windy hardly visible track, with many alternative paths even if the direction appears constant. Wild winds or monsoonal rain sometimes induces sheer oblivion, and at other times progress may be slow. Stuff does happen! But usually even if walking is not easy or stopped (actually or metaphorically), thinking is possible, and emotions palpable – unless pharmaceutical efforts intrude far too much.

What tools are there? The machinery for exploration is in not so much the legs now (however fit!) but the mind, and the mind knows mountains (Wordsworth) and 'cliffs of fall'(Hopkins), sometimes clouds, but with lucidity between times.

Are there maps? No. Many have written much and taught much, and we are drowned with i*nformation* but information is not *knowledge* (which implies my grasping the information and making it my own), and knowledge is not *understanding*, which implies further interpretation, assiduous hermeneutic activity. The information I garnered in a lifetime has, then, to be sifted to retain only the significant (hard in the internet age), absorbed into my personal network of knowledge, and interpreted in the light of what else I know, until I have a grasp of its place in my world. Then, I need *wisdom* if the understanding has bearing on a task I am performing or a decision I must make – even if the decision I must make is an exercise of what Victor Frankl, a survivor of Auschwitz, called 'the last of human freedoms: to choose one's attitude in any given set of circumstances.'[5] It is easy to see why Solomon asked not for 'information', knowledge or understanding, but for *wisdom*.

But is not the philosophical tradition a guide to wisdom? Philosophers did indeed seek to enrich to ways of living: some more explicitly. Some contemporary philosophers offer guides to life, particularly late in life,[6,7] and popular philosophy abounds. But the deliberations even of distinguished philosophers often fail to nourish the ordinary person (or clinician) in mind or heart or engender wisdom, and frankly disappoint. We need to look elsewhere: but where? Where may wisdom be found now? Books are written about this! The late Harold Bloom, writing on this theme, recounted his near-death experience, noting that 'at the gates of death I did not seek interlocutors but poetry I remembered'.[8] This comment highlights the significance of poetry. It was the physician-poet William Carlos Williams who, highlighting the significance of late life context and of experience, left us these memorable words:

> It is difficult
> to get the news from poems
> yet men die miserably every day
> for lack
> of what is found there.[9]

What does 'experience' do to a person? How is the person I am now, both different and the same, as the person I was when being enthralled by the majesty of mountains as a medical student, or the vistas of ideas and knowledge available as a humanities student in Europe fifty years ago, or when scaling the cliffs of say professional competence, and then exercising responsibility in the middle years? Or, later, recognising that there are limitations to what can be achieved, some of them intrinsic to the self, others etched in the boundaries of context, others due to unrealistic dreams, while at the same time noting new horizons not previously seen because one was still in the valley?

What changes are wrought by the years?
The physiological changes are obvious – and here not worth further consideration: tomes are written, careers of gerontologist and geriatricians are vested in all this. What are the changes in my *person*? This is a critical question since my perspective is influenced not only by changes in my perception and capacity for interpretation but also by my context and standpoint: my ensuing personal *judgement* is an end result of all of this. At a time when artificial intelligence is in ascendency, the lineaments of personal judgement bear close scrutiny.[10]

2

Excursus: what is a 'person'? Further thoughts

First, I need an adequate notion of person. In 1967, when I was a young specialist internist, Jacob Needleman, in a communication of the New York Academy of Sciences stressed: '[w]hat medicine lacks is any fundamental notion of the nature of man and any remotely adequate understanding of that to which we refer as person'.[11] I thought I knew, because I had studied these things. What do philosophers and theologians and dictionaries – or even Wikipedia – say? There is a vast intellectual tradition concerning person, and some of it has been focussed on health care in our time.[12] But somehow this rich vein of thought proved little of practical use to me in my explorations. There didn't seem to be a concept of 'person' which could energise or frame either my experience of life in general or medical practice in particular.

At the time when Jacob Needleman was writing I was involved an investigation of the health of the Aboriginal people of Sydney, who afforded me the privilege of spending time in their homes in an attempt to learn how they lived and why their children were rumoured to be dying at alarming rates, even in Sydney hospitals.[13] In the course of this privileged experience I found myself trying to conceptualise how to understand an Aboriginal person. I built on the seminal ideas of John Apley, a paediatrician, who stated: 'a child is an ecological experiment' and developed what might be thought of as an ecological or relational model of 'person'. The core concept is that a person is *constituted* by relationships – with persons (including oneself), things, place, the past, and inheritance (biological and cultural), aspirations (through hope) – and with All-That-Is; these moieties are interiorised. The integrating principle during life of this whole complexus maybe what the 'soul' is. Human dignity is vested especially in the safeguarding of these constitutive relationships – torturers know that the breaking of these relationships is the path to the 'breaking' of a man or woman.[14,15] Human suffering is most precisely understood, after [Eric] Cassell, as a sense of impending personal disintegration: we know it colloquially as a sense of ' being about to go to pieces', and we even talk of 'breakdowns'.[16] This notion is in accord with the ecological concept of person with interiorised, indeed embodied, relationships.

The health care system, seeking explicitly to be 'person centred', should be founded on such concepts of 'person'. Levinas, well explicated in Australia by Desmond Manderson, has taught us that the philosophical basis of the duty of care, classically in the helping professions of law and medicine is not law or contract but the call of the other in need.[17] Threats to any of the constitutive relationships of a person renders a person needy, and this we, notably doctors, need to understand better, as we seek, as our core task, the safeguarding of the human good. The COVID-19 pandemic has highlighted specifically the fundamental role of personal relationships and how thriving depends on them: the realisation that these relations with place, persons, culture etc are not optional extras but constitutive of what we a*re* may give the needed extra spur to the redesign of procedures meant to restore or safeguard wellbeing throughout life (even at its close), and not only for aged persons.

Personal development (maybe better called 'evolution'?) over a lifetime has been extensively studied. Erik Erikson characterised life stages by stage-specific developmental tasks, the quality of fulfilment of which, in one stage, affects profoundly the capacity to address the tasks of the next and subsequent stages.[18] Other authors and researchers have differing formulations, but there appears agreement that life involves challenges and tasks which differ as life progresses, and even though patterns are discernible, each person is unique. Human complexity is manifest in manifold ways, not least in the diversity of evolutional patterns. The framing of personal evolution in stages may be enriched by a relational concept of person, already outlined.

Persons do change because the constitutive relations change! Relations are dynamic. Over time relationships ebb and flow, weaken and strengthen, any change from being positive to negative, with the impetus to engage turning from attraction to repulsion – but even if this occurs the pattern wrought by relations is still constitutive of that person. Over time, the relationship with place, with goods, with other persons, with inheritance, with biological roots, with culture – all evolve, fruitfully, happily, or painfully, destructively – and my story, my memory of the changes as well as items enters into the story which I am.

Persons change! What is constant? Persons are complex – and the complexity is in flux. The narrative is the continuity. One may muse that the *pattern* may be the constant – with the elements constituting the pattern changing inexorably over time. David Hume considered those who think they can find in themselves some perception of a self:

> But setting aside some metaphysicians of this kind, I may venture to affirm of the rest of mankind, that they are nothing but a bundle or collection of different perceptions, which succeed each other with an inconceivable rapidity, and are in perpetual flux and movement.[19]

And yet, there may be some resonance with Hume. Also, there may be some resonance here with the complexity theorists. In the early deliberations of theoretical biologist Stuart Kauffman concerning complexity, he wrote of 'non-equilibrium dissipative structures' as the basis of life.[20] It is consoling to see lack of equilibrium and complexity playing a positive role in the emergence of life, in creativity! – an idea worth pondering as a source of hope. He is consoling when he stresses 'life exists at the edge of chaos'.

What is certain is that the perspective of person as radically relational, and with the relations internalised, is fitting for an Australian today, for our first peoples, forebears on this land for over 60,000 years richly articulate human relationality and interconnectedness in a new key. Just one recent example: in an art exhibition of Saltwater Country, Northern Territory at The Maritime Museum Sydney a note attached to a painting read: 'Gumanti clan people say "I am from that water there, I am that water"'. And the accompanying note on the clan by Raymatta Marina read:

> The relationship is much more complete than just 'owning' or even 'caring for' the land. In the Yolnu world views there are two moieties – they are two halves of one whole. So everything in the world is holistic. The knowledge and the worldview is all

connected through the songs, the songs are connected to the people and the people is [sic], their connection is through songlines, stories, from stories to art, country and land through clans, through ... Everything in the world is interlinked.

And we thought Western philosophers like [Baruch] Spinoza were teaching something new!

How do I change as a whole person?
The pattern is constant – I remain responsible for what I did fifty years ago, for good or ill – as the law, as well as my memory and conscience recognise. But I, as a continuing person, a continuing narrative, a continuing yet ever-in-flux web of relationships do change: I know myself to be the same but changed, for good or ill, in complex ways. Actions done by me are what change me: just as the walking over new snow etches foot prints in the snow – but the changes wrought by my action leave ineradicable traces. I change not so much through what is done to me, but by action in response to what impinges on me. Actions include decisions, including the exercise of the last of human freedoms already mentioned (see Victor Frankl), 'to take an attitude in a given set of circumstances'. This last exercise of freedom is of increasing importance in late life, for obvious reasons: the stuff happening medically, the regular experience of loss with (as it were) increasing centrality, or the need to witness/ share a little and try to alleviate the distress of others. It is much harder to do that last one when old and experiencing the onset of uselessness than when one is an eager conscientious young doctor! The influence of context, pressures, previous ways of acting, cultural imperatives – all these and more influence the shape an action takes, but I do not accept that I am wholly determined: Spinoza offers balance on these matters. I quote Professor Genevieve Lloyd:

> Spinoza offers ... a vision of freedom as the joyful acceptance of what must be ... freedom derives from the active engagement of the mind with necessity, an engagement that flows from the understanding of the truth.[21]

I must *think* my way through to freedom.

In all, I am after all responsible for all I have done and who I have become – even if maybe I hope to be forgiven for some matters by compassionate if not merciful others, and by myself (crucial). If there has been no error, there may hardly have been life! Karl Popper's principle that advancement in knowledge is facilitated more rapidly by error and criticism than by success and praise is hard to apply to one's life long efforts in living – yet has to be true. We need to be kind to the self as the mistakes outweigh all else in the memory: it is the learnings which need to be etched in gold, not in black.

So, the person who is the late life explorer, brings to the task a complex array of capabilities as well as liabilities. Ideally these capabilities will be embodied in the capacity for wise judgement. Judgement implies issues to be addressed, and notably, questions to be faced. What are the issues, the questions, the challenges for such an explorer?

It may be that for oneself at least (maybe for others) evolution in the *questions* dominating thinking and action, manifest particularly in moments of reflection rather than in everyday occupational activities, may offer a way of considering the evolution of personal life.

I can surely recall the questions dominating concerns in early life, trying to abstract from the foreground (not background) noise of educational activities – school, university student years, junior medical training, postgraduate studies and so on? But what now?

The questions of lateness?
What now indeed? Late in the second decade of the twentieth century? It is somewhere recorded that the savant Gertrude Stein, when facing surgery from which she did not survive (and she knew the possibility) was asked, 'What is the answer?' She responded, 'What is the question?' Life is lived between questions. What indeed are the questions in situations, not of extremity, but lateness? Lateness of life cannot be denied now ... not by me.

Spinoza conceived the essence of a person as *conatus – striving to continue in being.* What can this mean in an individual life? especially in a time of lateness. What indeed?

Immanuel Kant's three questions in his *Critique of Pure Reason* may give structure to the discussion: What may I know? What should I do? In what may I hope? Maybe, as a start, one could add 'now' to the end of each of Kant's questions in order to focus more clearly on the tasks of late life – and the way we can facilitate each other in the fulfilment of these tasks.

What may I know – now?
The universe of information is limitless! The digital world shouts that truth. My capacity for retaining knowledge – information after digestion – is limited. What may I know? What should I seek to know?

First of all, the guide is, what do I want to know? Is my instinct for wonder dead? Surely not ... Let me dream of the stars, consider the shards of archaeological ruins, explore the shape of a new language, investigate patterns of new art or new music. My instinct is my guide ... Maybe. Some of us ageing persons like books, not electronic screens! Note the implications for ensuring access of older persons to libraries and art galleries. This screams caution against ageism in the arts and sciences, and educational opportunities.

Then there is another contentious issue in some cultures. I should have all the information I wish about my own situation, notably my physical status and prognosis for survival and wellbeing – more important usually – carefully explained. The information is primarily mine, not the possession of health or other professionals. This principle is not accepted in all cultures and subcultures, where persons can be shielded (for beneficent motives) from such existential truths.

What is more contentious in practice, though not in principle, is the priority needing to be given to the maintenance of cognitive capacity in the face of some morbidity. The overuse of psychotropic drugs in the elderly, blunting cognition or affect, sometimes deliberately is a moral travesty. Precise use of therapeutics is a *moral* necessity.

What should I do – now?
It is obvious that one of the things to be done is to fold up one's tent, to try to bring order into the chaos of one's material and personal world – for the sake of not burdening others. It is obvious but oh so difficult, daunting and hard to face. There is forgiveness to seek (maybe to offer), gratitude to express, recompense to pay (but one cannot ever do it really), even 'uselessness' to accept and no end in sight. Stuart Kauffman, in his investigations concerning complexity stresses that alongside Darwinian selection there is a capacity of complex structures to self-organise: 'sources of order in the biosphere include both selection and self-organisation' and that this occurs at the edge of chaos. Such notions should urge one to be calmer about the tasks of lateness which seem at times to be not only chaotic but overwhelming.

Of more immediate interest is the issue of the maximising of the maintenance and use of capacities ... Obvious, but whose responsibility?

It must be recognised that the care of dependent persons (including us, the very elderly) is a serious burden for society. At issue is the place in society of those who can no longer contribute to the economic goods – and are dependent now on life savings or the public purse – or even worse, on considerable contribution from publicly funded services for continuing life. The Nazis disparaged the 'socially unproductive', the 'useless eaters'.[22] In 1920, legal and medical authorities, [Karl] Binding and [Alfred] Hoche, published a small book outlining for Germany the case for the destruction of life 'not worthy to be lived'. In Germany, less than two decades after the publication of that book, centres were set up for the 'elimination of the burdensome' – to kill incurably ill, physically or mentally disabled, emotionally distraught, and elderly people: the T4 program: all this before the Holocaust. We must never forget.

Leo Alexander, an observer at the Nuremberg trials of Nazi doctors, tried to analyse the roots of the moral collapse of some of the most eminent medical academic leaders, and in a 1949 paper pinned the beginning on a shift in *attitude* to the non-rehabilitatable sick – a caution for our own times and forever:

> The beginnings at first were merely a subtle shift in emphasis in the basic attitude of the physicians. It started with the acceptance of the attitude, that there is such a thing as a life not worthy to be lived. This attitude in its early stages concerned itself merely with the severely and chronically sick. Gradually the sphere of those to be included in this category was enlarged to encompass the socially unproductive, the ideologically unwanted, the racially unwanted and finally all non-Germans. But it is important to realise the infinitely small wedged-in lever

from which this entire trend of mind received its impetus was the attitude toward the non-rehabilitatable sick.[23]

This is not a dead issue: ethical arguments even in the course of COVID-19 regarding economics in relation to morbidity and even mortality of the frail echo matters foreshadowed by past controversy and unspeakable tragedy.

It is said that the quality of a society and its institutions and personnel maybe gauged by its care of the most vulnerable – they have value and place an obligation on the rest of society. In the Judeo-Christian tradition this is a deeply rooted concept. See for instance in Jewish law provisions for orphans, widows and the poor, the observance of Sabbath being rest for all, the concept of jubilee with a special impact on the ownership and management of land; the freeing of slaves and more.

There may be another dimension of care, namely 'education' and it is Erik Erikson who has stressed it in a lecture for psychoanalysts:

> Parenthood is, for most, the first and for many, the prime generative encounter yet the perpetuation of mankind challenges the generative ingenuity of workers and thinkers of many kinds. And man *needs* to teach, not only for the fulfillment of his identity, but because facts are kept alive by being told, logic by being demonstrated, truth by being professed ... Every mature adult knows the satisfaction of explaining what is dear to him and of being understood by a groping mind.

And further, Erikson notes 'man's love for his works and ideas as well as for his children'. He goes on to consider these notions in relation to the very last stage of life:

> Any span of the cycle lived without vigorous meaning, at the beginning, in the middle, or at the end, endangers the sense of life and the meaning of death in all whose

life stages are intertwined ... [E]ach generation must find the wisdom of the ages in the form of its own wisdom. Wisdom ... is detached concern with life itself, in the face of death itself. It maintains and conveys the integrity of experience, in spite of the decline of bodily and mental functions. It responds to the need of the on-coming generation for an integrated heritage and yet remains aware of the relativity of all knowledge.[24]

Erikson, in stressing education as an aspect of the care that even one who is approaching the end of life can offer to others less close to the close of life, has offered a new dimension of responsibility – a new task for lateness, indeed. Or fanciful? (It may also be noted that, as Erikson points it out, individuality is maximum in old age – and diversity of modes of not only thought but also action is to be expected: but care arrangements and public policy may not reflect this reality.)

So what can the late life person *do* of any real use to society? Power of effective action is surely with the young and middle aged, and the younger elderly. Educator? Now? Maybe one's role is after all to learn to listen, to minimise the burden one is, to soak up the stress, to be at the edges of society when life at the centre gets impossible – to be safe places, to be sanctuaries, now there is the rub, to be a place for the holy, after all. And all this needs to be thought about in a new way in the midst of a pandemic where caseloads are immense – and the dying elderly are truly places of lament, but also may be places where humanness is laid bare in a way this world will not forget.

What may I hope? Now?
The third question of Kant is by far the most difficult to ask and to answer of oneself and of another.

Old age is often a time of frailty. Frailty, individual or communal is a common human experience. It implies the perceived inadequacy of responsive capacity, weakness, tenuous possibility of response, fragility in the face of threat ... all the antithesis of robustness.

Yet frailty is part of the human condition, and for persons accustomed to robustness, maybe a trigger for anxiety, apprehension or even despair if the challenge to be faced is perceived to be disproportionately strong.

The last stage of life, as the first, is likely to be an experience of frailty, with opportunities for a perception of frailty at really all stages of life as a result of events like trauma, sickness, pandemic,[25] imprisonment, disgrace (deserved or undeserved), shame, ridicule ... Some individuals and communities have excesses of such experiences: men and women in war, refugees, women in childbirth in ages past – and still in some parts of the world – orphans, the aged, communities exposed to starvation, European Jewish communities over centuries. French psychoanalyst Frantz Fanon wrote about the 'wretched of the earth' in his eponymous book.[26] Wretchedness is still present though with some new patterns of distribution: COVID-19 in our own time has highlighted inequities, some sadly old (and ignored), some of them new or unexpected.

At the last stage of life (at any age), but maybe at any time of frailty, there is, in Erikson's formulation, an opportunity for the person to move towards either despair or to integrity, that is, wholeness and acceptance of one's space and time. It is critically important to recognise that frailty does not take away the possibility of integrity – radical wholeness. indeed, such conceptualisation of wholeness, may be a condition for the emergence of hope. But there may also be the possibility of hope even in a state of brokenness; some of the most powerful liturgical experiences incorporate images of brokenness within which new possibility is found. Hope appears to involve a dynamic towards the future, and a going out from the depths of the self, a facing outward, a facing toward the Other.

Then what can engender hope in a situation of frailty?

i An adequate notion of integrity – acceptance of one's space and time.
ii Perception of the possibility that the disproportionate threat will go away.
iii Perception that frailty will be alleviated by influx of power.
iv Perception of a new meaning – reinterpretation of the present, recognition of the present as being part of a larger meaningful pattern (e.g. the history of the individual or community).

Note that the engendering of hope requires knowledge or perception of other reality – by remembering, or imagining. The preservation and maximising of cognition must be a central medical task in the frail.

Towards a conclusion?

Is there any more to say? Maybe.

Let us return to the relational view of person mentioned at the beginning of this essay: 'person' is conceived as a relational reality – constituted by relations with elements of the present environment (persons, place, things), with the past (historicity), with inheritance (biological and cultural), all in dynamic but fragile equilibrium. The land in which I live, my place, has been trodden by human feet for over 60,000 years and our forebears in this land, whose culture is the oldest continuous living culture on earth, epitomise the relational view of personhood set forth in this essay. Our indigenous peoples incorporated the land, their kin, and all of nature; the interiorisation of the relation with land, with 'country', is a feature of their being – and the fracture of this and other interiorised relations wrought by colonisers' policies is one of the wounds of this nation, Australia. But I as a contemporary Australian whose immediate ancestors came from afar, have in my midst persons who may teach me how to find the meaning of personhood.

'Human dignity' involves respect for every constitutive relation. 'Suffering' implies threats to the integrity of the (fragile) whole, nearing a tipping point, for which triggers may be named. 'Hope' as action may be thought of as a thrust out of a closed system (with potential for lock in). Hope as object may be conceived as the terminus influencing the direction of the thrust towards an Other (which could be within the self) – but hope-as-action is surely primary, integrating transcendence, moving us to become what we are, uniquely: hope is labour yielding new life. Stuart Kauffman would add that even on the edge of chaos we have within us the capacity to create, to generate something new.

So, in what may I, as individual – and unique, hope? For intactness of non-violated relationships (with present, past – by memory, inheritance – cultural and biological) in which my dignity rests; for coherence – that the centre may hold; for becoming who I am, be a flame of my own like [Georg] Hegel said, sing my own song. And all of this in the end by facing if not praising the Other. What is the source of the thrust to the Other which is hope? That which integrates the whole, that which sustains life, that which has as its source whatever is added to the dust in the making of man. Maybe in hope we humans are continually drawing on as well as reconstructing god.

Maybe there can be no conclusion to my thought. Spinoza, not holding for personal immortality held that, on death, when the body can no longer sustain the mind, one's thought entered into the slip stream of eternal mind – a world parallel, as it were, to the material universe – a peace inducing notion for one with a restless mind.[27] So, while life endures, my thinking may continue to evolve – with no conclusion of which I can be aware. Others may try to make sense of what I have articulated, but I may not: I as a person have truly passed away and can think no more.

So, the tasks of late life maybe, like the rest of life, basically to respond to questions. To live in the in-between, between questions, in the midst of the encounter with others and the whole of nature. And to BE a question, and not just to myself. Maybe the answer to Gertrude Stein's 'What is the question?' is that the question is me ... who am I? And I must go to my death being just that.

But maybe the quest does not end there. While there is life, *thinking* – that weird colloquy within the self – goes on. Kant, after all, only asked three questions! *What could be the fourth question?* Surely: *what may I love?* –and, in the perspective of extreme lateness, *What may I love, now?*

In extreme lateness, notably if also a time of frailty, the time is long past for fastening the energy of love on the acquisition of goods, or of achievements, or even recognition of them, or of influence, or on 'usefulness'. Or experiences of music and the arts – for such experiences become rare or more tenuous, and even perception may be more and more dimmed, even while the inner self thrives. And even the persons one has loved have often gone elsewhere because of commitments or death – living only, however vividly, in the memory. So what is there to love now? – to yield to in love, as one did in adolescence, in that first spring?

Maybe the notion of spring is the clue!

The mind may, in its roaming, rest on the words of Augustine, in his *Confessions*: 'Late have I loved you, O beauty ever ancient and ever new'. Augustine's ideas on many matters may not resonate but one senses the beat of his heart. Could the notions of Spinoza relate? Spinoza, profoundly secular but steeped in the Jewish tradition, regarded the highest human activity is to gaze on god, wholly immanent in all Nature, and his perspectives may offer us a handhold for our time. Not for Spinoza the notion of an interventionist God, but, as radically Jewish and grounded in the seminal ideas expressed in Genesis, he would have had the conviction (as I do) that what is (including the human, even myself) is not vitiated but radically *good*.

The *order within the whole, the unity of the whole:* this, for Spinoza (and for me) is the wholly immanent 'God'. This is the order manifest in the smallest garden: the seed, given water/ nutrients/ warmth, becomes a seedling, and then, according to its particularity, continues to grow into buds, flowers, fruit – and so on. The laws within all being, the order – surely this calls for not only amazement but paeans of praise – and yes, love. And the awareness that this same *order* within reality encompasses also myself: it is this ever-growing awareness which may prompt not fear but loving surrender, like to that of adolescence, again.

So, in lateness, after all, the circle of life may be made complete – and the gaze finds its place of rest. And that surely is enough.

REFERENCES

1. Said E., *On Late Style*, Bloomsbury, London, 2006.
2. Bloom H., *Till I End My Song: A Gathering of Last Poems*, Harper, New York, 2010.
3. Eliot TS., 'East Coker' – from *The Four Quartets*.
4. Eliot G., *Daniel Deronda*, 1876.
5. Frankl V., *Man's Search for Meaning*, 1946.
6. Hadot P., *Philosophy as a Way of life*, Trans M Chase, Wiley, Oxford, 1995.
7. Putnam H., *Jewish Philosophy as a Guide to Life*, Indiana University Press, Bloomimgton, 2008.

8 Bloom H., *Where Shall Wisdom be Found?*, Penguin Putnam, New York, 2004.
9 William, CW., 'That Greeny Flower', in Asphodel, *That Greeny Flower and Other Love Poems*, New York, New Directions, 1995.
10 Lindstrom R. and Wojtowicz A. (eds), *Human Judgement*, University of Tasmania, Hobart 2016.
11 Needleman J., 'The perception of mortality', *Annals NY Academy of Sciences*, 1969, 164:733–738.
12 Thomasma DC, Weisstub D N., Herve C. (eds), *Personhood and Health Care*, Kluwer, Dordrecht, 2001.
13 Lickiss JN., *The Aboriginal People of Sydney with Special Reference to the Health of Their Children: A Study in Human Ecology*, MD Thesis University of Sydney, 1972.
14 Lickiss N., 'On human dignity: fragments of an exploration' in Malpas J. and Lickiss N. (eds) *Perspectives on Human Dignity*, Springer Dordrecht, 2007, p 27–41.
15 Lickiss N., 'Facing human suffering', in Malpas J. and Lickiss N. (eds) *Perspectives on Human Suffering*, Springer, Dordrecht, 2012. p 245–60.
16 Cassell E., 'The nature of suffering and the goals of medicine', *New England Journal Medicine*, 1982, 306: 639–645.
17 Manderson D., Levinas, *Proximity and the Soul of Law*, McGill, Montreal, 2007.
18 Erikson EH., *Identity and the life cycle. Psychological Issues Monograph*, New York International Universities Press, 1965.
19 Hume A., *Treatise on Human Nature*, Book 1, Section VI 'Of personal identity' (p252 in Oxford Edition, ed by LA Selby-Bigge).
20 Kauffman S., *At Home in the Universe*, Penguin, Harmondsworth, 1996, p20.
21 Lloyd G., *Providence Lost*, Harvard University Press, Cambridge Mass, 2008, p200 ff.
22 Binding K. and Hoche A., 'Allowing the Destruction of Life Unworthy of Life: its Measure and Form', (1920) trans Modak C. *Policy intersections Research Center* 2012–15 pub by Suseteo Enterprises.
23 Alexander L., 'Medical science under dictatorship', *New England Journal of Medicine*, 241, 1949, 39–47.
24 Erikson EH., *Insight and Responsibility*, 1964, Norton NY, p130.
25 Lickiss N., 'COVID Time', *Hectoen International Journal*, 2020 (hekint.org/2020/08/COVID-time).
26 Fanon F., *The Wretched of the Earth* (1963), trans Richard Philcox, Grove Press, New York, 2004.
27 Lickiss N., 'Spinoza and medical practice: can the Philosophy of Spinoza Enrich the Thinking of Doctors?', *Hektoen International Journal*, Fall 2019.

VI
COVID TIME
2020

Hektoen International, 2020

>Who will be the chronicler of this?
>of how the tower fell,
>of how the tolling bell
>sounded the world's crying.
>
>And how the darkness fell,
>how deep the night, how bare
>the city streets, how hard
>to count and lay the dead.
>
>And how the distanced other
>ached for touch and how
>the crowded ones still loved
>and held the ones who died.
>
>And how the shielded ones
>so cared for those who lived
>and died with some who died.
>We weep and fear the tide …
>
>How hard to wait this dawn!
>Who can be the chronicler of this?

VII
On Poetry
2021

> It is difficult
> to get the news from poems
> yet men die miserably every day
> for lack
> of what is found there.
> —*William Carlos Williams*[1]

But what *is* found there? First thoughts.

1. In poems we may find *questions* and *fragments of responses*.

    Questions are the stuff of life – the matrix within which we have our human being.

    a) Look at the many questions in Genesis, the foundation document of Western civilisation, for example: To Adam: Where are you? To God from Cain: Am I my brother's keeper? To Hagar from God: Where are you going?

    b) Look at the questions of [Immanuel] Kant:[2] What can I know? What should I do? In what may I hope?

    or

    c) Ernst Bloch, in the opening lines of The Principle of Hope,[3] Who are we? Where do we come from? What are we waiting for?

    These questions, and more, are articulated by thinkers of all ages, embedded in literature and the arts, and in my view, finely focussed in poetry – as are fragments of response. In fact the 'fragments of response' may be suggested answers to the question, or may be a nudge towards a changed view of the question or of the landscape in which the question has emerged, new ways of seeing ('perspectives') or new perceptions of possibility.

The questions are always contextualised and so are the responses – in the times, the culture, in the person of the questioner and/or the responder, but also the questions and the fragments of response endure beyond time, culture, circumstance. The human web is not only spatial but temporal. We are all connected not only in substance but in mind (which itself is best conceived as embedded in material reality).

2   Poetry indeed offers *new perspectives* on experienced realities (things, events, persons), new ways of seeing.

Can an orange tree look the same after reading John Shaw Neilson's 'The Orange Tree' – or a daffodil after [William] Wordsworth, or the hills of Bondi after reading Christopher Brennan? Each person will have had perspectives changed forever by contact with a particular poem.

Poetry is a perspective about the particular – but the perspective brought may smack of the universal. As metaphor ('metaphor' in Greek is fundamentally a vehicle for conveying something from one place to another – pointed out by poet David Mason) the poem may connect the particular with the universal – may open up the particular to the universal, and may thus express the radical truth that all reality is one web of being and that as an individual, I am part of the whole, a perspective emphasised by 17C philosopher Baruch Spinoza.[4] Or the particular may be seem simply in a new light, as particular, with its own inherent value, meaning, dignity, or mystery.

3   Poetry may presage, suggest, infer *new horizons* – new boundaries for one's vision, new challenges for one's journeying, new evocations for the spirit: will you come? or try to come, here? There may be a hint of a new land long searched for, or a safe harbour longed for, or a glimpse of a person agonised for – or a mirage to be faced. Whatever of these, it is a stretching out of the self which is called for. And a poem can do this by questions, (How far is it to Babylon? ...) by innuendo, or by the power of evoked emotion as a poetic image lights up the deep memory. As a wise medico (a professor of anatomy indeed), deploring the dangers of a mind 'closed by science or religion', remarked: 'In a mind still open, a mind if not without conviction at least without prejudice, the universe has oceans yet uncharted, shorelines etched upon distant, beckoning horizons and glimpses of another hinterland.'[5] He could have been speaking of poetry.

The new horizon may point to a new questioning, even painful questioning, of what has been considered foundational, trustworthy, and complete, and as such may stir passion, engender strife not peace, and lead not to calm but disquiet. A poem may be dangerous and destructive, but also may heal and show a path forward into human flourishing. The responsibility of a poet (like that of any artist) for the well-being of others, then, may be extreme. Words matter, and words in poetry bear extra freight.

4   A poem may bring *closure* – maybe after opening up wounds ... even 'cliffs of fall'; as the poet after turbulence finds calm, so may the receiver of the poem find peace of soul after journeying with the poet awhile. A poem is not infrequently an articulated inner migration – from one place to another, even though the landmarks are subtle and inferred though not clearly articulated. And the poet may

prefer to leave impressions rather than readily readable images or signs. And the receiver of the poem may prefer not to articulate the whole which is received or perceived. The conversation which the poem is may remain, thus, private – and woe betide an educator who seeks to explain the meaning of the utterance. In any case even the poet may not be able to or wish to make more explicit the 'meaning' of the pattern of words spoken or written. The interior colloquium of the poet is to be respected; it is enough that a pattern of words has been uttered. The pattern of words has entered Karl Popper's 'world 3',[6] and is henceforth part of the world beyond the poet, with a life of its own and is free to be interpreted by whoever encounters it – this is the hazard of art.

5   There is a sense in which what may be found will be *what a finder seeks*, but the finding will be dependent up recognition of some shared imagery or symbolism. Poems belong, like ancient cave art, in the symbolic universe – belonging to which is a mark of humanness.

We do not know when poetry became part of the human heritage – certainly long before there was writing. The Epic of Gilgamesh dates from about 3000 BCE, but is surely a late manifestation of a very old oral tradition. Ancient cave art which as far as we know, became really prominent in Lower Pleistocene (c30000 BCE), has defied explanation. Was it a manifestation of shamanism, or what? There is a vast literature – see some discussion elsewhere.[7] One interpretation is that parietal art became possible as brain function (not size) changed – a new flexibility appeared enabling concepts to be related together in new ways. I have expressed the thought that the ancient concept of *conatus* which the philosopher Spinoza made central to his thought as 'the striving to continue in being'[8] – may be at the root of the appearance of art on the human scene: to strive to continue in being may demand that we continually burst the bounds of our being. It may be that to be human is to be creative – and those amongst us who give us what we call art or literature or poetry express more richly than the rest of us the essence of humanness. There is much to ponder there.

6 But why do men, persons, 'die miserably every day for lack of what is found' in poems?

There is need to probe more deeply into what we mean by 'person'. For a start we may note, an articulation of what Heidi Ravven called the self beyond the self? Ravven discusses the insight that 'a person is an open system in relation to other open systems, natural and cultural'.[9] But she built on a rich tradition of thought outlined elsewhere.[10]

Poet Walt Whitman (*Song of Myself*) noted that 'I am not contained between my hat and my boots'. I, as a person, am more than that. 'Person' is a relational term (like father, son): with actions/memories etc as additional facts to be taken into account when gazing at an individual, a richer view of person is available. Relations with other persons, place, the past, cultural inheritance, and with one's aspirations/hope and with All-That-Is (however named) may be best seen as interiorised, as constitutive of 'person' – just as the filaments of a spider's web constitute the web. What holds such constituent elements together, what is the principle of integration? Maybe we could call it 'soul'. Cassell's landmark definition of suffering[11] as a 'sense of impending personal disintegration' fits well with this notion.

What is it in poems which nourish the soul? and prevent or relieve suffering/disintegration? It may be that poems articulate one or more of the constitutive relations – with persons, place, things, memory, cultural imperatives or treasures, aspirations – or with All-That-Is, and thereby enrich (even repair) the person as one whole. 'Dying miserably' implies not the peaceful conclusion of life as a completed whole, but suffering. What is implied by all this is that poetry may facilitate flourishing, not personal disintegration. At least a space is opened up for consideration.

So, what may be found in poems? Why is it a *medical* poet who asks the question? and made the comment that every day men die for lack of what is found there? What is the connection? Why draw attention to it?

There are many possibilities. Maybe, just maybe, these questions arise for doctors because of an intense familiarity with the limit experiences of the human condition, not in words but in the raw: birth, becoming, dying and death, strength and weakness, darkness and light, illness, despair and hope, suffering and healing, regression and transformation, with some of these jumbled together in our patients and ourselves and in the space between where so much happens. Doctors know the *what* and *how* of human being, but stumble at the *why*. Doctors in general are not wordsmiths, nor fountains of wisdom, just replete with often unspoken and unanswered questions.

Dying for lack of what is found there? Doctors know the experience of 'lack', despair of soul, 'burn out', and have a high suicide rate. We are, of all men and women, seekers after meaning, seekers of order within chaos. Yet doctors hold on to the road, however dark. Mostly. We do not speak of, but *know* failure of our dreams – we trample on our own dreams; we know how the soul (the principle of coherence of the constituents of the self?) may languish – since Cassell's landmark paper we call it 'suffering', or may even die. And we know (though maybe not understand) what nourishes the soul, what heals.

So, what may be found in poems? An expression of the human quest for shaping questions as well as responses? An attempt to map the unmapped country within the self? ('There is a great deal of unmapped country within us which would have to be taken into account in an explanation of our gusts and storms', wrote George Eliot).[12] Or, the search for a new road– Emily Dickinson: 'Death is a wild Night and a new Road'?[13] Or simply the thirst for meaning in the place where one finds oneself? Or, maybe all of these – or none? That may be the question.

REFERENCES

1 Williams WC., 'That Greeny Flower', in Asphodel, *That Greeny Flower and Other Love Poems*.
2 Kant I., *Critique of Pure Reason*, 1781–87.
3 Bloch E., *The Principle of Hope* (1938–47, revised 1953 and1959), Trans N Plaice, S Plaice and P Knight Blackwell, Oxford, 1986, Introduction, p3.
4 Lloyd G., *Part of Nature*. Cornell University Press, New York, 1994.
5 Mortimer K., 'The impossible profession: the doctor –priest relationship', *Proc. Aust. Assoc. Geront*, 2(2) 1974.
6 Popper, K. 'How I see Philosophy.' in *Philosophers on Their Own Work*, vol.3 (ed. A. Mercier and M. Svilar) Peter Lane, Berne, Frankfurt am Main, Las Vegas, 1977.
7 Lickiss N., *Art, Personal Care and the Jewish Tradition*.
8 Lloyd G., *Spinoza and the Ethics*, Routledge, New York, 1996.
9 Ravven H., *The Self Beyond the Self*, The New Press, New York, 2013, p402.
10 Lickiss N., 'Facing Human Suffering', in Jeff Malpas and Norelle Lickiss (eds), *Perspectives on Human Suffering*.
11 Cassell E., 'The nature of suffering and the goals of medicine', *New England Journal of Medicine*, 306 (1982),639–645.
12 Eliot G., *Daniel Deronda*: Book 3, Chapter 24.
13 Dickenson E., *Letter to Perez*, D Cowan, October, 1869.

VIII
Medicine as Art? Reflections in COVID Time
2021

Human history (oral and written) is replete with chronicles of disaster! Floods, plagues, pestilence and a myriad of other disasters have wrought havoc on the people. Historian William McNeill authored a classic account of the shifting balance between human hosts and infectious organisms, and concluded: 'Infectious disease which antedated the emergence of humankind will last as long as humanity itself, and will surely remain, as it has been hitherto, one of the fundamental parameters of human history'.[1]

On the occasion of the COVID–19 pandemic, first named as such in 2020, another catastrophe has fallen (*casus* – a fall) on humanity, there is almost fixation on various aspects of medicine as a solution to the global tsunami of distress. Hardly a day goes by without media mention of medical matters. A spotlight has been thrown on medicine in all its dimensions – from public health to clinical medicine and health service administration, to finer aspects of laboratory-based sciences, notably virology, immunology, and fundamentals of ethics. It would be tedious to attempt to list the manifest problems and achievements, but mention should be made of the moral aspects, not only from the facing of searing global, national and local inequities but also from the radical moral challenge of needing to offer, in times of scarcity, resources according to *need* has had to give way to offering in terms of potential benefit, hoping that first the most needy comfort can be assured if not life 'saved'. That is classic 'triage procedure' associated with battlefield, not with hospitals even in affluent nations: a truly radical challenge.

The fact that medicine is science, and a human science at that – is cast in high relief. But traditionally medicine is also spoken of as 'art'. Is this simply testimony to a craft? Or fiction, or metaphor, or a glib way of stressing some of the complexities and intuition involved in medicine? Is that all? Or is there something justifying exploration in these strange times? Maybe. Medicine as 'art'! Words have weight. There may be a case for exploring this notion, rather like a stranger in unfamiliar terrain searching for resonances with one's homeland. There are several perspectives to consider.

1
What is art?

There is a vast history of ideas concerning art and aesthetics! I refer here only to a relatively recent and useful (to a medico) discussion. The late Denis Dutton, a philosopher of art who died in New Zealand in 2010, noted first that, by 'art' and 'arts' he meant artefacts (sculptures, paintings, and decorated objects, such as tools or the human body, and scores and texts considered as objects) and performances (dances, music, and the composition and recitation of stories). Dutton then delineated a list of the signal characteristics of art considered as a universal cross-cultural category: he called them *cluster criteria)* found cross culturally in the arts. Very briefly the list (with the opening words of Dutton's discussion of each) is as follows:

1 *Direct pleasure.* The art object ... is valued as a source of immediate experiential pleasure in itself, and not essentially for its utility in producing something else that is either useful or pleasurable ...
2 *Skill and virtuosity.* The making of the object or performance requires and demonstrates the exercise of

special skills. These skills are learned in an apprentice tradition in some societies ...

3 *Style*. Objects and performances in all art forms are made in recognizable styles, according to rules of form, composition, or expression ...

4 *Novelty and creativity*. Art is valued, and praised, for its novelty, creativity, originality, and capacity to surprise an audience ...

5 *Criticism*. Wherever artistic forms are found, they exist alongside some kind of critical language of judgement and appreciation, simple or, more likely, elaborate ...

6 *Representation*. In widely varying degrees of naturalism, art objects, including sculptures, paintings, and oral and written narratives, and sometimes even music, represent or imitate real and imaginary experiences of the world ...

7 *Special focus*. Works of art and artistic performances tend to be bracketed off from ordinary life, made a separate and dramatic focus of experience ...

8 *Expressive individuality*. The potential to express individual personality is generally latent in art practices, whether or not it is fully achieved ...

9 *Emotional saturation*. In varying degrees, the experience of works of art is shot through with emotion ...

10 *Intellectual challenge*. Works of art tend to be designed to utilize the combined variety of human perceptual and intellectual capacities to the full extent; indeed, the best works stretch them beyond ordinary limits ...

Dutton considered art in relation to evolution as his overall frame and emphasised art as an *instinct* of survival value.[2] There may be some kinship here with 17C philosopher Spinoza's notion of *conatus*[3] – that striving to continue in being which may be in play in the appearance of art in the early aeons of human history.

Is it totally ridiculous to consider medicine from these perspectives? Some of the 'characteristics' seem alien, but other notions have resonance when carefully considered. Anyone steeped in practice has experienced some elements of many of the matters Dutton raises. At the very least the perspectives he introduces may prompt further thought – and in our time there is room for deep reflection concerning medicine and its place in the human condition, and not just in our own time. Art is ancient, and so is medicine in its core idea that some in the community would be trusted/authorised to care for others, even in extremis.

2
Medicine is a human science
It is not trite to insist that medicine is not a 'natural science'[4] but a 'human science' – a matter of significant theoretical and practical moment.

i) *What is the mark of humanness?*
Thinkers of all times have contemplated this question!

Ernst Cassirer, a philosopher who flourished in Germany in the first decades of 20C, and later in USA until his death in 1944, is being increasingly appreciated in our time. Cassirer held that to be human is fundamentally to be a symbol maker: homo sapiens might be better named *homo symbolicus*.[5] Art belongs (with language and religion) to the world of symbols. Human history demonstrates an association with art, with making symbols, with performances not related to utility. A notable and moving Australian discovery was the finding that the remains of Mungo Man, the earliest known burial of modern man – over 30000 years ago – bore traces of decorative ochre.[6]

ii) The human body has long been a significant theme of art.
Living tissues are beautiful! Cells and tissues seen through a microscope are often exquisitely beautiful. Biologists know this and even hardened medical students can be reduced to awe. Likewise surgeons faced with anatomical intricacies. The sheer beauty is sometimes overwhelming. But we doctors do not often speak of these things, being mindful of other things, most of the time.

But other artists do ... and archaeologists know well the wonder of discovery of the beautiful. Ancient figurines depict the human form. Art history demonstrates that each period and each culture had different nuances: in accord with the fact that the body of each individual is unique, as is each culture in every dimension – physical, emotional, intellectual, spiritual. Some works seem to transcend time and cultural context, maybe because they offer traces of a human universal or at least, for the one experiencing the art, lead to a response which impinges on fundamental human truths.

The 'Prisoners' of Michelangelo depict the human body emerging as it were out of the stone – unfinished. Memorable. *As if life itself is a work of art* – and the task of life is to emerge from one's context, into a new freedom: a powerful metaphor indeed with many possible interpretations. What did the sculptor have in mind? Personal development occurs while life lasts; and psychologists (such as Erikson) stress that growth spurts occur at times of crisis – in which doctors are often deeply involved There are many ways of thinking about a person in our care: maybe we should add the concept that (like ourselves) the patient is a work of art, a work in progress, in which we may (unwittingly) play a part, like a sculptor.

iii) The human person as image of god? Now?
The relation between human and god(s) is the stuff of much mythology and takes many forms. The idea of the human as

the *image* of god is particularly to be found in the Hebrew scriptures, in Genesis, the book of origins, which borrowed much from the ancient near east but had unique features. This writing which undoubtedly articulated ancient oral traditions was probably finalised in the third or second century BCE. The idea of man as the image of God figured strongly thereafter in the Jewish (and later Christian) theological tradition – but what could it mean now in a secular age?

In part this depends on the prevailing concept or concepts of 'God', and there is a long history concerning that matter. It is being increasingly recognised that 17C thinker Baruch Spinoza is a significant figure in this tradition: Spinoza outlines the concept not of a transcendent being, but of god as wholly immanent, co-extensive with all-that-is; all in nature is in god and god is in all nature (technically panentheism). As a recent thinker remarked, after Spinoza there is no going back. With such a concept of god can we see the power of the idea that the human is image of the whole – a statement of human possibility which stretches the mind and heart.

But Spinoza stressed something else: the human person is *part* of nature, wholly interconnected. Such a notion (which COVID is drastically demonstrating) is an antidote to the travesty of individualism. Can medicine resonate with that? Can this notion of radical interconnectedness not only counterbalance individualism but also, if truly grasped, replenish the spirit and alleviate the depression deep in our affluent societies? even in our young?

3
A note on the 'sublime'
The aesthetics tradition, concerned with the history of perception by the senses, received much attention in the eighteenth century, the century of the so called 'Enlightenment'

which shaped European thought, and influenced the early decades of the European settlement of Australia.[7] The significance continues to be pondered by Australian philosophers.[8] Edmund Burke, the same who decades later (1790) gave us *'Reflections on the Revolution in France'*, influenced the development of thought concerning aesthetics through his work, *Philosophical Inquiry into the Origin of Our Ideas of the Sublime and the Beautiful (*1756). Burke distinguished the beautiful from what he termed the sublime.

Cassirer wrote extensively concerning the intellectual history of the 18C, the zenith of the Enlightenment, and considered the aesthetics tradition of that period, and considered Burke's ideas. His words in his early writings, in the first decades of the twentieth century are noteworthy:

> The contemplation of beauty as harmonious proportion and strict unity of form does not awaken in us the deepest emotions of the soul or the most intense artistic experiences. A different and stronger emotional effect appears when, instead of unity of form, we are confronted with its disintegration, or even its complete dissolution. Not only form in the classical sense, but distortion, has aesthetic value and a rightful place in aesthetics. Not only that which is governed by rules, but that which is not subject to rules, not only that which can be measured by certain standards whatever can please. This phenomenon, which shatters the conceptual framework of previous aesthetic systems, is called by Burke the sublime. The sublime defies the aesthetic demand for proportionality; for transcendence of all mere proportionality constitutes its real character. The sublime consists precisely in this transcendence and derives its effectiveness from it. Not only what we form and shape within in pure intuition affects us, but also that which eludes any such attempt, which

overwhelms us instead of being formed and controlled by us. We are never more powerfully moved than by this incomprehensible element of experience; never do we feel the power of nature and of art so much as when we are confronted with the terrible. That we do not succumb to the terrible, but that we maintain ourselves against it and that we actually feel an exaltation and intensification of our powers in its presence – these are the elements of the phenomenon of the sublime and the basis of its deepest aesthetic effect. The sublime removes the boundaries of the finite. The ego, however, does not experience this removal as a destruction, but as a kind of exaltation and liberation.[9]

These are extraordinary words! The idea that confrontation with almost overwhelming reality may intensify our inner selves! Interiority, so impaired by some aspects of our contemporary experience as Sebastian Smee has noted,[10] may be strengthened by such an encounter? The note of 'pleasure' is surely not essential for an object or performance to be recognised as art (aesthetics, as noted above, is concerned not with pleasure but sensory experience): but, apart from this jarring note, these ideas concerning the sublime justify further reflection.

The matter of a sense of powerlessness as well as intensified interiority in the face of an overwhelming reality – an element in the response to the sublime – merits further pondering with reference to the everyday practice of medicine. We clinicians *know* that the experience of patients in extreme distress (as well as the witness of it) may be almost overwhelming, with (for a witness) an element of awe. Something stirs our core, intensifying our very being. And, if Cassirer's words ring true, somehow something to do with the interiority from which art springs may be there.

In mid twentieth century psychiatrist Viktor Frankl wrote of the experience in Auschwitz in his classic, *Man's Search for Meaning*.[11] He noted that the almost unimaginable horrors of daily life led in some prisoners at least to an intensification of inner life manifested in an appreciation of the beauty of art and nature. Since that time there have been, in various parts of the world, almost unspeakable natural as well as man-made disasters – and also now COVID affecting almost the whole of humanity, everywhere. COVID has stressed doctors and nurses as well as patients and families in ways unimagined, at least outside war time. Countless professional (as well as non-professional) carers have died from COVID–19, a matter too deep for tears. They have been part of scenarios almost beyond credibility – the use of lifts in a NYC hospital to store the bodies (as described by a traumatised nurse forced to walk up flights of stairs) – is almost beyond belief, as were scenes in Bergamo, India and elsewhere – and it goes on. Care of others who are suffering, in limit situations, may, like the vision of the sublime, force one to plumb one's own depths. Yes, there is bonding with others who are involved in the same tasks (the 'team'), but the exploration into the depths of the self is a lone experience. And yes, we as doctors fail often, and we may falter when even slight heroism is asked of us for the sake of another, but at least we are aware that we fail and become more conscious of this element of our frailty as the years pass.

There may be resonance here with the philosophy of Emmanuel Levinas, as discussed by Manderson. Levinas stressed that the philosophical basis of the duty of care cannot be merely law, or contract, but the call of the other. *Why* do our doctors and nurses care for patients with COVID, even at risk of their lives? Mention should also at least be made of the medical scientists whose labours and artistry gave humanity the vaccines. Why do they not all just walk away? Maybe

Levinas was right. Maybe, in the face of such tremendous pressures, they may have dug so deep into their profoundest selves that they *must* work and care as an expression of their striving to continue in being. Just as an artist cannot but make art, these heroic doctors (and nurses and all the rest immersed in the sea of distress) are (tragically) artists – authentic artists, even to the end. Is *this* a dimension of medicine as art? And what of survivors – those whose lives they saved? Those of us who have been spared the burden: how do we live on knowing of such a price? and of such global and even local inequities?

So, what will be the effects of the overwhelming COVID experience on humanity, (individually and collectively), and particularly on doctors (individually and collectively). Death? – that is the case for many. For those who contracted COVID, prolonged morbidity? Post-traumatic stress persisting for the rest of life? Unspeakable bereavement? Enduring survivor guilt? But could there be also a new sensitivity to human possibility for good or ill? a new perception of the good? of what matters? a new capacity? Is it possible that not only the conventional artists among us will be key interpreters of what humanity has experienced, but that medicine as art will find a new impetus?

Conclusion?

Can there be any conclusion or adequate responses to any of the questions raised or implied? Maybe not yet. We are still immersed in the COVID experience – and the pain of the global inequities so manifest. In this time when the noise of this world (including the digital world) is so intrusive, and reflection so difficult, we each of us (and especially doctors) need, somehow to foster interiority, to enhance (or revive) our inner capacities. It may be that we as individuals may need to plumb our own depths by becoming more *aware*, gazing again at the 'sublime' wherever it may be found, in the faces of those we may encounter, in the wildness of our bushland, in the violence of storms (human or otherwise), in the scenarios we can hardly bear to witness even on a screen, and in the silence wherever it may be found. And all this in the face of complexities beyond our fathoming in this strange time, a time which may in hindsight prove to be a caesura in the history of humanity.

But there may be another note worth mentioning. Edmund Burke, reflecting on the French revolution which, like COVID, reverberated throughout much of the world:

> All the decent drapery of life is to be torn off. All the superadded ideas, furnished from the wardrobe of a *moral imagination*, which the heart owns, and the understanding ratifies, as necessary to cover the defects of our naked shivering nature, and to raise it to dignity in our own estimation, are to be exploded as a ridiculous, absurd and antiquated fashion.[13] (my emphases)

Dutton stressed the note of imaginative experience as one of the characteristics of art. *Moral imaginative experience* may be one of the hallmarks of COVID time. It will mark medicine forever. And this at a time when there is widespread moral collapse of institutions hitherto trusted.

A distinguished NZ anatomist (Kingsley Mortimer) wrote that 'the task of medicine is to emancipate man's interior splendour'.[14] It may be a worthy task to reflect on what that splendour may be, on the limits of human possibility embedded, not in extending physical prowess (as in the Olympics) but notably in the *capacity for imagination of the not yet* – and maybe with Burke, include *moral* imagination? Is it the capacity for moral imagination – the capacity (despite our recognition of our own flaws and frailty) to envisage a *moral possibility* for each of us and our world, a moral felicity which is *not yet* ... Is it this which maybe at the root of the hope we know in medicine, energising the way forward to respond to the call of the other in need, no matter what? And is the exercise of moral leadership based in profound understanding of person and the human condition and the unfailing commitment to beneficence, even in or especially in hard times: is this after all, the soul of medicine?

References

1. McNeill WH., *Plagues and Peoples*, Random House, New York, 1978.
2. Dutton D., *The Art Instinct*, Oxford, Oxford University Press, 2009.
3. Lloyd G., *Spinoza and the Ethics*, Routledge, Milton Park, 1996.
4. Curthoys J. (ed), *Medicine is a Human Science and other essays* by Norelle Lickiss, Ginninderra, Adelaide. 2022.
5. Cassirer E., *An Essay on Man*, New Haven, Yale University Press, 1944.
6. Flood J., *The Original Australians: Story of the Aboriginal People*, Allen and Unwin, Crows Nest, 2006.
7. Gasgoigne J., *The Enlightenment and the Origins of European Australia*, Cambridge University Press, Cambridge, 2002.
8. Lloyd G., *Enlightenment Shadows*, Oxford, Oxford University Press, 2013.
9. Cassirer E., *The Philosophy of the Enlightenment* (1932) trans FCA Koelln and JP Pettigrove, Princeton University Press, Princeton, 1979, pp328–329.
10. Smee S., 'Net Loss: The Inner Life in the Digital Age', *Quarterly Essay*, No 72, 2018.
11. Frankl V., *Man's Search for Meaning*, 1946, Trans I Lasch, Rider, London, 2004.
12. Manderson D., *Proximity, Levinas, and the Soul of Law*, McGill-Queens Press, Montreal, 2007.
13. Burke E., 'Reflections on the Revolution in France 1790', in G Himmelfarb, *The Moral Imagination*, London, Souvenir Press, 2006, p90.
14. Mortimer K., 'The Impossible Profession: The Doctor-Priest Relationship', *Proceedings of the Australian Association of Gerontology*, 2 (1974), p81.

IX
ON BEING BEREAVED LATE
2021

Bereavement is part of human life (and the lives of other animals), commonly experienced, variously expressed and ritualised, and it has been exhaustively explored in the arts as well as academia. There are well charted recommendations for the care of the bereaved – even specifically elderly bereaved.[1]

So is there place for further comment in relation to the experience of bereavement in lateness? Maybe. At least to raise questions. It is to be noted that 'lateness' is not merely a matter of age: it is an issue of life stage.

I

Why is the loss of a significant object, notably a person, so painful? The acute awareness of loss may cause death. Takotsubo syndrome – acute dilatation of the heart under the influence of an hormonal torrent related to sudden extreme stress – may be fatal. But what of the psychological pain ('my heart is breaking', 'I am falling apart') which may be extreme without obvious physiological manifestations?

It may be that the best explanation of this experience lies in a deep appreciation of a specific relational view of person, with the insistence that relations do not merely supplement but actually *constitute* the person (just as filaments *constitute* a spider's web). I have outlined this view elsewhere, and referred to it as an ecological view of person.[2]

Reference has been made to loss as pertaining to a significant object, notably a person. This comment calls for expansion. Each of us has a 'world' and many elements of that world may and do constitute us as persons. Place, our perception of ourselves (as say, not frail), other persons, articles, culture – all may inhabit, or better – construct our current world. But so does the past – our personal history, so does the future as construed in our aspirations, expectations and hopes, and so does the whole cosmos as I perceive it. We not only express but also construct this world through symbols, which include art and myths and language and religion, and scientific theories: the whole thought-world.

The structure of one's world is fragile. Certain elements of this world are so critical, that loss (by whatever cause) can threaten disintegration – I may have a sense of being about to go to pieces (a wholly subjective phenomenon). Cassell called this 'suffering'[3] which is wholly subjective – a very different matter from 'distress' which may be objectively observable. It is possible for a person to experience extreme distress (say a fractured leg) without having 'a sense of personal disintegration', that is, *'suffering'*.

Whether or not a particular experience of *distress* leads to suffering depends on many other factors in the person's 'make-up' as we say: Post-traumatic Stress Disorder (PTSD) is a classic example where a particular stimulus (a say a minor noise in the street) might evoke extreme suffering in a previously traumatised person. So, similarly different losses will have differing personal consequences. Loss of 'place', say place of residence, may lead to unbearable personal suffering for one person – yet be of little consequence to another, just minor distress perhaps. The same will apply to loss of a thing like a house or a significant ring, or one's artefact (like a garden, a painting, a poem, a design, a language …). Or to loss of a culturally significant ritual. Even mentioning these things highlights the cost of some events of history to displaced or otherwise traumatised peoples: the losses are immense and the burden of bereavement almost beyond the imagination. And such losses still continue to afflict many persons, near and far.

All this is of extreme relevance to a person late in life: the upheavals related to changing care needs can be expected to be diversely catastrophic, with generalisations dangerous if not impossible. But also, so is the loss of persons central (for any reason) to the person's structure.

II

If the loss is of one element central to the structure of a particular person, what are the possibilities of personal repair and renovation, now? Has this way of thinking about person anything to offer?

Maybe yes? What would an architect think if a critical structure of a building were suddenly compromised? Transfer this thinking to a person feeling 'about to go to pieces' in the grip of acute bereavement, say on the death of a partner. What are the consequences of such transposition? What guidelines would emerge – for thoughtful action? Some may be:

i No personal strain; expect nothing heroic of this person for a while, little agency to be exercised. Attend to basic physiological needs – rest food and shelter. (Maslow's hierarchy is relevant).

ii Strengthen existing relations – with place, persons, things, the past, culture, the whole.

iii Encourage signs of reconstruction, manifest in the exercise of initiative, of agency, of the rebirth of imagination – and assist the person in achieving goals.

Scholars like anthropologist Roy Rappaport[4] have emphasised that ritual has a critical role to play in many aspects of personal life, but very obviously at a time of loss, especially at the time of death. Every culture has relevant customs, sometimes obvious to an observer, at other times less so. It is noteworthy that in the Jewish tradition the steps delineated above are precisely mirrored in ritual (after a funeral as soon as possible after the death):

a) sitting *shiva* – staying in place for a week while others fulfil needs for care,
b) *sheloshim* for the rest of that first month, and,
c) at one year after the death, fixing a headstone or other memorial, and as possible and appropriate in intimate circles, *yahrtzeit* – commemoration (*remembering*) of the annual anniversary.

III

What is distinctive about bereavement late in life (at any age)?

First, there is urgency: time is limited, and so may be energy (physical, psychological and spiritual). The reconstruction will be demanding of both, and will require gentleness on the part of any concerned, as well as firmness of vision. This may be the last reconstruction and renewal within the lifelong task of becoming oneself. 'To thine own self be true' ... true to one's possibility. It is as if a sculptor had limited time to take a piece of art as far as it can go. But the sculptor is the self, the whole person, incorporating (embodying) still all the constitutive relations which are the pattern, the web, which one is.

Second, there is the unknown shape of the final possibility of oneself. Can the narcissism be corrected in this rebuild? Can beneficence finally rule the moral compass? Can true tolerance and kindness, not masquerades, prevail? Can shame give way to gladness? Can light master the dark? And can even desiring and gratitude give way to wonder at it all, to praise (the core of *Kaddish*)? At last?

There is a lot at stake, the *quality* of a life, when 'last drinks' are being called.

...

Bereavement is the frame for grieving. And grieving then, is a human activity, in response to loss (or threat of loss) – an activity not of 'adaptation' but of personal reconstruction. The person who emerges from such a process will not wholly be 'the old self'. It is in the new possibility that one in pain may take heart, and find strength, even in frailty.

REFERENCES

1 See publications of International Working Group on Death, Dying, and Bereavement, and volumes such as JD Morgan (Ed) *Ethical Issues in the Care of the Dying and Bereaved Aged*. Baywood, Amityville, New York 1996. *Oxford Textbook of Palliative Medicine* (many editions).
2 Various books related to the Hobart International Interdisciplinary Colloquium (Joske Colloquium): such as: 'On human dignity' in *Perspectives on Human Dignity ed Jeff Malpas and Norelle Lickiss*, Springer, Dordrecht 2007; 'On facing human suffering', in Jeff Malpas and Norelle Lickiss (eds), *Perspectives on Human Suffering*, Springer, Dordrecht, 2012; Randall Lindstrom and Amanda Wojtowicz (eds), *On Human Language*. University of Tasmania, Hobart, 2019. Also in Jean Curthoys (ed), *Medicine as a human science: selected essays of Norelle Lickiss*.
3 Cassell E J., The nature of suffering and the goals of medicine, *New England Journal of Medicine* 306: 639–645.
4 Rappaport R., *Ritual and Religion in the Making of Humanity*, Cambridge University Press, Cambridge, 1999.

10

ON HOSPITALITY AND MEDICINE: A NOTE

2022

'Hospitality in the 21st Century Hospital' was the theme of ethicist Xavier Symons in the 24th Annual Lecture of the Sydney based Plunkett Centre for Ethics, July 2022.[1] He outlined (with apposite references to contemporary thinkers) the concept of humans as wayfarers, sometimes made to feel strange and isolated by illness, and the possibilities within a hospital for alleviating this situation, with awareness of the challenges involved in doing so. He stressed the need and opportunity for doctors to offer spiritual care (in the broad sense – not equated with religion) or to refer to others (such as chaplains) to assist in such essential care.

Such a presentation stirs the mind even of the most anergic and lethargic of listeners. The following comments arose as a result of overnight musings, as a contribution to further discussion and action.

I
What is hospitality?
and what does it look like?

The word hospitality is rooted in the Latin *hospes,* guest, and is clearly related to words such as 'hospice' originally a safe place for pilgrims on a dangerous path, 'hospitality' and 'hospital.' 'Host' is one who gives hospitality. The history of hospitals alludes to such concepts as foundational.

What does hospitality look like?

A glance at the tale of Abraham and the visitors at Mamre in the Hebrew scriptures (Genesis 18) might be rewarding:

> And the Lord appeared unto him in the plains of Mamre: and he sat in the tent door in the heat of the day. And he lift up his eyes and looked, and lo, three men stood by him: and when he saw them, he ran to meet them from the tent door, and bowed himself toward the ground.
> (King James Version)

Robert Alter, in a recent three volume translation of the Hebrew Scriptures,[2] offers further nuances:

> And the Lord appeared to him in the Terebinths of Mamre when he was sitting by the tent flap in the heat of the day. And he raised his eyes and saw, and look, three men were standing before him. He ran toward them from the tent flap and bowed to the ground.

Abraham went on to offer generous hospitality to the strangers who arrived unannounced as he was resting in the heat of the day. There is even a medical twist: the preceding verse (in Chapter 17) suggests that Abraham had just been circumcised (presumably with no anaesthetic). Maybe the one offering hospitality was himself 'wounded', in some distress! Maybe burnout?

But there are some deep aspects of this presumably mythical story – as is the case for most myths. Deep human truths are to be found.

i) It is stressed that the visitors were *strangers*.

The theme of mindful graciousness towards strangers is almost a mantra in later (post Exodus) Hebrew tradition, but here under the tree at Mamre we have an earlier depiction.

The kindness *of* strangers is a later nuance regarding the relationship with strangers, depicted so memorably by Tennessee Williams in the *Streetcar Named Desire*, but also central in considerations of the practice of care, including medical care.[3]

ii) The identity of the strangers is tinged with mystery, with the overall impression that they were in some way redolent of divinity – the opening words of the story emphasise this. The tale of the arrival of the messengers or angels to Sodom which is in continuity with the experience of Abraham at Mamre emphasised the unworldly dimension to this whole story.

Whatever is understood of 'God' may have been present in the mysterious encounter. Certainly, an immanent rather than transcendent concept of God, fits comfortably with the notion that the strangers were indeed a manifestation of God in that place at that time. Contemporary Jewish thinkers such as Rabbi Arthur Green would be in accord with such notions.[4]

There is a current commonly expressed in some considerations of care – that somehow, caring for this patient is energised if seen as done in the name of God. The New Testament passage ... offering the words of Jesus: 'Inasmuch as you have done it for the least of these you have done it for me' is a clear Christian statement of this idea.

Later Christian thought laid more layers of interpretation onto the encounter at Mamre. Rublev's 15C icon 'The trinity' depicts three human figures at the table (with Sarah hiding in the background) with the central figure holding a chalice, clearly a eucharistic scene.

Some comments are in order concerning the Abraham encounter with the strangers, considered in its original form as part of the Hebrew scriptures. In particular it is wise to recognise the danger of caring for the patient in the name of God or Jesus (or as an exercise of charity or justice or even as a mitzvah); the danger is the failure to value this individual human being as such, in all his or her particularity. Humanists would rightly insist on this point.

II
Hospitality is twice blessed

Professor Bernardette Tobin, Director of the Plunkett Centre, suggested that, like mercy ('The quality of mercy is twice blessed')[5] the act of hospitality blesses the giver and the receiver.

But what do we mean by blessing? Is this an expression of augmentation of human flourishing, of enhancement of the human good of this individual person? Human good – in whose eyes?

Much ink (and blood) has been spilt regarding what is the 'good' – for example, the work of Bengt Brülde, a Scandinavian scholar.[6] What is certain is that no doctor can assume to specify what is the good for this individual patient. This is particularly significant when patients express (maybe to the consternation of carers) the wish to die, and even to refuse to accept treatments or interventions with a reasonable chance of prolonging life.

It must not be assumed that such a wish is a manifestation of despondency or depression, or inability to sustain any further a burdensome illness or to be a burden on others. At other life stages it is normal for a person to wish for a partner, parenthood, and so on; a wish to die may be an expression of an equally valid instinct of the fittingness of dying. Obviously, such an assertion does not obviate the cogency of efforts to maximise comfort (by unfailing respect, freedom from major symptoms, and the provision of care), nor is it in any way an apologia for suicide or euthanasia, but may suggest the need for consistently wise judgement and humility in the presence of the other.

III
The doctor as guest

There is another perspective maybe worthy of consideration in the clinical context: namely that it is the patient who by the act of seeking assistance is offering hospitality to the doctor. The patient is opening the door to his or her personal even bodily presence to the (authorised by society) doctor who enters as guest. The patient is opening the door to a sanctuary, and the doctor, bound by a code of conduct to respect privacy etc. should recognise that he or she is treading on holy ground – and take off the shoes. There is indeed a code of conduct (ethics) and there is no place for arrogance in any of its disguises. The situation is even more fraught (with the danger of arrogance) if the patient is suffering in Cassell's terms,[7] that is with 'a sense of impending personal disintegration'.

An adequate understanding of what we mean by 'person' is essential and has been discussed for clinicians elsewhere; in brief, a relational view of person appears crucial – with (I think) the relations essential to person – such as place, things, other persons, the past through memory, aspirations/hope, culture and with the whole, all interiorised and constitutive of 'person', not just add-ons. If, as I have suggested elsewhere, the spirit is best understood as the principle of integration[8] then an adequate understanding of 'spiritual care' needs to be grounded in an adequate understanding of 'person', and has little to do with 'religion' and is certainly not grounded in religious concepts or practice. Religious concepts and practice associated with well recognised religious traditions may, in particular patients, be a part of spiritual care but are not essential nor central. In fact there are many and diverse traditions relevant to the life of the spirit, including a radical humanism, which Erich Fromm noted is 'one of the main stages of the evolution of the Jewish tradition'.[9] There is need to recognise the 'spiritual privacy' of each patient – a difficult task for some fine persons confident in their grasp of the true and the good. There is much need for reflection on this matter.

What are the responsibilities of the doctor as guest? In hospital, clinic, ER, in disaster situations (in addition to being thoroughly competent in relevant clinical sciences)?

a) Be mindful of the extraordinary privilege of being admitted to the patient's sacred ground;

b) Minimise any harm related to the problem besetting the patient or interventions designed to alleviate it;

c) Maximise the good – as perceived by the patient – and ascertained by 'active listening' (*dadirri*);

d) Practice justice – toward the individual, and towards others needing to share the resources available; recognise that when resources are scarce triage principles may need to be applied – to offer the resource not to the ones in most need but to the ones who will likely to benefit;

e) Act with unfailing integrity and according to a well-informed conscience in all clinical decision-making and implementation of clinical interventions.

Obviously, the above remarks are redolent of the ideas of 20C medical ethicists. The Australian Aboriginal concept of *dadirri* is a precious gift to contemporary Australians[10] and critical in interpersonal exchange which is 'hospitality'.

So, hospitality from many perspectives is a foundational concept for clinical practice – in all contexts, but especially in contemporary hospitals, large or small. For the concept is embedded not in the walls of the hospital but in the relationships between patients and those who care for them.

I have focussed especially on doctors who still have the role of healers, leaders, and advocates of the weak. Above all doctors are 'educators' (expressing both the Latin *educere* – to lead out, and *educare*, to nourish) with the responsibility to lead others (including staff and patients) out from where they are to a new place, and to support them during the journey.

Hospitality, generically, implies the making of space available to another. Clearly there are physical dimensions to this notion – demonstrated tragically in COVID time – visions of persons dying in the streets will not fade. But the notion of space is more than that. Care of another manifest as hospitality calls for the sharing of self, the making available of the space within oneself, a space threatened in our time. Many wise thinkers, including Australian Sebastian Smee,[11] have alerted us to the dangers of the digital world as potential invader of gracious interiority. The space within each giver and receiver of hospitality needs guarding, even in a modern hospital: it is sacred ground.

References

1. Symons X., 'Welcome to the Stranger: Rediscovering the art of hospitality in a 21st Century Hospital'. Plunkett Centre Annual Lecture, 28 July 2022.
    (The Sydney based Plunkett Centre for Ethics, situated on the Darlinghurst campus of St Vincent's Hospital, is a joint venture of Australian Catholic University, St Vincent's Health Australia, and Calvary Health Care. It is devoted to the study and teaching of ethics in clinical practice and biomedical research.)
2. Alter R, *The Hebrew Bible: A translation with Commentary*. Norton, New York, 2019.
3. Lickiss N., (ed Curthoys J), *Medicine as a Human Science: Essays by Norelle Lickiss*. Ginninderra Press, Adelaide, 2022.
4. Green A., *Radical Judaism: Rethinking God and Tradition*. Yale University Press, New Haven, 2010.
5. Shakespeare., *The Merchant of Venice*, Act IV Scene 1.
6. Brülde B., *The Human Good*. Acta Universtatis Gothoburgensis, Göteborg, 1998.
7. Cassell EJ., 'The nature of suffering and the goals of medicine'. *New England Journal of Medicine*, 1982 306: pp 639–645.
8. Lickiss N., On the occasion of COVID-19 pandemic: consideration of the personal. In Lickiss N., *On the Kindness of Strangers and Other Essays*, p 579–600.
9. Fromm E., *You Shall Be As Gods: A Radical Interpretation of the Old Testament and its Tradition* (1966). Holt, New York, 1991, p12.
10. Stockton E., *The Aboriginal gift: Spirituality for a Nation* (1995) Revised edition. Blue Mountains Education and Research Trust, Lawson. 2015.
11. Smee S., 'Net Loss: the Inner Life in the Digital Age'. *Quarterly Essay* 72, 2018 Black Inc. Carlton, Victoria.

11

ON THE OCCASION OF COVID-19 PANDEMIC: CONSIDERATIONS OF THE PERSONAL

2022

It is not yet possible to understand the human impact of the present pandemic but some matters are already clear: fissures in the fabric of global and local human society have been laid bare. But measures taken to curb the pandemic, notably isolation procedures, have highlighted human interconnectedness, and the cost of separation. The development of digital communication has been remarkably accelerated, with demonstration of possibilities for good or ill as well as limitations. All these matters call for reflection. But one issue is central – namely, the personal.

Always in human communities there have been persons to whom others turned for help with certain deeply personal matters, especially those afflicting the body. Such special persons were in more recent times known, at least in the west, as 'doctors'. The patient (the one suffering – from the Latin *patiens*) has been variously considered as subject (subordinate – one who obeys the medicine man or doctor), employer (with doctor even as slave for a time in ancient Greece), partner, customer or client (in some business models), and as person.[1] One of the traditional tasks of doctors in society is advocacy for the weak, the powerless. But the *central* task of medicine, on which all else depends, is that of healing – the preservation or restoration of individual persons afflicted by disease or trauma – *personal reconstruction*, even when life is slowly or rapidly drawing to a close. The deliberations of medical scientists, for example as epidemiologists or developers of vaccines can profitably be seen in this light. The contribution of doctors to the healing of a troubled, even fractured world begins with the healing of persons. So the understanding of persons is critical.

In sum, the experience of COVID-19 has emphasised the need to understand in a new key (and with new urgency) the lineaments of persons, what this means for so called 'person-centred care', and what we should seek to salvage for and with persons, even *in extremis*. A renewed (or recapitulated) focus on the personal appears more than justified at this time, not to bring forth new facts but to search for richer perspectives, particularly in relation to medical practice. Thinking may be enriched thereby for practitioners (and educators), with subsequently wiser decisions and procedures for the benefit of all, including health care personnel on the front line of disasters.

COVID-19 has impinged on several aspects of personal life, quite apart from, in many societies, massive suffering and death, and the personal consequences of impoverishment.

Three dimensions of the personal are particularly highlighted by this pandemic:
1. The interconnectedness of persons.
2. The person in relation to digital communication.
3. The fundamental being of persons.

These three matters are interrelated and distinguished only for convenience; the first two will be introduced briefly, but the third – a fundamental matter of medical moment will be explored at greater length. The COVID-19 pandemic experience may assist in clarifying thought, or at least in making clear perspectives which are useful for clinicians however stressed and indeed stretched in extreme situations as well as in everyday scenarios. Such thinking may contribute also to more effective care of the self (a not insignificant matter in the face of widespread 'burnout' of clinicians).

i) *The interconnectedness of persons*

The people have shown the central role of interconnectedness, notably in the rather privileged situations where mandated isolation is possible. Denial of this, rampant individualism, has major consequences in medical practice (as well as in the streets). Individualism has a history: in the West the trend is traceable in the last few centuries, but there are other intellectual traditions emphasising our connectedness. The pandemic points out where the truth lies, not merely because the probable cause of COVID-19, the spread from wild animals to man, may be rooted in the upheavals in environmental ecology, but also in the almost desperate yearning manifest for togetherness when real contact with other humans is made impossible. [Baruch] Spinoza, the 17C philosopher whose relevance to our times is being increasingly recognised, put forth a formulation of the human as *part* of nature[2] – implying radical interconnectedness which has at least in part been rediscovered in COVID-time. We are radically connected with the rest and wither if isolated. This has been *felt* in our time. And online connectedness, though precious, is a faint shadow of the possible.

ii) *The person in relation to digital communication*

The pandemic has dramatically accelerated developments in digital communication, but also has thrown into relief some of the differences between bodily and virtual presence, and highlighted some of the threats to humanness offered by some cultural trends, including the overreliance on the digital world and other depersonalising practices. The replacement of co-located 'in person' communication by digital has obvious advantages for convenience in the world of commerce, and in some aspects of education (notably, transfer of information) and, indeed, medical practice. But the limitations are serious and far reaching for individuals and society, and are of serious moment quite apart from technical matters like equity of access: the *personal* limitations require scrutiny.

Thomas Fuchs, psychiatrist and philosopher of Heidelberg, has (with awareness of the pandemic) offered recently a profound study of these matters. On his consideration of 'empathy in the age of virtuality' he notes:

> It is precisely through the contrast with digital communication that we can recognise what bodily presence really means:
>
>> it does not merely consist of the alternating exchange of messages but also enables simultaneous communication, namely *active listening* with the signs of attention, questioning, or confirmation through glances or nods;
>>
>> added to this is the empathic perception of expression, enabling *mutual bodily resonance*;

> the experience of the *direct encounter of the gaze*, in which the embodied intentionality of the person condenses;
>
> the possibility of *touching and being touched*;
>
> finally, the atmospheric feeling of the presence of the other, which is based on the synaesthetic interaction of the senses. This shows itself not least in shared silence as one of the most intensive forms of physical co-presence, which is inaccessible to technically mediated communication.[3]

Caution is needed therefore regarding any attempt to substitute digital communication for bodily co-location in any activity founded on interpersonal communication. For example, care is needed in medical education, at its core an interpersonal activity fostering personal growth as well as the acquisition of facts and concepts, and growth in clinical judgement and wisdom. Furthermore, caution is also needed in reliance on tele-consultation or tele-therapy, especially in the absence of a strong interpersonal connection previously established by in-person communication. The doctor-as-comforter, a traditional role still essential, is seriously hampered by solely virtual presence to a distressed patient. The evaluation of suffering, a wholly subjective state, is surely seriously inadequate, yet is being considered as sufficient in some nations to fulfil bureaucratic requirements concerning even eligibility for physician assisted suicide or euthanasia – surely an erroneous (and frightening) judgement.

The digital world also has implications for the relationship of person and place. The dislocation is profound and basic. An internet address is not a nurturing place. A GPS 'location' is *impersonal*. There is far more to be conceptualised in the face of the flourishing of the digital space. Is that really where the human is 'placed' now? in the virtual world?

The points made by Fuchs (and others) are of crucial importance for planners and administrators. *Re-personalisation* should be the explicit norm guiding reconstruction or individual and societal function post COVID; the depersonalisation undertaken for 'efficiency' may have gone too far. The educational implications are surely obvious.

iii) *What do we mean by 'person'? What **is** a person?*

The gauntlet was laid down by philosopher Jacob Needleman in a communication with New York Academy of Sciences in 1969 – in globally turbulent times:

> What medicine lacks is any fundamental notion of the nature of man and any remotely adequate understanding of that to which we refer as a person.[4]

Many cognate terms are used, and usage varies in time and place. It may be wise to note that the term 'self' is best understood as 'the particular being any person is':[5] person is the generic term. The term 'subject' is so variously understood that it may be wise to refrain from considering this in the present context. The focus here is on the notion of 'person'.

Philosophy does not stand still, and it is not fair to see it as merely footnotes to Plato, and this must be particularly true in a multicultural society such as Australia where there is potential to juxtapose to the western tradition the riches of our indigenous tradition and that of our more recent immigrants notably from Asia. Only the Western tradition will be noted here save to note that Western writers are aware of Chinese thinkers such as Mencius (pupil of Confucius) as increasingly recognised to have relevance, for example in ethics.

a) *A note on 'person' in Western thought*

There have been many concepts of 'person' in the history of Western thought. Readers versed in the humanities will recognise the difficulty of doing justice to this richness. It could be worth noting that John Locke, the English philosopher and physician, rather confounded the whole matter – he thought that a 'person' need not be a human being and characterised a person as a thinking, intelligent being, that has reason and reflection and is aware of its own identity over time, but Locke did link personhood with moral responsibility. We clinicians can generate strange ideas at times, but there is an obligation to contribute in some way to our intellectual tradition.

Indeed, recent writing in medical contexts has made available useful accounts of relevant contemporary thought, coming from diverse traditions and perspectives. The collection of 30 essays edited by [David] Thomasma and colleagues is a rich resource focussed precisely on the implications for health care of the varying notions about persons and personhood. Further consideration of the western tradition, could be useful, however limited in contemporary global perspectives.[6]

The Western thought tradition is vast and complex, though merely part of the whole thought traditions of humankind. Those with formal education in philosophy, theology (especially) and the other 'humanities' continue to mine its riches and develop new ways of explication of personhood, relevant to the new questions of our day. Yet, however erudite the Western intellectual tradition, notably in the philosophical and theological strands, there appears room for developing a concept which will offer a foothold or a handhold for clinical practice. In any case, it is asserted by some that medicine is a source of food for philosophy: clinicians do have privileged, even if closely focussed, immersion in the human condition. Australian philosopher, Jeff Malpas has made remarks relevant to this point:

> Whatever conclusions we may finally arrive at, and wherever we may suppose we end up, the place in

which we begin our philosophy, the place in which philosophical questioning first arises, is the place in which we find ourselves – that place is not an abstract world of ideas, not a world of sense data or 'impressions', not a world of theoretical 'objects' nor of mere causal relata. Finding ourselves 'in' the world, we find ourselves already 'in' a place, already given over to and involved with things, with persons, with our lives. On this basis the central questions of philosophy, questions of being and existence, as well as of ethics and virtue, must themselves take their determination and their starting point from this same place.[7]

b) *Towards a concept of persons for clinicians: an ecological concept of 'person'*

The foregoing currents of thought, patchily mentioned but articulated in humanities circles elsewhere, introduce ideas of value, but not readily accessible or applicable for a busy clinician whose core commitment is to persons. The rich complexity, and even the language, is overwhelming! The challenge of [Jacob] Needleman remains: is there need to explore another articulation? Maybe there remains a residual need for a concept (a way of thinking) of 'person' which is not only readily accessible, intellectually and emotionally, but also applicable to everyday medical practice, furniture for the mind worth carrying into the clinic, hospital and emergency room. Omission of any account even of the key ideas within the Western tradition should not be seen as a devaluing of complexity or precision but an attempt to provide a framework for thought. What follows is first an account of the evolution of such a concept, and sketches of some implications of such a concept for everyday medical practice. Finally, there some consideration of the implications for medical education.

Clinical practice over many years involves rich experience of the human condition and it is to be expected that our concepts evolve in the course of a clinician's life, not in accord with scholarly humanities traditions but in ways which express our increasing awareness of the real. Over several decades I gradually developed a way of thinking about persons, an ecological concept, not just with respect to the connectedness with all Nature, and the most proximate relationships, but also as a way of thinking of the interior landscape of a person.

The genesis of an idea can be traced to the late 1960s when I returned from specialist education in Europe, soon after the National Referendum (1967) which at last conferred citizenship on our first people. There were rumours that Aboriginal children were dying in Sydney hospitals. In 1968–70 I, as a newly fledged internist, temporarily unable to undertake conventional clinical work, undertook an inquiry into some aspects of the health of Aboriginal children in Sydney with the background support of Aboriginal leaders such as Charles Perkins.

At that time the science of ecology was ascendant. Living things were seen in relation to their environments: the concept of *ecology* was ripe for expansion. In the course of this inquiry, I encountered the thinking of John Apley, a paediatrician.[8] Apley wrote of a child as a 'unique ecological experiment', and produced a simple diagram of child and environment: the concept was powerful and timely and proved seminal for me in my own reflections on what I was experiencing in privileged contact with the Aboriginal people of Sydney.

It was quickly apparent to me that in the case of the Sydney Aboriginal people an historical dimension was essential for understanding the present. At that time it was thought that Aboriginal people had been in the land now called 'Australia' for only about 10,000 years: now it is known that the figure should be at least 60,000 years. Indigenous thought and social patterns were ignored for the most part, though appreciated as curiosities, and the brutality of their experience after the arrival of the British was not common knowledge. But at least it was clear to me then that the past of each person, and the inheritance (both biological and cultural) should be recognised as significant elements in the ecology of each individual person. So, Apley's concept was enhanced and the bare bones of an *ecological concept of 'person'*, with an accompanying schema, was laid down in what became a doctorate thesis,[9] followed on resuming clinical responsibilities by occasional published reflection on the precious excursus into the indigenous milieu in Sydney.[10] The ecological concept of 'person', deeply embedded so to speak in my psyche, influenced my subsequent activity from 1970 in Tasmania as clinician, researcher and medical educator as part of the first decade of the fledgling medical school of the University of Tasmania.

My clinical work as an internist changed from 1985 when I returned to Sydney as Director of Palliative Care at Royal Prince Alfred Hospital, a metropolitan teaching hospital affiliated with the University of Sydney, with appointment also to the Prince of Wales Hospital and Royal Hospital for Women, affiliated with the University of New South Wales. Most of the several thousands of patients (most but not all with some form of cancer) seen in the next 25 years in consultation in Sydney (and some regional centres in the countryside) had incurable disease with major symptoms needing relief; some were close to death. It was possible to improve the quality of life of the vast majority of these patients and the experience was precious, and formative.

The training of future specialists in several medical fields was a feature of these years, and many thousands of patients were encountered, mainly but not only in major metropolitan

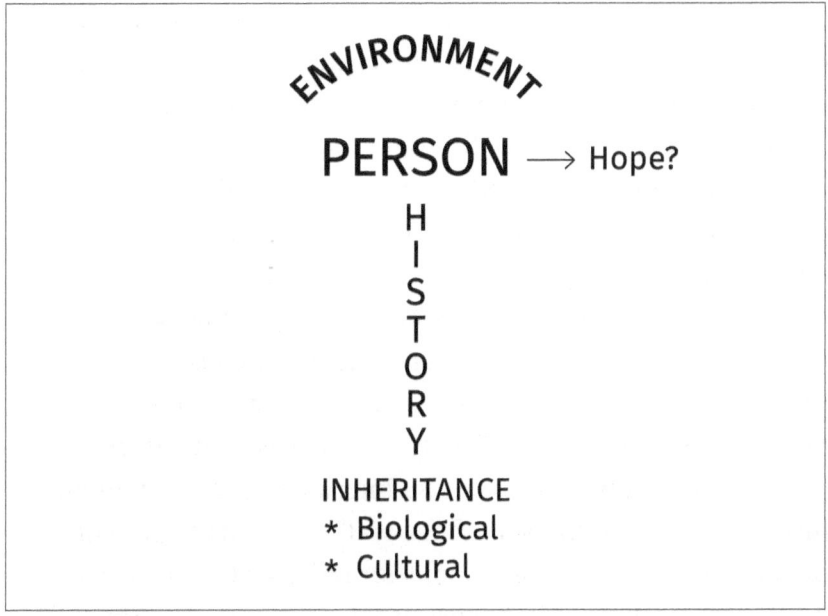

Figure 1: Ecological Model of Person

hospitals but also in regional clinics, small hospitals, nursing homes and suburban homes, since the context of the training influences experience.

The patients truly were my *educators* in the sense of roots of that word – *educere* – to lead and *educare* to nourish; they led me out into new places of understanding and nourished me as I travelled. The patients, their families and the young specialists in training (as well as my senior colleagues) helped me realise that the concept as expressed was, as it were, a closed system, and that the aspiration of the patient – hope, is a vector leading out of that system. So hope found place in the schema (Fig.1). If one could understand what the patient most hoped for now, how they formulated their desire – and in what their hope now rested, then one, as a doctor, could (after gently assisting the patient to settle on a reasonably realistic goal) focus all medical action (and the action of one's team members) far more effectively. International medical education, including bedside teaching of oncologists in teaching hospitals in China and Iran confirmed my growing conviction that an ecological concept of person was fruitful for clinicians.

As the years passed and experience and reflection deepened, it seemed that the relations already noted, including that expressed in hope, may be thought of as interiorised; the relations may be not add-ons but *constitutive* of person. Just as the filaments of a spider's web are what the web *is*, or the layers of an onion are what the onion *is*, so the identifiable relations mentioned above may not merely characterise but *constitute* a person. The notion here is of an interior architecture, of an interior *ecology* of 'person'. This would explain the pain of loss: of place (by removal/alienation/desecration), persons (isolation/death, etc), of things (say a bushfire/theft), of comfort (by pain/regret/ bullying, etc), one's past (as memory is lessened for any reason – including disease/drugs), or loss of culture. There is a temporal dimension to each constitutive relation: all is in flux, with each relation subject to change.

Each of the relations which together constitute the web a person *is* justify focussed exploration, and have received this, as separate entities, in distinct scholarly traditions. They are simply noted here:

> Place? There is a world of scholarship about place, essentially personalised space. There are several senses of the word 'place' – but one of these concerns simply the geographic material notion of land – sometimes expressed as 'my place' and relevant not only to indigenous persons in Australia but also to more recent immigrants in whom there may be profoundly conflicting concepts of place – sites in Australia being just one of the places of significance interiorised in the complex immigrant psyche.

Other persons? – and the space between in which creativity and healing may occur, tense with concern about what we owe to each other and the priority of proximity in defining obligation. One can 'go to pieces' in sustaining the pressure of interiorised personal relations, or the loss of them.

The self as the other – within. Intrapersonal dialogue may displace all else in some circumstances, notably in a dying person who may appear to be moving away from concern with and attention to, not only mundane affairs, but also other persons: it may be like a boat casting off moorings, and the distancing needs to be understood and accepted for what it is, a final phase of growth as a person becomes what he or she may be. But the sense of the movement from the shore as it were, may cause dismay, even grief to the one left behind.

Things? All that can be perceived of the matrix within which this person is embodied; perceptions, albeit in flux, which are immanent in the evolving self. Things may be part of the symbolic universe within the self. Things may bear much freight.

The past? – accessible through memory, including the memories etched in the body; cells, tissues, organs, not just the mind, bear traces of past experience. Memory can be heightened by events triggering 'reminiscence', and dulled by mood, distraction, but also by drugs.

Culture? Culture is a complex reality and has been variously defined. The cultural matrix in which a child is born, and continues to be embedded, includes not only, what has been termed the 'womb of language' but so much else which will not only influence what happens to this developing person, but how this person will interpret what happens – and all this includes disease and illness and treatment, and health care, and this has been widely researched. Clifford Geertz[11] mentioned that Kluckhorn in his monumental introduction to anthropology, included at least 10 definitions of culture: including, 'the total way of life of a people, the social legacy the individual acquires from his group, and a way of thinking, feeling, and believing. Geertz, instead, espoused another way of conceiving culture: 'Believing, with Max Weber, that man is an animal suspended in webs of significance he himself has spun, I take culture to be those webs, and the analysis of it ... is interpretative ... in search of meaning.' This richer view of Geertz appears to resonate well with the ecological concept of person.

So persons are always in flux – and yet there is continuity. A clinician, keeping the above ideas in mind might fasten on the notion that it is the pattern of the complexus which persists, despite changes in all constitutive elements and their interactions. Strengthening and diminishment of relations are inevitable over time. Hope and articulated aspiration – what the person radically desires – may change shape over time. Changes may result from experience (the word is related to 'peril') with favourable or unfavourable outcomes, from immersion in language through conversations, reading and so on. Conversation within the self (the interior colloquium) is a powerful means of change. So is an experience of bonding, especially if wrought in fragile state. But despite all this the pattern may continue to be discernible: it is as if a person is a work of art! It is noteworthy that the patient holds it all together through *narrative*. Notions of personal development prompted by personal crises, such as in the schema of Erikson[12,13] fit comfortably within this framework. However, despite many currents of scholarship there is much about persons which is not comprehensible within our current conceptual framework.

Could such a concept of 'person' cast light on the matter of spiritual dimensions of care?

Controversies, or at least worrying conversations, were occasionally encountered during my busy clinical years (notably at multidisciplinary conferences) about 'spiritual care', with even moves to measure 'spiritual health'. There were concerns about the relationship between 'spirituality' and 'religion', with some unease as well as impetus to respect varying positions and the persons holding them. Australia is a secular nation, and religion is regarded as a private matter. But doctors, being not only individuals with personal opinions and cultural practice, but also often as leaders or others having much influence on the culture of health services, had need of some clarity in these matters. How to understand what is meant by 'spirit' and 'spiritual' dimensions of care – especially if one is 'not very religious'? There is extensive recent literature on these matters, but there seems a place for a unifying concept, and the emerging concept of person seemed to have merit. Could the relation between person and the whole of reality (All-That-Is) complete the schema?

Each of us has, necessarily, some concept of the whole reality in which we are immersed – All-That-Is – even if we are not constantly aware of this. Some experiences may awaken this awareness. We may say 'it takes us out of ourselves' … Ecstasy is precisely just that. Freud talked of the 'oceanic' feeling. We have often ways of experiencing, recognising or articulating this relation to the whole; we may gaze at the sea, walk in the wilderness, gaze at the wonders in a garden – or in a child's face, listen to music, make love, become 'absorbed' (we say) in art, in tasks. But we may also experience and express this same openness to and awareness of the whole of reality in religious rituals. [Roy] Rappaport emphasised, from the perspective of a distinguished anthropologist, the critical role of religion in the development of humanness (not 'human evolution')[14]: he may well, if he wrote now, have broadened his focus to include rituals expressing the awareness of the whole, however named. Some name the whole, All-That-Is, 'God'. God talk is to be found in many places, including clinical contexts, with patients raising hard questions. Maybe it is possible to stay with the notion that All-That-Is may be named 'God', accepting that there are many ways that God may be conceived – as transcendent (outside all the reality we can know) and creator, sustainer and carer of All-That-Is, or (alternatively) not transcendent but wholly immanent, present within All-That-Is. In the first instance (God as a transcendent being) petitionary prayer for intervention would suppose the possibility of suspension of the laws of the material universe. The alternative view would imply that miracles are not possible but that prayer is an expression of the awareness of All-That-Is on the part of the one praying. In either instance, the activity of prayer (and other religious acts) is recognised as befitting the human person. The philosopher [Baruch] Spinoza, who favoured the latter view, regarded the intellectual love of god (as he conceived god) as the highest human activity … and many thinkers with roots in the Jewish tradition, would insist that Spinoza's god was indeed the god of Moses and Abraham – as it were, the presence of transcendence within immanence. It is to be stressed that, as in all cultural traditions, conceptual pluralism is notable in the Jewish tradition and vigorous argument continues, including concerning Spinoza.[15]

It is appropriate that respect be paid to those who would prefer that the word 'god' not be used, not because of the sacredness of the name (precluding use in traditional Judaism), but in view of unfortunate connotations, and the unspeakable violence done to persons done in the name of god in the West – a travesty deplored by the wise among us such as Jonathan Sacks.[16] But the word remains prominent in Western parlance. As already adumbrated, there is a wide spectrum of understandings of the concept of 'god' ranging from a being transcending all of nature, to a process immanent within nature, energising the whole or the unity within All-That-Is, the experience of which may for some persons be overwhelming. There is a vast literature on this matter, bearing traces of the ponderings of men and women searching for meaning regarding the whole of reality within which we are embedded, and the challenge of perceiving the whole as radically beneficent or maleficent. Others, less restless, see no need for such a search – nature just *is*. Abandonment of the term 'god' appears unwise, but there is room for continuing exploration and care to recognise plurality of views.

Attention has been paid to the concept of 'god'. It is impossible to avoid some attention to what we mean by 'spirit' or 'soul'. Again, there is a long history and a vast literature, including works by such persons as contemporary medical historian Roy Porter.[17] Clinicians are immersed in the reality of the bodily embeddedness of persons and in the world of personal complexity – and there is increasing awareness of 'burnout' affecting clinicians (a whole person experience indeed with sometimes specific mention of matters of spirit). There is confusion and disquiet (however masked) – and clinical conversations usually avoid these profound matters – and yet they are at the core of humanness. Some traditions stress personal immortality and specifically, the immortality of the soul: the influence of Descartes of 17C Amsterdam continues to be strong. Others draw attention to the power of the concepts of Spinoza (interestingly, a near contemporary in Amsterdam of [René] Descartes in that turbulent century) who asserts the immortality not of the soul but of the expressions of the mind: Spinoza considered that what we have contributed to the world of thought endures after our death.

Maybe there are simpler ways of considering even the aspect, in personal reality, of 'spirit' or 'soul'. I have suggested elsewhere that the spirit or soul may be the name of the principle of integration: that is, in the face of the complexity of a person, whatever holds that complexity together and ceases at death: after death the 'person' is no longer there where the body lies. The 'person' has passed away – the folk saying may be correct and profound.

Ideas set forth in these lines have resonance with some powerful aspects of the human condition, notable the notions of human dignity and human suffering. Respect for the whole complexus is inherent in respect for human dignity.[18] The notion put forward in these lines is in accord also with the notion of [Eric] Cassell who in 1982, published what would prove to be a landmark paper on the nature of human suffering:[19] he postulated that an operational definition of suffering is 'a sense of impending personal disintegration' – which (I think) in common parlance may be 'a sense of being about to go to pieces'. Patients who are suffering in this way, 'feeling about to go to pieces', 'losing it', 'breaking up' – note the nuances of such terms – are frequently able to name a cause or 'trigger'; interventions may reduce (or needlessly increase) the impact of such a factor.[20]

Doctors with finely honed clinical skills have potentially critical roles in society as healers, leaders, educators, advocates for the powerless, and comforters. The central point of this present discussion is the contention that doctors with an adequate concept of person, in which relations with all that is other (persons, place, things, memory, culture, and All-That-Is, called by whatever name) are *embodied* (note the powerful nuance), may enhance their potential to be a source of comfort and healing in a fragmented, distressed world. Much to ponder. And as persons, to conjecture throughout all our days.

In sum, fundamental to the ecological concept of persons is the conviction that a person is a relational reality. Initially, the relation is recognized to exist with the current environment, personal and non-personal, in a continuous dialectic, with these constitutive relationships held together by what we may term spirit, but with the continuing possibility of fracture, evident as a sense of impending personal disintegration. Hope as aspiration for action or vested in a recognised reality or ideal is the arrow leading out of what could be a closed system. We may recognise indeed that not only the person exists as part of the complex ecology of nature, but what we call a personal network is best thought of as an ecological system. Furthermore the ontological structure of a person may be thought of as an ecology – indeed a fragile web capable of being affected by strain in one of its components, and threatened with a sense of impending personal disintegration if there is too much fracturing – the phenomenon which Cassell designated as 'suffering'. Kingsley Mortimer, a New Zealand professor of anatomy, wrote that, 'it is the task of medicine to emancipate man's interior splendour.'[21] Intriguing! It may be the task, then, of the enlightened clinician not only, as Cassell declared, to seek to relieve human suffering, but to unmask human splendour, aware of the interior architecture of the 'self', the particular person being encountered, even in great darkness.

This is not the place to consider the implications of the ecological concept of person (and considerations of complexity, including 'layering') for clinical practice or medical education – but they are clearly significant, even in the midst of catastrophe. But there is at least need to think again of pondering, as Needleman prompted, a far more adequate notion of person and the personal – as means to sounder approaches to all we do in the name of medicine, even *in extremis*. And, as [Alan]

Mittleman, in concluding his deliberations, noted, 'Our dignity is found in our activity – and ... in our potential for full personhood. Persons can help the hidden goodness, truth and significance of life to emerge.'[22] That sounds like a charter for clinicians! Everywhere, and at all times, even now.

Has the ecological concept of person set forth in this essay (this *exploration*) any value in thinking about the human impact of COVID-19? There is a place for studied reflection on the impact of the pandemic on one's relation to persons, place, things, oneself, one's past, culture, hopes and aspirations, and relation to the whole, however conceptualised and expressed. Obviously, the effects of the pandemic on each one of the identified constitutive relations of persons is profound and obvious, and hardly need explicating, and it would be tedious to do so, however instructive. However, clinical decision-making in the course of the pandemic deserves mention.

Moral and ethical dilemmas concerning persons and related values have been prominent in the pandemic. Traditional ethical principles have been tested. Tragic clinical situations forced decisions about the distribution of scarce resources to be decided not on the basis of need (the traditional ethic) but on the 'triage' basis of who would be most likely to benefit. At a societal level the debate about 'saving lives or saving the economy' has been a major issue, not only in Europe. There was more than a hint of regarding some lives as more expendable than others – and some deaths less consequential than others; frailty increases the likelihood of unpreventable death from COVID-19 but equal attention to the quality of care of each dying person is an ethical imperative. The trauma of not being able to give the usual quality of care has been widely expressed by distressed medical and nursing staff: the moral injury inflicted on thousands of doctors and other health care professionals is beyond words. The trauma has been exacerbated unspeakably by the death of colleagues. We clinicians who are bystanders can only be in awe.

A final word.

Human disruption associated with the pandemic has been and is continuing to be dramatic but is being assuaged by the development of effective vaccines, though global equity of access is sorely lacking. It will take time to assess and understand the human significance of this COVID-19 pandemic in the long march of human history.

However, another reality is casting a shadow. The pandemic is occurring at a time of unspeakable inter-human violence and suffering, occurring in many parts of the world, in 2022 (as I write), threatening to tear apart even a large part of the global community. Everything the COVID-19 pandemic has thrown into relief is amplified now in the horrors of war. We witness, even in real time, the separation of bonded persons, destruction of place, cultural icons, traces of inheritance, and the dashing of hope. We can only imagine the interior shattering of persons, and yet we glimpse the centre (of persons and communities) 'hold'. As words fail, silence (save for the sound of violence and suffering) may be the only response for now.

References

1 Ramsay P., *The Patient as Person: Explorations in Medical Ethics*, Yale, New Haven, 1970.
2 Lloyd G., *Part of Nature: Self-Knowledge in Spinoza's Ethics*, Cornell University Press, Ithaca, 1994.
3 Fuchs T., *In Defence of the Human Being.* Oxford University Press, Oxford, 2021, p99.
4 Needleman J., 'The perception of mortality', *Annals of the New York Academy of Sciences*, 164 (3),1969, pp733–738.
5 Seidel H., *The Idea of the Self: Thought and Experience in Western Europe since the Seventeenth Century*, Cambridge University Press, Cambridge, 2005.

6. Thomasma DC., Weisstub DN and Herve C (eds), *Personhood and Health Care*, Kluwer, Dordrecht, 2001.
7. Malpas J., *Heidegger's Typology: Being, Place*, World, MIT Press, Cambridge, Mass, 2006, p39.
8. Apley J., 'An ecology of childhood', *The Lancet* 1964 2:1.
9. Lickiss N., *The Aboriginal people of Sydney with special reference to the health of their children: a study in human ecology*, MD Thesis University of Sydney, 1972.
10. Lickiss J N., 'Health problems of urban aborigines with special reference to the Aboriginal people of Sydney', *Social Science and Medicine*, 1975, 9: pp313–318.
11. Geertz C., *The Interpretation of Cultures*. Selected Essays. Basic Books, New York, 1973.
12. Erikson EH., 'Identity and the Life Cycle. Psychological Issues', Monograph, New York, International Universities Press, 1969.
13. Erikson EH., *The Life Cycle Completed*: A Review, New York, Norton, 1982.
14. Rappaport RA., *Ritual and Religion in the Making of Humanity*, Cambridge University Press, Cambridge, 1999.
15. Bloom J., Goldstein A., Student G (eds) *Strauss, Spinoza and Sinai: Orthodox Judaism and Modern Questions of Faith*, Kodesh Press, New York, 2022.
16. Sacks J, *Not in God's Name*. Hodder and Stoughton, London 2015.
17. Porter R., *Flesh in the Age of Reason: the modern Foundations of Body and Soul*, W. W. Norton Company, 2003.
18. Lickiss N., 'On human dignity: fragments of an exploration', in Malpas J, Lickiss N (eds), *Perspectives on Human Dignity*. 2007, Springer, Dordrecht, pp27–41.
19. Cassell EJ., 'The nature of suffering and the goals of medicine', *New England Journal of Medicine*, 1982 306: pp639–645.
20. Lickiss N., 'On Facing Human Suffering', in Malpas J, Lickiss N (eds), *Perspectives on Human Suffering*, Springer, Dordrecht, 2012, pp245–260.
21. Mortimer K., 'The impossible profession: the doctor-priest relationship', *Proceedings of the Australian Association of Gerontology*, 1974, 2: pp81–82.
22. Mittleman AL., *Human Nature in Jewish Thought: Judaism's Case for Why Persons Matter*, Princeton University Press, New Jersey, 2015, p183.

12

THE VIEW FROM HERE: LATE NIGHT MUSINGS

2022

> Empty are the words of that philosopher who offers no therapy for human suffering. For just as there is no use in medical expertise if it does not give therapy for bodily diseases, so too there is no use in philosophy if it does not expel the suffering of the soul.
>
> —*Epicurus* (341–271)[1]

Hospital based physicians, notably retired elderly formerly hospital-based physicians still wondering about what they (we) have experienced of the human condition, may seem at times like fishers with rods at the ready, sitting wistfully beside a stream in which are to be found (like baubles) the thoughts of thinkers down the ages (and even in our own time). Suddenly one item looks attractive enough to snare – letting the rest go onwards undisturbed. Distinguished scholars, notably professional philosophers, know well and understand the whole stream: its history, its makeup, its patterns, its classification into various species, what items are worth retrieving and what are best ignored. But a musing physician, much to the annoyance of philosophers, might find just one idea a stimulus to reflection – and having hooked it, so to speak, may proceed to run with it into places far away from the frame of the thinkers. Such is the freedom of old age! These comments may be seen as musings at the end of a long day (or life) after prolonged fishing at the stream of human thought.

What is the view not from 'nowhere' but from 'here'? From here, in this place, at this time, at this particular juncture of place and time in long continuous history of humankind – and the view from here of this particular person, not another. Why here and now? A sense of nearness of the horizon? An issue of heightened awareness of the peaks and troughs, albeit a little shrouded in mist, of the road now travelled? And the hazardous terrain of the close world? Consciousness of the possible proximity of what [Gerard] Hopkins called 'cliffs of fall'? There is a place and time for 'musing' and such is what follows.

Some decades ago philosopher Thomas Nagel, in his classic *The View From Nowhere*, was concerned (he wrote), 'about a single problem: how to combine the perspective of a particular person inside the world with an objective view of this same world, the person and his viewpoint included,' and the difficulty of reconciling the two standpoints in the conduct of life as well as in thought. He conceded that these perspectives form a spectrum, but their integration is a challenge.[2] This is all worth considering for I, as a person (even an aged person) am a point of concurrence of many perspectives whether aware of them or not!

Objective perspectives, as Nagel conceived them, could well correspond with the perspectives of health care administrators, say, considering provisions of care for the aged or with the perspective of a fit runner (or scooter rider) passing an elderly person walking with a stick or frame! Objective perspectives on the situation of very elderly persons rightly concern probable care needs as the capacity for self-care is diminished, for one reason or another and in one form or another, as well as notions of their priorities. 'Assessments' based on objective perspectives and measures are occasionally in order and essential, however resisted.

The objective perspective concerning such matters and data emanating from it are essential for the good order of a compassionate society; administration is grounded in such information. But the subjective perspective usually dominates self-awareness, even if I try to keep the objective perspective in mind, and be 'balanced' in my approach. In what may I hope now? What is the shape of my responsibility now? How should I live now? It is not always easy to maintain (precisely named) 'equanimity': either the objective or subjective perspective may overwhelm. An example? As one ages, awareness of distress in the world impinges more and more on one's consciousness. The unspeakable suffering of persons from COVID-19 especially in resource poor countries, and the glimpses of the heroism of doctors and nurses may be (and have been) a major distress for a retired doctor conscious now of being unable to help. Similarly, the spectre of the continuing 'useless' suffering of people in war is almost unbearable – or images of fellow citizens battling natural disaster (like current catastrophic floods). Then, objective perspectives, by impinging on the subjective, may almost overwhelm the capacity of a person to remain integrated. 'Suffering' in the sense defined by [Eric] Cassell ('a sense of impending personal disintegration')[3] may ensue. The somewhat silent suffering of elderly persons about such matters may be underestimated. And the philosophers, even Epicurus, may be of little use. Comfort is a precious commodity.

There is nothing static or fixed about growing old. Advanced age is a phase of life which, like any other phase of life, has distinct characteristics. Traces of the tasks of earlier life stages (to use an [Erik] Eriksonian model) may emerge; the search for identity characteristic of adolescence, the thrust for generativity characteristic of adulthood, the thirst for wholeness of life – integrity – rather than despair; all of these and more. But there is one feature deserving of particular attention – the layer of loss in diverse forms. Gains are evident – a new-found interior freedom is one, and delight in the achievements of others notably the young – but the experience of even devastating loss is commonly a feature of the lives of very elderly persons.

'Person' is a composite and relational reality. Relations are not only features of personhood but may be considered in truth as constitutive of 'person' as I have discussed elsewhere.[4] Relations with place, other persons, oneself, one's past, culture and inheritance are in the course of life internalised, accessible usually by memory. Loss in each of these domains is almost inevitable in the course of a life, and losses may be compressed in one's later years in the face of changing individual circumstances, deaths of closely-bonded others, reduced physical capacity, loss of precious memorable things, social change or even catastrophe. Grieving for past or current loss may follow well-known patterns but is individualised – and sometimes fails to occur (so called 'disenfranchised grief') or takes pathological pathways. Triggers may be powerful – setting off severe distress in the face of a long past trauma. The power of symbols and symbolic action maybe incomprehensible to persons (including health professionals) a generation (or two or three) younger than this elderly person. These matters are profound and narratives concerning them are painfully powerful. The dramatic changes in social attitudes over several decades lead to a response of near incomprehensibility if not disbelief, when well-meaning young professionals encounter such narratives. Awe is in order.

What of responsibility now, for a maybe frail, very old person who feels powerless in the face of all that is being experienced, whether concerning others or the self? This sense of powerlessness may be especially acute in persons like physicians whose lives have featured competence to assist others. Yet, there are ways of looking at present possibilities for agency: radical passivity may be not be the only stance. A glance again at the constitutive relations of oneself offers glimpses of what one can do – in regard to place, other persons, things, culture, memories – and not just tidying up and preparing for closure! Imagination is called for: there are usually many more possibilities than are immediately apparent. And also a careful appraisal of the truth about all these matters. Spinoza urged that cognition, knowledge, at several levels (including intuitive knowledge), not willpower, should be the basis for action. When emotional turmoil arises there is a place, at all ages but especially in very old age, for the quiet question to be asked of oneself: 'What is the *truth*, now, about all this?'

But sometimes the sense of uselessness becomes ascendant. Simon Leys, translator of Confucius, called his late collection of essays *The Hall of Uselessness*.[5] Leys quotes Daoist Zhuang Zi, 'Everyone knows the usefulness of what is useful. But few know the usefulness of what is useless?'. The Chinese understood the value of 'uselessness' and saw opportunities for creative thinking in spaces thought useless. And such is true. For when one perceives the loss of opportunities for conventional agency, there is always the opportunity to be the gracious receiver of kindness, an active listener (practise *dadirri*), be a benign presence in a fraught situation, even a brake on a torrent of unwise words or actions careering downhill in a conversation or encounter one is privileged to share. Wisdom, honed by a life time of experience (including personal errors and failures as well as success), may be a rare find for a troubled other.

The creation of symbols is, according to early 20C German philosopher Ernst Cassirer, the mark of humanness. He was forced to flee Germany and eventually arrived at Yale where his ideas were much appreciated and a concise summary volume was prepared to make his ideas available.[6] His vast master work, *Symbolic Forms*, was eventually translated into English. Cassirer regarded language, myth and religion as 'symbolic forms', creations of mankind, in that order. Language and myth will be left aside in this note, as too complex for brief comment, but religion should have mention. As one ages ultimate issues become more prominent in the mind. Nagel was very concerned with 'religion' – and not only had much to say about it in his writing about the subjective in *The View from Nowhere* in 1988, but went back to it over 20 years later, then in his eighties, writing a fresh the title essay for his 2010 collection, concerned still with an adequate response to the 'cosmic question'.[7]

Nagel in his volume of 1988 remarked as follows, 'The wish to live so far as is possible in full recognition that one's position in the universe is not central has an element of the religious impulse about it', and 'I would rather lead an absurd life engaged in the particular than a seamless transcendental life immersed in the universal, or at least an acknowledgement of the question to which religion purports to supply an answer. A religious solution gives us a borrowed centrality through the concern of a supreme being'.

In his 2010 essay, *Secular Philosophy and the Religious Temperament*, Nagel defined the 'religious temperament' as 'the appropriate term for a disposition to seek a view of the world that can play a certain role in the inner life – a role that for some people is occupied by religion'. And he specified the cosmic question as 'How can one bring into one's individual life a full recognition of one's relation to the universe as a whole?' Indeed! And he noted that 'our awareness and its expansion as part of the history of life and our species are part of the natural evolution of the cosmos. This expands our sense of what a human life is'. His ideas resonate at least in part with those of medical doctor and biologist Stuart Kauffman published around that time. Kauffman stressed the emergent universe, with God as 'the fully natural, awesome creativity that surrounds us'. In his preface he noted, 'The vast tangled web of life – arose all on its own. This web of life, the most complex system we know in the universe, breaks no law of physics, yet is partly lawless, ceaselessly creative. So, too, are human history and human lives.'[8]

Nagel (who classed himself as an atheist) toyed with the idea of religion without a 'supreme being' – and noted religious (or at least spiritual) traditions such as Buddhism. He had difficulties in seeing humanism as compatible with his concept of 'religion'. Kauffman was not comfortable with the notion of secular humanism. But categories or labels do not really matter. Writers, the wordsmiths par excellence in symbolic space, may illuminate our quest. As Kauffman wrote, 'Sublime poetry, sublime literature, is a lens through which to view ourselves, our lives, and our world. It shows us the truth'.

There may be a way through this complexity by taking a more strictly subjective view, insisting on the *interiority* of the relations which constitute a 'person'. As creator of symbols I, if aware of my interior self – that which integrates me (my spirit), clothe such relations in forms/actions which I (and others) may call ritual. It is a small step for others to call my ritual a religion. Considerations of Aboriginal 'religious business' edited by philosopher Max Charlesworth,[9] and a penetrating study of Aboriginal thought and spirituality by renowned priest-archeologist, Eugene Stockton[10] are relevant to the present discussion; Australian Aboriginal people had very diverse concepts, but no notions approaching monotheism – their views were in fact somewhat closer to the panentheism of Spinoza who stressed not only that man is part of the whole of nature but also stressed the immanence of God.[11] Clare Carlisle, British philosopher and theologian has recently undertaken an analysis of the religious thought of [Baruch] Spinoza.[12] A notable anthropologist, Roy Rappaport, wrote of the essential role of ritual and religion in human development.[13] Incidentally, many thinkers have noted the hazards to interiority posed by the digital world (addiction to phone messages, and so on); it is to be noted that Fuchs, professor of philosophy and psychiatry at Heidelberg, wrote recently about the hazards posed by the digital revolution to human *being*.[14] A caution indeed for educators.

There are countless cultural traditions concerning these matters. The Hebrew Scriptures remain formative for European traditions and derived settler societies. It may be wise to keep in mind that in the encounter in the desert (Exodus 3.15) with an unusual phenomenon (the 'burning bush') when Moses had the consciousness of being addressed in some way (as I also felt alone in the desert in Israel one day in 1980), the response to his query about who might be addressing him was 'I am who I am' or 'I am Being'. Moses recognised the ground as sacred and took off his shoes. It is not surprising that there have been points of deep affinity between some Jewish people and Australian Aboriginal people. Kauffman stressed that it is a human privilege not just to recognise but to create the sacred. And it is worthy of note that the making sacred (consecration) of persons, place or time may, in this *modus cogitandi*, indicate not separation from but more intense awareness of and participation in the mundane whilst manifesting a radical orientation to the Whole: a somewhat a different notion from that found in traditional Christian monastic and other ascetic traditions.

If one considers persons as radically constituted by relations, including the relation with the whole/the cosmos, it is conceivable that a person lacking in a religious sense is in a way truncated or at least diminished. The person whose response to the cosmos is expressed in rapture at the wildness of a wilderness, or the sublimity of a mountain – or the face of a child, or in 'radical amazement' (Abraham Heschel) at consciousness of the unity of the energy within all reality – this person is more fully alive somehow than one who is not aware or cannot respond to such things. And each person may have a unique pattern of response to the Whole, maybe in conjunction with like-minded others, maybe not. This to me is a way of conceiving the 'religious sense', and it is intrinsic in the possibilities of personhood individually and collectively embodied in total personal being. I see such a concept of religion as clearly compatible with a new humanism. I believe my notions are in accord in large part with Nagel and Kauffman: at least we are musing in the same space. Jewish theologian and Rabbi Arthur Green identifies as a 'religious humanist' and 'panentheist': 'Transcendence dwells *within* immanence. There is no ultimate duality here, no 'God and world', no 'God, world, and self,' only one Being and its many faces'.[15] Shades of 17C Spinoza, indeed, and resonance with Australian Aboriginal thought which non-indigenous Australians are coming to respect and esteem.

The view from 'here' will change: the view may be different tomorrow. Yet I as a person have continuity during my lifetime (despite what some philosophers contend). A *pattern* endures, rooted not in the elements forming my body, nor even in the dictates of my genetic profile, but in the structure of my being wrought by the myriad relations which constitute me as person. The pattern somehow endures, and with it, my responsibility for what I do, and my accountability to all the rest of nature of which I am part. Personal immortality, a cherished notion for some, may not be human truth. But my thoughts may endure, in the stream of thought which Spinoza called the eternity of the mind when I as a person am no longer here, in this place.

So, what should I do here, now? How should I live? Spinoza (reviving an ancient term) in the Ethics wrote of the *conatus* within all things, the striving to continue in *being*.[16] When the horizon of life is clearly drawing closer, and may be very near, what can it mean to strive to continue in being? It surely cannot mean to strive for immortality. No, my 'being' is concerned with the everyday, and every moment of every day. It may be that whereas at other times my deepest desire was to learn, or wander and wonder, or to find an immortal soul mate or to achieve objectives, now my project is simply to respond, in ways outlined above, to the reality within which I am embodied and within it to create the sacred – in space and time. To quote Nagel again, 'We may think of reality as a set of concentric spheres, progressively revealed as we detach gradually from the contingencies of the self'. The day may come when my striving is consciously to be merged now with the rest of nature – to take my last breath. And one can hope that others accept that such is in accord with nature – and care for me as I, as a person, pass away. And such is life, after all.

And what of the task at the close of life? In the utter powerlessness of being close to death? Maybe, for an individual, dying marks the completion of the human task, an entering into interconnectedness, into one's roots, in a complete way. Dying finally expresses the radical reality of inter-connectedness and coherence, and the final discovery. And maybe that is it. And enough.

References

1. Epicurus in Gottlieb A, *The Dream of Reason*, Penguin, London, 2016, p283.
2. Nagel T., *The View from Nowhere*, Oxford University Press, New York, 1988.
3. Cassell E., 'The nature of suffering and the goals of medicine.', *New England Journal of Medicine*, 1982, 306: pp639–645.
4. Lickiss N., 'On Facing Human Suffering', in Malpas J, Lickiss N (eds), *Perspectives on Human Suffering*. Springer, Dordrecht, 2012, pp245–260.
5. Leys S., *The Hall of Uselessness*, Black Inc, Collingwood, 2011.
6. Cassirer E., *An Essay on Man*, Yale University Press, New Haven, 1944.
7. Nagel T., *Secular Philosophy and the Religious Temperament*, Oxford University Press. Oxford, 2010, p6.
8. Kauffman S., *Reinventing the Sacred*, Basic Books, New York, 2008.
9. Charlesworth M. (ed), *Religious Business: Essays on Aboriginal Spirituality*, Cambridge University Press, Cambridge,1998.
10. Stockton E., *The Aboriginal Gift: Spirituality for a Nation*, Millennium Books, Alexandria (Sydney), 1995.
11. Lloyd G., *Part of nature: Self Knowledge in Spinoza's Ethics*, Cornell University Press, Ithica, 1994.
12. Carlisle C., *Spinoza's Religion*, Princeton University Press, Princeton, 2021.
13. Rappaport R., *Ritual and Religion in the Development of Humanity*, Cambridge University Press, Cambridge,1999.
14. Fuchs T., *In Defense of the Human Being*, Oxford University Press, Oxford, 2021.
15. Green A., *Radical Judaism: Rethinking God and Tradition*, Yale University Press, New Haven, 2010.
16. Lloyd G., *Spinoza and the Ethics*, Routledge, Abingdon, 1996.

Epilogue

> Do you think I would take so much trouble ... in writing ... if I were not preparing – with a rather shaky hand – a labyrinth into which I can venture, in which I can move my discourse, opening up underground passages ... in which I can lose myself and appear at last to eyes that I will never have to meet again ... Do not ask who I am and do not ask me to remain the same ...
>
> —*Iris Murdoch* (1919–1999)
>
> Oxford philosopher – one of four renowned Oxford woman philosophers, wrote these words in 1954 in her novel *Under the Net*

Her compatriot of the 19C, George Eliot (1819–1880), would surely have been in accord with Murdoch when she wrote in her last novel *Daniel Deronda* that, 'There is a great deal of unmapped country within us which would have to be taken into account in an explanation of our gusts and storms'.

These essays bear testimony to gusts and storms of the mind of one clinician over many years of adventure in the human condition, sometimes witnessing or experiencing its limits. They offer no answers, but just may point to questions worth considering or to fields worth examining maybe for a second time.

And there must always be questioning. The matter of understanding the human condition is never closed – I (like Isaiah Berlin) distrust completion of exploration or a conviction of certainty except in those matters which are the bedrock of our capacity to live together – and sages down the ages have formulated these rules for life.

Radical availability, at the core of medical practice, has a cost: competence is hard won and workloads may be almost unspeakable – as healer, as guardian of dignity, as leader, as educators, as advocate of the weak, and as comforter always. As a consequence of these responsibilities, doctors have sometimes lived and worked in silos, alienated from the thought currents sweeping through society. Previously powerful sources of moral guidance have little credibility in contemporary society. But now, at a time of bewilderment with widespread loss of trust in institutions and in expertise, doctors on the whole continue to be trusted as committed to beneficence: there is need now for the *wisdom* of doctors to be expressed in the halls of power as well as in private spaces.

But we also need to recognise the limits of our wisdom. And maybe it may come too late. Umberto Eco (1932–2016), at the end of his novel, *Foucault's Pendulum* – at the end of the long search, wrote:

> Where have I read that at the end, when life, surface upon surface, has become completely encrusted with experience, you know everything, the secret, the power, and the glory, why you were born, why you are dying, and how it all could have been different? You are wise. But the greatest wisdom, at that moment, is knowing that

your wisdom is too late. You understand everything when there is no longer anything to understand.

But it is never too late to be learning! Or to be questioning.

Modern Australia with its extraordinary beauty, natural resources and human achievements, has at its core, deep suffering, manifest in many ways including appalling rates of suicide and domestic violence. Its dark almost inexplicable colonial history is not truly known: some say that Australia will not find its soul until that history is properly revealed and acknowledged.

But there are springs of hope. There is growing awareness of the legacy which our first people are making known and sharing: Archie Roach, indigenous songman and peacemaker who died (July 29, 2022) as this collection of writings was being concluded, was interviewed in 2018 on ABC: a memorable interview replayed after his death. In response to a question concerning how, as a creative musician, he could blot out negativity, he remarked that his way was to realise that we are all part of humanity, 'I go to the river of all humanity where that consciousness is, and drink there'. The metaphor of a river is powerful; its source is higher ground, and (unless it dries out), it flows eventually into larger water and is lost in it. So is the pattern not only of the whole of humanity but of each individual person.

I have drunk at that river and I am grateful.

Last Word

But maybe poetry should have the last say:

> DO NOT CAGE ME
>
> Do not cage me in your categories,
> bind me in your gridlock, name me
> in your universe, or seek to comprehend
> me or my boundaries.
>
> Just leave me, let me be
> outside the gates of your city –
> beyond the pale if you prefer –
> and let my spirit know the wind.
>
> When my wings are broken, done,
> maybe, could you fold me to the earth
> quietly, using no words or names,
> or yield me to the fire, then. Bless you!
>
> (2002)

Norelle Lickiss AO

Citation for award, Doctor of Medical Science (honoris causa) University of Sydney 2017 (cf p 150)

Dr Lickiss is a graduate of the University of Sydney Medical School. After postgraduate studies in Europe, she undertook community based research in Sydney and was awarded MD in 1971, her doctorate thesis being on *The Aboriginal People of Sydney with Special reference to the Health of their Children: a study in Human Ecology.* Dr Lickiss is a Fellow of the Royal Australasian College of Physicians and Honorary Professor of University of Sydney and University Associate in the School of Medicine at the University of Tasmania.

Dr Lickiss is a medical academic who has undertaken a variety of scholarly activities during her career that span the full spectrum of health care. Her published research has covered such diverse topics as the epidemiologic aspects of myeloproliferative and lymphoproliferative disorders; in vitro drug selection in antineoplastic chemotherapy, and the role of alcohol in the etiology of hypertension. She has written and contributed to several academic publications, including

Perspectives on Human Dignity (2007), Perspectives on Human Suffering (2012) and most recently On Human Complexity (2014).

Dr Lickiss is also a respected clinician, with several decades of experience as consultant physician in clinical practice in Hobart and Sydney. She joined University of Tasmania in 1970 as lecturer in medicine and in 1985 became Acting Head of Medicine and concurrently was appointed as Foundation Professor of Community Health (the first woman to be appointed Professor in the University of Tasmania). Her clinical practice was focussed particularly on cancer medicine.

In 1985, Dr Lickiss was invited to return to Sydney to become Director of Palliative Care at Royal Prince Alfred Hospital: this marked the beginning of an association which endured until 2009. During this period Dr Lickiss was also Clinical Associate Professor and later Clinical Professor at the University of Sydney. She also had a conjoint appointment as Director of Palliative Care at Prince of Wales Hospital and Royal Hospital for Women, and was, for 8 years, Associate Professor at the University of NSW. Whilst in these roles, she not only developed innovative modes of clinical service but also contributed significantly to the development of the clinical science of palliative medicine as an integral part of mainstream clinical practice as well as a specialty.

Dr Lickiss is recognised internationally as a medical educator. Her international educational and consultancy activity has included most Asian countries, particularly Iran and China, and it continues to this day. She has lectured in The Netherlands, Belgium, Austria and Argentina concerning palliative medicine as a constitutive part of the care of women with gynaecological cancer. To advance her educational objectives, she established the Sydney Institute of Palliative Medicine which continues 25 years later, and established a major training program in that discipline. Former trainees are now clinical leaders not only in Australia but also Hong Kong and Iran. She assisted the health authorities of both Indonesia and Iran to formulate national plans for cancer pain relief and palliative care. Dr Lickiss was World Health Organisation consultant to China in 1996 concerning cancer pain relief, and during the mid 90s, was one of two western doctors invited to Japan to celebrate the 400 year anniversary of the coming of Western thought to Japan.

Dr Lickiss has a long standing interest in the humanities, notably philosophy, and in interdisciplinary activities, particularly in the concept that persons from diverse intellectual backgrounds working together may enrich understanding of problematic aspects of the human condition. In the early 2000s, as Honorary Research Professor, UTAS she initiated a collaborative effort with Jeff Malpas, Head of the School of Philosophy at the University of Tasmania, in the form of an Interdisciplinary Colloquium Program which continues to flourish.

Her service to the development of palliative medicine was recognised in the Queen's Birthday Honours in 2003, with her being made an Officer of the Order of Australia (AO).

Acknowledgements

May I express gratitude to all those persons, teachers and institutions responsible for my privileged education in Australia and Europe. Teachers include not only formal educators in many disciplines, but also patients (and their families), medical students and registrars, and medical and nursing colleagues in Australia and elsewhere: all of these enhanced my knowledge, understanding, experience and awareness of the human condition – and, in some instances in recent years, skilfully cared for me and gave me the gift of a longer life.

Many friends have given me, at various times over my many years, crucial support as I struggled to find my roots. They know who they are and I am indebted to them. Truly, no woman is an island ... I owe a debt of gratitude also to the many thinkers I have encountered over the years in many times and places – either in person or in their writings: any thoughts of mine are based on theirs.

The present collection of writings was made possible by the expertise and commitment of Anita Hansen who reduced a chaotic collection of manuscripts into some order. Thanks are also due to Rosemary Scott for proofreading the manuscript.

Earlier editorial assistance and encouragement of Barbara Grunseit and Vera Ranki with regard to some of the essays is also gratefully acknowledged. I acknowledge also the assistance of those medical and other colleagues who generously helped appraise some of the included pieces: notably Barbara Grunseit, Neville Hacker, Roger Kimber, Frank Nicklason, Pam Schindler and Peter Sullivan.

A debt of gratitude is owed to Arthur Conigrave who meticulously read all of the pieces in this compilation and made valuable suggestions. I must take personal responsibility for the shortcomings in the final form of these attempts at articulation of matters which exercised my mind over many decades.

Finally, I thank Max Bingham for more than I can say.

www.ingramcontent.com/pod-product-compliance
Lightning Source LLC
Chambersburg PA
CBHW032020290426
44110CB00012B/612